Ethnicity, Immigration, and Psychopathology

The Plenum Series on Stress and Coping

Series Editor:
Donald Meichenbaum, *University of Waterloo, Waterloo, Ontario, Canada*

Current Volumes in the Series:

BEYOND TRAUMA
Cultural and Societal Dynamics
Edited by Rolf J. Kleber, Charles R. Figley, and Berthold P. R. Gersons

COMMUTING STRESS
Causes, Effects, and Methods of Coping
Meni Koslowsky, Avraham N. Kluger, and Mordechai Reich

COPING WITH CHRONIC STRESS
Edited by Benjamin H. Gottlieb

COPING WITH WAR-INDUCED STRESS
The Gulf War and the Israeli Response
Zahava Solomon

ETHNICITY, IMMIGRATION, AND PSYCHOPATHOLOGY
Edited by Ihsan Al-Issa and Michel Tousignant

HANDBOOK OF SOCIAL SUPPORT AND THE FAMILY
Edited by Gregory R. Pierce, Barbara R. Sarason, and Irwin G. Sarason

PSYCHOTRAUMATOLOGY
Key Papers and Core Concepts in Post-Traumatic Stress
Edited by George S. Everly, Jr. and Jeffrey M. Lating

STRESS AND MENTAL HEALTH
Contemporary Issues and Prospects for the Future
Edited by William R. Avison and Ian H. Gotlib

TRAUMATIC STRESS
From Theory to Practice
Edited by John R. Freedy and Stevan E. Hobfoll

A Continuation Order Plan is available for this series. A continuation order will bring delivery of each new volume immediately upon publication. Volumes are billed only upon actual shipment. For further information please contact the publisher.

Ethnicity, Immigration, and Psychopathology

Edited by

Ihsan Al-Issa
University of Calgary
Calgary, Alberta, Canada

and

Michel Tousignant
University of Quebec at Montreal
Montreal, Quebec, Canada

PLENUM PRESS • NEW YORK AND LONDON

Library of Congress Cataloging-in-Publication Data

Ethnicity, immigration, and psychopathology / edited by Ihsan Al-Issa and Michel Tousignant.
p. cm. -- (The Plenum series on stress and coping)
Includes bibliographical references and index.
ISBN 0-306-45479-3
1. Minorities--Mental health. 2. Immigrants--Mental health. 3. Refugees--Mental health. 4. Cultural psychiatry. I. Al-Issa, Ihsan. II. Tousignant, Michel. III. Series.
RC451.5.A2E84 1997
616.89--dc21 97-14149
CIP

ISBN 0-306-45479-3

A Division of Plenum Publishing Corporation
233 Spring Street, New York, N. Y. 10013

http://www.plenum.com

10 9 8 7 6 5 4 3 2 1

Printed in the United States of America

Contributors

Victor R. Adebimpe, 320 Fort Duquesne Boulevard, Pittsburgh, Pennsylvania 15222-1616

Ihsan Al-Issa, Department of Psychology, University of Calgary, Calgary, Alberta, Canada T2N 1N4

Christopher Bagley, Department of Social Work Studies, University of Southampton, Southampton, SO17 1BJ, United Kingdom

Morton Beiser, Department of Psychiatry, University of Toronto, and Department of Culture, Community, and Health Studies, Clarke Institute of Psychiatry, Toronto, Ontario, Canada M5T 1R8

Yoram Bilu, Department of Psychology, and Department of Sociology and Anthropology, The Hebrew University of Jerusalem, Jerusalem 91905, Israel

A. Gailly, Centrum Welzijnszorg, E. Delvastraat 35, 1020 Brussels, Belgium

Peter J. Guarnaccia, Department of Human Ecology, Institute for Health, Health Care Policy, and Aging Research, Rutgers University, New Brunswick, New Jersey 08903

Ilene Hyman, Department of Culture, Community, and Health Studies, Clarke Institute of Psychiatry, Toronto, Ontario, Canada M5T 1R8

Perminder Sachdev, School of Psychiatry, University of New South Wales, and Neuropsychiatric Institute, The Prince Henry Hospital, Sydney, Australia

Harry Schröder, Department of Clinical and Health Psychology, Institute of Applied Psychology, Leipzig University, 04275 Leipzig, Germany

Peter H. Stephenson, Department of Anthropology, University of Victoria, Victoria, British Columbia, Canada V8W 2Y2

Michel Tousignant, Laboratory for Research in Human and Social Ecology, University of Quebec at Montreal, Montreal, Quebec, Canada H3C 3P8

Gabrielle Tyrnauer, Refugee Research Project, McGill University, Montreal, Quebec, Canada H3A 2A5

James Waldram, Department of Native Studies, University of Saskatchewan, Saskatoon, Saskatchewan, Canada S7N 5E6

Eliezer Witztum, Mental Health Center, Ben-Gurion University of the Negev, Beer-Sheva 84170, Israel

Preface

With political upheaval, wars, and economic disparity between Western and non-Western nations, the second half of this century has witnessed massive movement of immigrants and refugees—particularly from Africa, Asia, and Latin America—to Western countries. The Nazi atrocities against Gypsies, Jews, and other minorities during World War II and the rise of ethnic consciousness during the 1960s and 1970s have resulted in legislation for the protection of human rights. Yet, the 1990s are witnessing a revival of right-wing ideologies associated with racism and prejudice as well as an increase in ethnic and racial conflicts. This volume presents some of the contributions of mental health professionals to the understanding of the stresses experienced by ethnic minorities, migrants, and refugees.

Although immigrants and ethnic minorities experience stressors common to all members of society (stressful life events and daily hassles), they also face stressors unique to them that are related to their cultural background and their experience within the majority culture. Minority groups share the stressful experiences of persons from lower socioeconomic status in the general population, as they tend to be overrepresented among the poor. Their degree of acculturation and assimilation brings about problems related to identity and intergenerational conflicts. In addition to daily individual experience of racial abuse, discrimination, and oppression in the host culture, there are historical forces and antecedent conditions (colonization, slavery, traumas of the Holocaust, torture, and concentration camp experiences) that may indirectly affect ethnic group members.

All groups discussed in the volume share the common experience of prejudice and discrimination. Chapter 2 (Al-Issa) shows how individual, social, and institutional factors could nourish and support bigotry against ethnic minorities. Other chapters discussed in Chapter 1 (Al-Issa) show that ethnic groups and migrants have their own unique experiences. Chapter 3 (Beiser and Hyman) on Southeast Asians in Canada, Chapter 4 (Tousignant) on immigrants and refugees in Quebec, and Chapter 5 (Guarnaccia) on Latin Americans in the United States reveal how sociocultural background, premigration stressors, as well as those during the migration journey interact with aversive experiences in the host culture in determining vulnerability to mental illness of both adults and children. Chapter 6 (Adebimpe) on African Americans and Chapter 13 (Bagley) on Jamaican children and adolescents demonstrate how race could play an important role in the development of self-concept or could result in psychiatric bias in the diagnosis and treatment of mental illness. A history of slavery interacts with current factors in breeding prejudice and discrimination based on skin color. Similarly, Chapter 9 (Al-Issa and Tousignant) indicates how the colonial experience that devalued and attempted to destroy North African culture cannot be separated from the problems of Muslims in France. North Africans provide an excellent example of how an institutional policy of assimilation by the French government and the experience of social exclusion that are practiced simultaneously in France result in stress and conflicts. Turkish guest workers in Belgium discussed in Chapter 10 (Gailly) share the same rural background and Muslim religion with North Africans in France. They share with North Africans similar experiences of cultural conflict, discrimination, and rejection by the indigenous population. Both groups pay a heavy price in psychological and physical ailments.

The only similarity between Jews in Chapter 14 (Bilu and Witztum) and Gypsies in Chapter 15 (Tyrnauer) is that both groups were exposed to prejudice and experienced the Nazi Holocaust. While Chapter 14 discusses the mental health of Jewish people inside and outside Israel, Chapter 15 depicts the struggle of the Gypsies to survive the pressure of marginalization and exclusion in Europe. Chapters 11 (Waldram) and 12 (Sachdev) describe the devastating mental health consequences of the destruction of native culture and the marginalization of its people in North America and New Zealand, respectively. Chapter 7 (Stephenson) deals with the mental health of the Hutterites, who chose a separate communal living but continued a link with North American technological society. Finally, Chapter 8 (Schröder) on East German migrants indicates that a similarity to West Germans in ethnic and cultural background does not provide immunity against the stresses of migration.

Although migration or ethnic minority status is a common factor among all the groups discussed in the chapters, the volume provides the reader with various possibilities of human diversity and potential in coping and adaptation. In recent years, there has been an increasing awareness among mental health professionals of the need to take into consideration the cultural and ethnic factors in research and training in psychiatry, clinical psychology, and counseling. It is hoped that the present volume will introduce students and professionals to major issues of mental health in our multicultural society.

Ihsan Al-Issa
Michel Tousignant

Contents

I. INTRODUCTION

VI. EPILOGUE

I

Introduction

1

Ethnicity, Immigration, and Psychopathology

IHSAN AL-ISSA

The concept of ethnicity refers to a social–psychological sense of belongingness in which members of a group share a unique social and cultural heritage. Ethnicity overlaps with the concept of race and culture. Race is a socially constructed category that specifies the identification of group members and is based on physical characteristics. Culture is those parts of the environment that are human-made, consisting of artifacts (objective aspects) as well as beliefs, values, and norms (subjective aspects) that are shared by the group. The term *culture* is often confused with race, and people who are seen as racially different may be assumed to have a different culture. The bond that brings members of an ethnic group together may be defined in terms of either racial or cultural similarities or both (Al-Issa, 1995). The term *migration* is used to refer to movement of populations between as well as within nations. The difference between immigrants and ethnic groups is generational, and when children of first-generation immigrants settle in a country they usually maintain a membership in an ethnic group. Although immigrants in a new country have their own unique problems, they also share many problems with ethnic groups that have been settled in the host country for a long time. It should also be pointed out that religion may not determine ethnicity, even though it may form the cultural basis for an ethnic identity. For example, North Africans in France who are

---

IHSAN AL-ISSA • Department of Psychology, University of Calgary, Calgary, Alberta, Canada T2N 1N4.

Ethnicity, Immigration, and Psychopathology, edited by Ihsan Al-Issa and Michel Tousignant. Plenum Press, New York, 1997.

Muslims are identified on the basis of their country of origin and not because they are Muslims. Similarly, Jewish people in Israel are divided into ethnic groups on the basis of their countries of origin.

ETHNICITY, IMMIGRATION, AND STRESS

The selection hypothesis and stress hypothesis have been suggested to explain the relationship between migration and psychopathology. The selection hypothesis indicates that those who are vulnerable to mental illness or those who are already mentally ill tend to migrate. In contrast, the stress hypothesis suggests that psychosocial stressors related to migration are responsible for the mental breakdown of immigrants.

One stressful aspect of migration is social isolation and loss of social networks that provide both emotional and instrumental supports. Stress may also result from culture shock, the clash of one's norms and values with those of the host culture. Culture shock may result in confusion and loss of discriminative stimuli that provide the contextual framework for behavior.

Stress may be caused by goal striving, which is defined as the discrepancy between one's aspirations and actual achievement in the host country. This type of stress is great when the motivation for migration is economical. Loss of occupational status where one's skills and training become redundant and dysfunctional may be traumatic for immigrants. The devaluation of the immigrant's occupational or mental abilities is more stressful when it is based on ethnic background or racial characteristics rather than actual performance.

Cultural change that results in the devaluation of the immigrant's culture by the host society may become another source of stress. One source of stress is the pressure on immigrants and minority groups to give up their culture and assimilate into the new culture. Rejection of some basic elements of an ethnic culture by the majority group may increase identification with the minority culture and withdrawal from the major culture (Dion, 1979, 1986). For example, both the Salman Rushdie affair in Britain with its multicultural policy and the scarf or *foulard* affair (to be discussed later) in France with its assimilation policy have created resentment among Muslims in these countries and increased polarization between them and the native population (Bottery, 1992; Chapter 9, this volume).

The nature of the migration itself may be stressful when it is involuntary. Many East Europeans during the communist rule, as well as African, Asian, and Latin Americans, have escaped oppression and violence in their home countries. Some of these immigrants may continue grieving the loss of their culture for the rest of their life. This is particularly true for those who, because of the political system, cannot return to their country for even a visit for the rest of their life. Male members of the family may migrate first, leaving the spouse at home, such as in the case of guest workers from Turkey and North Africa in Europe and migratory labor from Latin America to the United States (see Chapters 5 and 9).

Characteristics of the host culture and its treatment of immigrants may mediate the stress response and may determine adaptation to the new environment. The greater the difference between the host culture and the immigrant's culture, the greater the culture shock and social isolation. A buffer against culture shock is the presence of a subcommunity. Prejudice and discrimination of the receiving population may also be a source of stress (see Chapters 3 and 5, this volume).

ACCULTURATION AND ACCULTURATIVE STRESS

Acculturation is defined as cultural change resulting from direct contact between two cultural groups. Immigrants and ethnic groups adapt to cultural change resulting from contact with the dominant group by using one of four strategies: assimilation, integration, separation, and marginalization (Berry, 1992). Assimilation is the relinquishing of one's own ethnic identity and adopting that of the dominant society. The American "melting pot" concept is an example of assimilation. Integration is the incorporation of part of the other culture but maintaining one's own cultural identity. The end result is a multicultural society with a number of distinctive ethnic groups within a larger social system. The third option is separation, when the ethnic group withdraws from the larger society. Separation may take the form of segregation when it is imposed by the dominant group. Finally, marginalization is when the group or individual loses contact with its own culture as well as with that of the culture of the majority and is usually characterized by alienation and loss of identity.

A combination of the acculturation experience and life change events during migration and contact with the dominant group result in acculturative stress (Berry, 1992). The manifestations of this kind of stress are

> lowered mental health status (particularly anxiety, depression), feelings of marginality and alienation, and heightened psychosomatic and psychological symptom level. Acculturative stress is thus a phenomenon that may underlie poor adaptation, including a reduction in the health status of individuals, identity confusion and problems in daily life with family, work and school. (p. 75)

Chapter 2 of this volume presents a discussion of prejudice and discrimination, which are major sources of acculturative stress to ethnic minorities. Other chapters emphasize the acculturative stressful experiences of a variety of ethnic groups, immigrants, and refugees in North America, Europe, and New Zealand.

PREJUDICE AND DISCRIMINATION

The expression of prejudice and discrimination has undergone important changes in Europe and North America during the 20th century (Chapter 2, this volume). In the first half of the century, prejudice was blatantly open against ethnic minorities, as indicated in studies of ethnic stereotypes (e.g., Gilbert, 1951) and biographical accounts (Malcolm X & Haley, 1965; Wright, 1937). However, the human rights movement of the 1960s and legislation against racial prejudice may have relatively reduced open prejudice and discrimination but have brought about aversive racism, a subtle, indirect type that is more difficult to confront and combat. Discrimination now may be justified on the basis that members of ethnic minorities violate cherished social or religious values and traditions (such as Christianity, democracy, and the law) of Western culture.

Personality and cognitive theories reveal how psychological factors predispose the individual toward prejudice and discrimination (Chapter 2, this volume). After World War II, a team of Stanford University psychologists, including some members who were victims of Nazi concentrations camps, contributed to our understanding of ethnocentrism and anti-Semitism (Adorno, Frenkel-Brunswik, Levinson, & Sanford, 1950). It is important to understand how vulnerabilities to the development of prejudice and discrimination interact with cultural norms and institutional racism. More recently, the cognitive approach to prejudice and discrimination suggests that categorization, which underlies stereotyping, is a basic characteristic of human thinking and essential for individuals to deal with and survive in a complex social and physical environment. However, categorizing by itself is not prejudice; but the cognitive research reported in Chapter 2 shows that once we assign people to groups, we tend to exaggerate similarities within groups (i.e., become vulnerable to the development of stereotypes) and differences between groups (i.e., become vulnerable to the development of ethnocentrism and favoritism) (Wilder, 1978; Chapter 2, this volume). An important contribution of the cognitive theory of prejudice and discrimination discussed in Chapter 2 is that it explains how a member of an ethnic group is perceived, evaluated, and reacted to on the basis of distinctive characteristics and labels.

In order for multiculturation or assimilation to succeed, it is important that contact between groups should be based on cooperative interdependence, an egalitarian structure, normative support from authority figures, and the offering of members of different ethnic groups the opportunity to know each other as individuals or to have positive experiences during their interaction. Since the majority of ethnic groups and immigrants tend to be predominantly poor, with power in the hands of the dominant group (Aponte & Crouch, 1995), it is difficult to reduce prejudice on the basis of contact in the context of an unegalitarian structure (Cohen, 1982). Reducing prejudice requires a change in the whole system that provides privileges and power to dominant groups.

REFUGEES AND IMMIGRANTS IN CANADA

Refugees provide an excellent example of how premigration stressors related to political persecution or natural disasters interact with psychological factors and stressors in the host country in affecting mental health. It appears, however, that experiences during the first years of resettlement seem to have more of an effect on mental health than past experience before migration (Westermyer, Vang, & Neider, 1983a,b; Beiser, Turner, & Ganesan, 1989; Chapters 3 and 5, this volume). Despite the traumatic experience of Southeast Asian refugees before their arrival to Canada, they tend to show similar or even lower rates of depression than their Canadian counterparts. Both the selection and the density (the presence of ethniclike community) hypotheses may explain the good health of Southeast Asians (Chapter 3, this volume). Data on these refugees indicate that the stereotype of associating psychopathology with migration cannot be generalized to all immigrants and ethnic groups.

Among Southeast Asians as well as migrant workers in Europe and the United States (see Chapters 3, 5, and 9, this volume), single males are the most vulnerable because of greater stressors of resettlement; they have to fulfill the obligation of financially helping the family in the home country. In some cases, the source of stress may not be the loss of status, lower self-esteem, and loss of social contact, but rather the financial obligation toward others. Thus, sociocultural and situational factors interact in determining stress (see Chapter 3, this volume). Refugees separated from their families or who have no access to their own ethnic community have the highest risk for depression. Such risk is reduced with ethnic density, since the presence of ethniclike community provides social support and buttresses self-esteem. Ethnic density, while reducing vulnerability to depression, has not been shown to reduce the risk of schizophrenia among immigrants (Cockrane, 1995). Another source of stress on refugees is sexual exploitation or proselytization by the host society (Chapter 3, this volume).

Adolescent refugees in Quebec tend to have high risk for emotional disorders when separated from their parents or exposed to hunger and bad treatment in the camps before arrival to Canada (Chapter 4, this volume). A father's unemployment is another important risk factor. Among ethnic groups, different acculturation strategies are related to high self-esteem. For example, among Greeks, high self-esteem is related to separation, while among the Vietnamese it is related to assimilation. Among the Haitians, however, better self-esteem is related to identification with both the host culture and their own culture. Even a separationist strategy could be adaptive if it is supported by a cohesive group, such as in the case of the Hutterites and Gypsies (Chapters 7 and 15, this volume). Attempts for assimilation also may not be the best choice: some Indian and Haitian women who attempted assimilation showed more symptoms than other women and felt distant from Canadian society, respectively (Chapter 4, this volume).

Many barriers may reduce the use of mental health service by refugees and ethnic groups: the stigma attached to mental health services, language problems, and lack of information about these services (Sue, Chun, & Gee, 1995). Overall, both premigration and postmigration stress interact with the sociodemographic characteristics (personal and social resources) in determining the mental health of refugees (Chapters 3 and 4, this volume).

LATIN AMERICAN IMMIGRANTS AND REFUGEES

Latin Americans in the United States come from different countries as immigrants and refugees. Many Latin Americans are also long-established citizens who have been living in the United States for generations. They are, therefore, subject to common stressors as well as specific ones, depending on their country of origin. Stressors related to lower socioeconomic status are related to psychopathology among Mexicans and Puerto Ricans as well as other Latin American groups. In addition, natural disasters are predominant among Puerto Ricans. Perceived threat of discrimination, racism, and lack of social support tend to have more negative effects on the mental health of Haitians than other groups. Salvadorians and Central American refugees are not only influenced by stressors during resettlement but also by traumatic experiences at home, as well as sexual and financial exploitation on their way to the United States. Cuban refugees and immigrants seem to benefit from community support.

Thus, the experience of both Latin Americans and Southeast Asians in the United States and Canada, respectively, fits an interactional model in which the interaction between individual characteristics, sociocultural background, and the context of exit and reception determine the level of distress and the help-seeking behavior of immigrants and refugees (see Chapters 3 and 5 for details).

AFRO-AMERICANS AND JAMAICANS

Afro-Americans and Jamaicans are exposed to stressors based on the negative evaluation of their skin color. Similar to American and New Zealand natives, black persons tend to be misdiagnosed, overrepresented in public psychiatric institutions, and prescribed higher drug doses (Wedenoja, 1995; Chapter 6, this volume). There is a tendency among mental health professionals to medicalize their social problems (Mercer, 1984). Results of high rates of mental illness of black persons and other minorities are often confounded by socioeconomic status (Chapter 6, this volume). Afro-American overrepresentation in prisons (Chapter 6, this volume) seems to be inconsistent with the finding that they show no significant difference from whites in antipersonality disorder and may reflect biases in the legal system against ethnic groups or lower social class persons. A positive note is that many sociocultural factors such as social support systems, spirituality, and religion tend to be a buffer against stress and reduce the risk of mental illness among Afro-Americans.

Negative self-concepts may increase vulnerability to the development of psychopathology (Brown & Harris, 1978; Chapter 12, this volume). Black children are faced with the negative conflict of choosing between an identification with whites, who represent the dominant culture, or with a subordinate ingroup black culture; a difficult choice between the denial of their own identity and accepting themselves as being of less worth (Bottery, 1992).

In the standard assessment of self-concept, black children typically identify with and choose a white over a black doll. This is more so in Jamaican society, which is based on a color–class pyramid structure. However, with the "black" consciousness in the 1960s and the "black is beautiful" movement, we are witnessing some change in favor of choosing a black doll over a white doll among black children (Milner, 1983). Indeed, in Toronto, Canada, where schools tend to be dominated by an ethnic mixture, black children show an improved self-concept compared with children in Jamaica. However, in cultures where black persons belong to the dominant group with no discrimination against them (e.g., Ghana), color is not involved in the development of self-image and does not become a source of stress (Chapter 12, this volume).

NORTH AFRICANS IN FRANCE AND TURKISH IMMIGRANTS IN BELGIUM

North African immigrants in France are of particular interest, since they are exposed to the French government assimilation policy that tends to intensify their culture shock. Following this policy, young girls, for example, cannot wear the traditional scarf in school (Chapter 9, this volume). The French assimilation policy seems to be incompatible with the life conditions of North Africans; they are "forced" to live in poorer suburban areas with high rates of unemployment, drug abuse, and violence (Jazouli, 1994). The manifestation of symptoms of depression and other psychopathology in this group may reflect social exclusion and rejection by the French society. The similarity between the experience of exclusion of North Africans in France and that of Afro-Americans in the United States is striking:

> Human beings who are forced to live under ghetto conditions and whose daily experience tells them that almost nowhere in society are they respected and granted the ordinary dignity and courtesy afforded to others, will, as a matter of course, begin to doubt their own worth.... These doubts become the seeds of a pernicious self- and group-hatred, the Negro's complex and debilitating prejudice against himself. (Clark, 1965, pp. 63–64)

The prevalence of "delusions" of persecution among North Africans may reflect in part their social exclusion in French society (Lemert, 1962). They also may reflect cultural differences between North African immigrants and the French population, making the former more vulnerable to "aliens" paranoid reactions in which new immigrants or foreign students develop "delusions" as a result of cultural misunderstanding (Murphy, 1967).

Turkish immigrants in Belgium share the Muslim religion with North African immigrants in France. The practice of Islamic rituals has created social and psychological problems for both groups in their new European secular environment. Both groups also predominantly come from a rural background in their native countries. However, Turkish immigrants had not experienced colonization and are less familiar with European culture in comparison with North Africans. While most North African immigrants speak French, Turkish immigrants are not familiar with the languages of the host European countries. These factors result in unique problems related to adaptation and acculturation among Turkish immigrants. Since their number is relatively small in Belgium, they tend to be more visible and more excluded from the majority society (see Chapter 10, this volume). The exclusion of non-Western immigrants and the creation of "illiterate ghettos" in major European cities have resulted in identity problems and have further increased conflicts between ethnic minorities and the host population (see Chapters 9 and 10, this volume).

GYPSIES

The Gypsies have a unique position among ethnic groups discussed in this volume (Chapter 15). In order to protect themselves as a distinct group within a society, they try to keep specific ethnic boundaries and isolate themselves from the majority society in Europe. Their history shows that they continually have practiced self-employment (Okley, 1983) and have refused to integrate within the capitalist system. Although they are similar to migrant workers where their greatest opportunities lie in those jobs others are unwilling to undertake, they differ from them in being self-employed and mobile. Unlike other nomads who may be independent for subsistence, the Gypsies' economy is directly dependent on the wider economy of Western society. A major source of stress for Gypsies is the political and legal constraints set by the larger society on their use of land for residence, work, and travel. Their helplessness and lack of control over their basic daily lifestyle made them one of the most stressed minority groups. Flight is used by them as a major strategy in coping with stressors.

Gypsies are often compared with Jews because between a quarter and a half million of them were exterminated by the Nazis. However, unlike Jews, there has been no break in their persecution after World War II, and the German government has refused to give reparation to many Gypsy survivors (Kendrick & Puxon, 1972; Chapter 15, this volume). Similar to foreign asylum refugees and Turkish migrant workers in Germany, they became targets of skinheads and neo-Nazis (Chapter 15, this volume). Prejudice and discrimination against Gypsies is not limited to Germany but is prevalent in other European countries (Okley, 1983).

JEWS INSIDE AND OUTSIDE ISRAEL

Unlike Gypsies, who refused to relinquish their urban nomadic style of life, Jewish people have been an integral part of the culture and societies in which they live. However, similar to other minorities such as African Americans and American and New Zealand natives, they were stereotyped by Western clinicians and researchers. Research in Israel shows that it is difficult to generalize about the mental health of Jewish people (Chapter 14, this volume). Demographic factors such as social class and gender result in wide differences in the manifestation of psychopathology in Israel, and idioms of distress are quite different among disturbed Jews from Western Europe, Iran, Morocco, Ethiopia, and Russia (Bilu, 1995; Chapter 14, this volume).

Israel is a natural laboratory for the study of stressful life experience associated with ethnic diversity and traumatic life events. This is demonstrated in research on immigrants from the ex-Soviet Union and Ethiopia, the Holocaust victims, and the recent wars in Lebanon and the Persian Gulf (Chapter 14, this volume; Freedy & Hobfoll, 1994; Milgram, 1994). Although ex-Soviet immigrants in Israel were demoralized and suffered from culture shock, they fared better than their counterparts in the United States, suggesting that minority status is more stressful than being part of the majority culture.

Ethiopian Jewish immigrants are not only the most traditional and culturally distant from the average Israeli, but their skin color makes them more visible than others, adding to the stressful migration experience. It is therefore not surprising that one quarter of them suffered from severe symptoms of psychopathology and a high rate of suicide. Ethiopian Jews in Israel provide an example of how stressful experiences during premigration and postmigration interact with other factors in the development of psychopathology. The Zionist dream of Israel as a "therapeutic milieu" for Jews of the Diaspora has not been realized in providing immunity against stressors. Ethnocentrism seems to be universal, and Israel is not an exception despite the common destiny of its people and the Jewish ideals shared by its various ethnic groups.

AMERICAN AND NEW ZEALAND NATIVES

The study of American and New Zealand natives demonstrates how attempts to destroy a culture and impose another culture on its people bring about many stressors and result in both negative physical and mental health. Studies of Native Americans reveal high rates of alcoholism, drug abuse, accidents, violent death, and suicide. Stress-related mental disorders such as neuroticism, anxiety, and depression are also relatively high among this group. These social and psychological pathologies have been associated with many chronic stressors such as "unresolved grief," extensive family disruption caused by alcohol, forced assimilation of youngsters in residential schools, removal of family members, sexual abuse, and identity problems (Chapter 11, this volume). Many of the risk factors related to psychological disturbance and chronic illnesses are shared by Native Americans and the Maori of New Zealand. Chapters 11 and 12 (this volume) describe the struggle of a culture for survival, with many physical and psychological costs.

THE HUTTERITES

The Hutterites chose to integrate economically within the capitalist system but kept a separate communal identity (Chapter 7, this volume). However, communal living and the abolishment of social class distinctions do not seem to provide the Hutterites with immunity against stress or mental illness. Indeed, social cohesion and its concomitant social support have not protected these people from a relatively high rate of depression. Communal responsibilities are a major source of stress in the life of the Hutterites: stressors inherent in contemporary commercial farming, such as decisions related to prices, unpredictable weather, and other insecurities associated with modern agricultural life. However, social support protects the individual in the Hutterite community from isolation and loneliness, which is typical of individualistic societies (cf. East German migrants, Chapter 8, this volume). Coping with stress is facilitated by communal obligations to share the suffering of others rather than blame individuals for their illness. However, some risk factors for psychophysiological disorders tend to be related to social norms and communal living (fat diet, little exercise in a mechanized agriculture) and may be difficult to change in order to lower individual vulnerability in the Hutterite society.

EAST GERMAN MIGRANTS

Risk factors associated with the migration of East Germans to the western part of Germany are quite similar to those found in studies of external migration (Chapter 8, this volume). Loss of social networks (family and friends) or being without a partner or employment were significantly associated with the physical and mental health of the resettlers in West Germany. The more lonely these migrants were, the higher was their experience of anxiety and depression. Many groups who remained in East Germany also suffered in the aftermath of German unification. Social and political changes had increased the risk of many groups. For example, the downward social mobility of the old political elites in former East Germany was reflected in relatively more depression, psychosomatic disorders, and psychotic behavior than in the general population. Other high-risk groups in East Germany were senior citizens, single mothers, young unemployed adults, and those who were forced to take an early retirement. Although East German migrants belonged to the majority ethnic culture and were not stigmatized because of their color or religion, they had similar stressful experiences as foreign migrants and refugees.

SUMMARY AND CONCLUSION

Ethnic groups and immigrants are exposed to the same stressful experiences (major life events and daily hassles) as members of majority groups. However, because of the process of migration and their minority status, they experience acculturative stressors that are unique to them. They not only experience the loss of a spouse or a job or other major life events, but they may grieve a loss of and separation from a whole family, social networks, and their own whole culture. Chapters in this volume indicate that premigration experiences, migration, and resettlement stressors may have negative effects on physical and mental health, but at the same time they demonstrate human resilience against and potential for coping with adversity. Although, in general, there are more emotional and social problems among ethnic minorities, there are also many exceptions. Some immigrants and ethnic minorities may have limited resources to deal with stressors, but the extended family and community social supports may provide immunity against mental illness.

Ethnic groups and immigrants discussed in the present volume may choose voluntarily or are forced to adopt one of the adaptation strategies of assimilation, integration, separation, and marginalization. Such strategies are determined by the interaction between the experiences and the characteristics of the immigrants or ethnic groups on the one hand and the social and cultural setting in the host country on the other. Factors related to the success of adaptation strategies and their relationship to mental health require further investigation.

REFERENCES

Adorno, T. W., Frenkel-Brunswik, E., Levinson, D. J., & Sanford, R. N. (1950). *The authoritarian personality.* New York: Harper & Row.

Al-Issa, I. (1995). Culture and mental illness in an international perspective. In I. Al-Issa (Ed.), *Culture and mental illness: An international perspective* (pp. 3–49). Madison, CT: International Universities Press.

Aponte, J. F., & Crouch, R. T. (1995). The changing ethnic profile in the United States. In J. F. Aponte, R. Y. Rivers, & J. Wohl (Eds.), *Psychological interventions and cultural diversity* (pp. 1–18). Boston: Allyn and Bacon.

Beiser, M., Turner, R. J., & Ganesan, S. (1989). Catastrophic stress and factors affecting its consequences among Southeast Asian refugees. *Social Science and Medicine, 28,* 183–194.

Berry, J. W. (1992). Acculturation and adaptation in a new society. *International Migrations, 30,* 69–85.

Bilu, Y. (1995). Culture and mental illness among Jews in Israel. In I. Al-Issa (Ed.), *Handbook of culture and mental illness: An international perspective* (pp. 129–146). Madison, CT: International Universities Press.

Bottery, M. (1992). Values education and attitude change: The need for an interdependent approach. In J. Lynch, C. Modgil, & S. Modgil (Eds.), *Cultural diversity and the schools: Prejudice, polemic or progress* (Vol. 2, pp. 275–291). London: Palmer Press.

Brown, G. W., & Harris, T. O. (1978). *Social origins of depression: A study of psychiatric disorders in women.* London: Tavistock.

Clark, K. (1965). *Dark ghetto.* London: Gottanz.

Cockrane, R. (1995). Mental health among minorities and immigrants in Britain. In I. Al-Issa (Ed.), *Culture and mental illness: An international perspective* (pp. 347–360). Madison, CT: International Universities Press.

Cohen, E. G. (1982). Expectation status and interracial interaction in school settings. *Annual Review of Sociology, 8,* 209–235.

Dion, K. L. (1979). Intergroup conflict and intercohesiveness. In W. G. Austin & S. Worchel (Eds.), *The social psychology of intergroup relations* (pp. 211–224). Belmont, CA: Brooks/Cole.

Dion, K. L. (1986). Responses to perceived discrimination and relative deprivation. In J. M. Olson, C. P. Herman, & M. P. Zanna (Eds.), *Relative deprivation and social comparison: The Ontario symposium* (vol. 4, pp. 159–179). Hillsdale, NJ: Erlbaum.

Freedy, J. R., & Hobfoll, S. E. (1994). Life events, war and adjustment: Lessons from the Middle East. *Anxiety, Stress and Coping, 7,* 191–203.

Gilbert, G. M. (1951). Stereotype persistence and change among college students. *Journal of Abnormal and Social Psychology, 46,* 245–254.

Jazouli, A. (1994). Un silence d'hôtages [A silence of hostages]. *Le Nouvel Observateur, 1570,* 14.

Kendrick, D., & Puxon, G. (1972). *The destiny of Europe's Gypsies.* London: Heineman.

Lemert, E. M. (1962). Paranoia and the dynamics of exclusion. *Sociometry, 25,* 2–20.

Malcolm X, & Haley, A. (1965). *Autobiography of Malcolm X.* New York: Ballantine Books.

Mercer, K. (1984). Black communities experience of psychiatric services. *International Journal of Social Psychiatry, 301,* 22–27.

Milgram, N. (1994). Israel and the Gulf War. *Anxiety, Stress and Coping, 7,* 205–215.

Milner, D. (1983). *Children and race ten years on.* London: Ward Lock.

Murphy, H. B. M. (1967). Cultural aspects of the delusion. *Studium Generale, 11,* 684–692.

Okley, J. (1983). *The traveller-Gypsies.* Cambridge, England: Cambridge University Press.

Sue, S., Chun, C., & Gee, K. (1995). Ethnic minority intervention and treatment research. In J. F. Aponte, R. Y. Rivers, & J. Wohl (Eds.), *Psychological interventions and cultural diversity* (pp. 266–282). Boston: Allyn and Bacon.

Wedenoja, W. (1995). Social and cultural psychiatry of Jamaicans, at home and abroad. In I. Al-Issa

(Ed.), *Handbook of culture and mental illness* (pp. 215–230). Madison, CT: International Universities Press.

Westermeyer, J., Vang, T. F., & Neider, J. (1983a). Migration and mental health among refugees: Association of pre- and post-migration factors with self-rating scales. *Journal of Nervous and Mental Disease, 171,* 92–96.

Westermeyer, J., Vang, T. F., & Neider, J. (1983b). Refugees who do and do not seek psychiatric care: An analysis of pre-migratory and post-migratory characteristics. *Journal of Nervous and Mental Disease, 171,* 86–91.

Wilder, D. A. (1978). Perceiving persons as a group: Effect on attributions of causality and beliefs. *Social Psychology, 41,* 13–23.

Wright, R. (1937). *Black boy.* New York: Harper & Row.

2

The Psychology of Prejudice and Discrimination

IHSAN AL-ISSA

Prejudice against ethnic minorities and immigrants seems to have reached an epidemic proportion in the world today. Although prejudice is almost universal and is not limited to one group or followers of a specific political ideology or religion, it tends to vary from one individual or one group to another. However, because of massive movement of populations from Africa, Asia, and Latin America to Europe and North America during the second half of the 20th century, prejudice toward ethnic minorities and immigrants has become a major social and political problem in almost every Western nation.

Prejudice and discrimination are the roots of ethnic and religious conflicts. This chapter aims to contribute to the psychological understanding of these phenomena and could serve as an introduction to other chapters of this volume, which deal with ethnic minorities and immigrants. First, the chapter deals with the definition of prejudice, discrimination, racism, and related concepts, followed by discussions of theories of prejudice, aversive racism, the psychological effects of discrimination, and finally the effects of intergroup contact on reducing prejudice.

Note: I use the term "black" instead of African American throughout the chapter in order to be consistent with the same label used by researchers in the eighties and earlier.

IHSAN AL-ISSA • Department of Psychology, University of Calgary, Calgary, Alberta, Canada T2N 1N4.

Ethnicity, Immigration, and Psychopathology, edited by Ihsan Al-Issa and Michel Tousignant. Plenum Press, New York, 1997.

DEFINITION OF PREJUDICE, DISCRIMINATION, AND RACISM

Allport (1954) defined prejudice as "an antipathy based on faulty and inflexible generalization. It may be felt or expressed. It may be directed toward a group as a whole, or toward an individual because he is a member of that group" (p. 9). Prejudice is an attitude that involves the evaluation of an object. Such evaluation has three components: a cognitive component, consisting of beliefs about the object; a behavioral component, such as experiences or actions exhibited toward the object; and an affective component, consisting of feelings or emotions associated with the object (Esses, Haddock, & Zanna, 1993). The cognitive component involves two types of beliefs associated with prejudice (Esses et al., 1993). One type is trait based, related to the characteristics of group members, and is called a *stereotype.* The other type is value based or symbolic and is concerned with certain beliefs that the attainment of cherished social values and traditions may be violated by one group or promoted by another group (Zanna, 1994).

The behavioral component of prejudice is usually expressed in discrimination, a selectively unjustified negative behavior toward members of a target group and often takes the form of excluding them from some activity or from a group (Allport, 1954; Dovidio & Gaertner, 1986). However, prejudice and discrimination are not always related to each other. An early classic study by LaPierre (1934) demonstrated that specific behavior directed toward an ethnic minority in a specific situation, such as admission of members of that group to a restaurant, may not be consistent with negative attitudes toward the same group as measured by tests of attitudes at a more global level. That members of an ethnic minority may be discriminated against in one situation but not in another reflects attitude–behavior inconsistency.

Affect or negative emotions such as hostility and anxiety may play a major role in prejudice. Displaced hostility, for example, has been suggested as an explanation of prejudice against minority groups (Dollard, Doob, Miller, Mowrer, & Sears, 1939). Anxiety as measured by physiological responses also tends to be associated with the degree of prejudice (Vidulich & Krevanick, 1966; Dijker, 1987). Anxiety is aroused when one interacts with others who hold a different worldview that causes uncertainty and unpredictability (Barna, 1983).

Racism involves the assumption of inherent superiority of one group and the consequent discrimination against others. Jones (1972) described three types of racism: individual, institutional, and cultural. Individual racism is based on biological characteristics of the victim and overlaps with prejudice because it refers to individual attitudes. Institutional racism refers to the establishment of institutional policies that unfairly restrict the opportunities of particular groups of people. Finally, cultural racism includes both individual and institutional expression of the superiority of the culture of one race over another. However, prejudice and discrimination should be distinguished from racism; they could be part of racism, but they may be practiced without a racist ideology. However, racial characteristics of groups such as skin color may intensify prejudice and discrimination.

THEORIES OF PREJUDICE

There have been many conceptual approaches to prejudice (Dovidio & Gaertner, 1986). Theories may be divided into those dealing with prejudice and discrimination on the social and interpersonal level (social conflict theory and social learning theory) or on the individual process level (including personality and cognitive theories).

Social Conflict Theory

One version of the conflict theory is the realistic conflict theory suggested by Sherif (1967). This theory considers prejudice to be a result of intergroup competition for scarce resources. However, Tajfel (1981) suggested that conflict of interest is not a necessary condition for intergroup discrimination. Tajfel and Billig (1974) demonstrated that simple categorization of people into two groups with no previous history of interaction could result in ethnocentrism, which is the expression of favoritism toward one's group and unfairness toward others. Such a group bias effect is seen more often in individualistic rather than communal societies (Gudykunst, 1989), where people identify more with all their peers and tend to treat everyone the same.

In contrast to the realistic conflict theory, Tajfel (Tajfel, 1981; Tajfel & Turner, 1985) suggested a social identity theory to explain in-group favoritism. Intergroup discrimination is assumed to reflect a competition for a positive social identity, which contributes to the self-concepts of group members. This theory is supported by the finding that subjects who discriminated against others had higher self-esteem than those who did not (Oakes & Turner, 1980; Lemyre & Smith, 1985).

Social Learning Theory

This theory suggests that prejudice and stereotypes are either based on social influences such as mass media, schools, parents, and peer groups or are the result of observation of actual differences between groups in a society. Parents play an important role in transmitting stereotypes by the information they provide their children or by serving as a role model in their behavior toward members of out-groups. They may demonstrate the typical form of interaction with out-groups and regulate contact with them. For example, forbidding a child from interacting with children of specific groups may give the impression to this child that they are bad. A child may also develop an early awareness of race by an increased preoccupation of parents with racial differences. Early awareness of race may make it more salient and may alert the child to cultural messages concerning race that could result in more prejudice (Albert & Darby, 1992). The mass media may also portray certain groups in a negative way such as the portrayal of blacks in subordinate positions, which reinforces ethnic stereotypes (Dovidio & Gaertner, 1986; Zuckerman, Singer, & Singer, 1980; Wirtenberg, 1978).

Eagly (1987) suggested that stereotypes may be the result of social roles that group members occupy when intergroup contacts occur. Social roles determine behavior of members of a group, which is observed by other people and may become the basis of stereotypes. For example, the repeated observation that women care for children may result in the belief that characteristics necessary for child care such as nurturance and warmth are typical of women. Indeed, many ethnic and racial stereotypes may be based on social structural differences. The content of ethnic stereotypes are often confounded by class differences, reflecting characteristics and behavior ascribed to different social classes (Stephan & Rosenfield, 1982).

Personality Theories

One version of personality theory is the scapegoat theory, which suggests that aggression toward out-groups is the result of displaced hostility from a powerful frustrated individual toward a powerless minority group. According to Dollard et al. (1939), aggressive behavior is a reaction to frustration when an individual is prevented from reaching an attractive goal. However, if the frustrator is powerful or cannot be identified, the aggression will be directed toward less powerful targets such as minority groups. Displaced aggression may be directed to certain groups but not others in society because of the higher visibility and/or powerlessness of these groups (Ashmore, 1970). For instance, after their defeat during World War I and the economic problems that followed, Germans vented their hostility on the Jews. During the medieval era, powerless women accused of witchcraft were the targets of persecution (Al-Issa, 1980). The theory may also explain the higher level of prejudice among the economically frustrated in Western Europe (Pettigrew & Meertens, 1991) and why the highest level of antiblack prejudice is found among lower-class whites (Greeley & Sheatsley, 1971).

Some personality characteristics such as the authoritarian personality are also related to prejudice (Adorno, Frenkel-Brunswik, Levinson, & Sanford, 1950). Adorno and co-workers found that ethnocentric people (those who believe in the superiority of their ethnic and cultural group and disdain other groups) tend to have authoritarian characteristics such as intolerance of weakness, excessive concern with power and status, intolerance of ambiguity, and a tendency to be submissive to those with power over them and aggressive or punitive toward those beneath them. Using a Right-Wing Authoritarian Scale, Altemeyer (1988, 1994) found that high right-wing authoritarians are extremely self-righteous individuals who feel threatened by outside groups; their fears and self-righteous hostilities tend to be expressed in prejudice. Using the same scale, Zanna (1994) found that high authoritarians show more prejudice than low authoritarians, and such a difference was more evident with the target groups that received the least favorable evaluations (Pakistanis and homosexuals). Zanna also reported that symbolic beliefs are particularly predictive of prejudice held by high authoritarians.

Pettigrew (1958) suggested that prejudice may simply reflect the sociocultural norms that operate in a given situation rather than personality. He found that regardless of authoritarian personality test scores, those who supported the Nationalist party and were influenced by the Afrikaan conservative tradition showed more intolerance of blacks. The effects of social norms were also demonstrated in studies where workers may accept integration at work but follow the segregation norms in their neighborhood (Reitzes, 1953; Minard, 1952). These findings suggest an interaction between individual, institutional, and cultural racism.

Cognitive Theory

The Effects of Categorization. Cognitive theories give less attention to the motivational aspects of prejudice than to how people process information about others and form social categories (Tajfel, 1969). Stereotypes, for example, are conceived as a result of the tendency to simplify a complex world by categorizing objects (social and physical) in the daily interaction with the environment. By categorizing people, we are able to think about them and predict their behavior more easily and effectively. The same process of categorizing, however, may bring group bias and discrimination.

Group membership may affect social perception by increasing the tendency to perceive out-group members as being more homogeneous in their characteristics and behavior than in-group members. Studies show that people of other races are perceived to be more alike than those of one's own race (Brigham & Williamson, 1979; Chance & Goldstein, 1981; Ellis, 1981), such as in the case of whites not being able to differentiate faces of blacks or vice versa (Bothwell, Brigham, & Malpass, 1989). Such bias seems to be unrelated to the perceiver's racial attitudes (Brigham & Malpass, 1985). However, the perception of out-group homogeneity is related to the tendency of perceivers to evaluate out-group members as more extreme on various psychological traits than members of an in-group (Hamilton & Trolier, 1986). Such a polarization effect is seen when a positively described person is evaluated more favorably and a negatively described person less favorably if that person belongs to an out-group than an in-group.

Stereotypes as Expectancies. Racial stereotypes influence the encoding of information and may serve as interpersonal expectancies. Studies indicate that when presented with information about others, subjects often form impressions consistent with these expectancies, and identical behavior is often perceived differently, depending on the target group membership (Langer & Abelson, 1974; Brigham, 1971; Farina, 1982).

How group memberships influence the perception and evaluation of behavior is shown by Sagar and Schofield (1980). They had cartoonlike stick figure drawings of children shown to a group of school children, along with verbal descriptions read by the investigator. The sketches depicted actors whose behavior toward the other child was ambiguous. One sketch, for example, showed two students sitting in the classroom, one behind the other, and was described as Mark sitting at his desk working on his assignment when David started poking him in the back. It was found that when the actor was black, his behavior was judged to be more mean, threatening, and less playful and friendly than if the actor was white. The same behavior was thus interpreted differently depending on the race of the person who was performing it. This finding replicates the findings of an earlier study by Duncan (1976) in which students were shown a video of one man lightly shoving another during a brief argument. When a white man shoved a black man, only 13% of the observers rated the act as "violent" and the shove was interpreted by the majority as "playing around" and "dramatizing." However, when the black man shoved the white man, 73% considered the act as "violent."

The effect of stereotypes on interpersonal behavior is demonstrated in studies of the self-fulfilling prophecy when

> one's stereotypic expectations guide one's behavior when interacting with a member of some social group and this expectancy-driven behavior in turn elicits behaviors from the target person that actually confirm the perceiver's initial stereotype. That is, one's behavior toward a member of the stereotyped group constrains the target's behavioral repertoire in such a way as to direct the person to behave in a stereotypic manner. (Hamilton & Trolier, 1985, p. 149)

In support of the self-fulfilling prophecy hypothesis, Word, Zanna, and Cooper (1974) have shown that black job applicants responded to a negative interview style by performing in a less effective and more nervous manner than those subjects responding to a positive interview style. Word et al. (1974) demonstrated that behavior guided by expectancies based on stereotyping may elicit actions from the target person that confirm the perceiver's stereotypes.

Distinctive Stimuli. Being different from others makes persons more noticeable, attracts more attention to them, and distorts the perception of them. Paying extra attention to distinct people creates the illusion that such people differ more from others than they really do. Langer and Imber (1980) found that when students were shown a video and were informed that the man they

may distort their response and obtain low scores on these measures of prejudice in order to appear egalitarian and unbiased in their judgment. However, physiological measures may be used to detect their negative attitudes. Devine, Monteith, Zuwerink, and Elliot (1991) found that whether subjects were high or low on measures of prejudice, they tended to have similar physiological reactions when interacting with African Americans, except that low-prejudice persons consciously suppress prejudicial thoughts and feelings. Thus, in certain cases prejudice seems to operate on the emotional rather on than the verbal conscious level.

In order to detect subtle prejudice, stereotypes could be measured by the associative strength of words as indicated in the reaction time to them. The assumption is that highly associated word pairs (doctor–nurse) produce faster reaction time than unassociated ones (doctor–butter). Using this technique, Gaertner and McLaughlin (1983) presented white American students with the words "blacks" and "whites," which were paired with negative (lazy, stupid) or positive (ambitious, smart) words. It was hypothesized that positive stereotypes toward whites and negative stereotypes toward blacks would result in subjects' responding more rapidly to positive characteristics when they are paired with whites than when they are paired with blacks. On the other hand, blacks paired with negative attributes yield faster reaction times than would whites paired with these same words. In this test, subjects are not directly asked to endorse the appropriateness of a specific word-pair combination, but only asked to indicate whether or not members of the pair are real or nonsense words. Results show that white subjects responded faster when positive traits were paired with whites than when they were paired with blacks. However, they responded as quickly to whites as to blacks paired with negative attributes. While blacks are not overtly described more negatively, these data suggest that they are considered by white subjects as less worthy than whites. Such results were obtained irrespective of the level of prejudice scores of these white college students.

THE PSYCHOLOGICAL EFFECTS OF DISCRIMINATION

Allport (1954) pointed out that discrimination may affect its victims in that "One's reputation, whether false or true, cannot be hammered, hammered, hammered into one's head without doing something to one's character" (p. 142). Allport summarized the effects of victimization into two types involving blaming oneself (withdrawal, self-hate, aggression against one's own group) or blaming external agents (fighting back, suspicion, increased group pride). In a chapter entitled "Reactions to Oppression," Pettigrew (1964) described three classes of responses: (1) moving toward the oppressor by seeking acceptance through integration, (2) moving against the oppressor by fighting back, and (3) moving away from the oppressor through flight or avoidance.

A person is stigmatized by belonging to a disadvantaged or a despised racial, ethnic, or religious group (Goffman, 1963). Crocker and Major (1994) pointed out that stigmatized individuals more often become targets of negative stereotypes, are generally devalued in the larger society, and receive disproportionately negative interpersonal and economic outcomes. The stigma tends to assumes a central role in the way a stigmatized individual construes his or her social world and reacts to others. The stigmatized persons often take it for granted that their stigma affects all behaviors of those who interact with them even when the stigma has no effect on the treatment they receive (Kleck & Strenta, 1980). Negative outcomes construed by the stigmatized (rejected for a job or in social relationships) may, of course, be due either to one's lack of personal deservingness or to the other person's reaction to the stigma. However, evidence shows that the stigmatized do indeed receive more negative evaluations and reactions than nonstigmatized persons and "attributing negative outcomes to the stigma or to prejudice and discrimination is not only plausible, it is often accurate" (Crocker & Major, 1994, p. 291).

Dion (Dion, 1986; Dion, Dion, & Pak, 1992; Dion & Earn, 1975) used the concept of psychosocial stress to explain the effects of "arbitrary" discrimination or perceiving oneself as a victim of discrimination by the majority group. He pointed out that since discrimination involves cognitive appraisal of threat, it is expected to have the same negative psychological consequences as other stressors (Dion & Giordano, 1990; Moritsugu & Sue, 1983). This model of discrimination also suggests that since an out-group threat tends to increase in-group identification (Dion, 1979), experiencing discrimination should also increase identification of the victims with their own groups. Furthermore, identifying with the in-group and obtaining its social support may result in reducing the level of stress from discrimination.

Support for the psychosocial stress hypothesis is reported by Dion and Earn (1975), who studied the emotional reaction and the stress symptoms resulting from anti-Semitism. Discrimination was associated with feeling more aggression, sadness, anxiety, and increased self-consciousness. Pak, Dion, and Dion (1991) also found that those Chinese students who reported the experience of racial discrimination obtained higher scores on psychological symptoms and expressed more positive attitudes toward the Chinese community than other Chinese students who reported no experience of discrimination. Another Canadian study by Kim (cited in Dion et al., 1992) also found that experiences of discrimination by Korean immigrants and Korean-Canadians in Toronto were positively related to higher levels of stress, anxiety, depression, phobic anxiety, paranoid ideation, psychoticism, hostility, and interpersonal sensitivity. Identification with Koreans was stronger among those who experienced discrimination than those who reported no discrimination, supporting the Dion model. Hardiness, which is defined in terms of self-esteem and personal control, seems to act as a buffer against discrimination-related stress (Dion et al., 1992; Kuo & Tsai, 1986). The data by Dion and his associates suggest that similar to other psychosocial stressors, discrimination could have both psychological and physical effects on its victims.

THE CONTACT HYPOTHESIS FOR REDUCING PREJUDICE

Although contact between groups has been often suggested for reducing prejudice, its effectiveness is related to certain conditions (Harrington & Miller, 1992). Contact between groups should involve cooperative interdependence in which the groups share common goals, rewards, or threats, with the aim of accomplishing tasks that require the efforts of the various groups for its accomplishment (Harrington & Miller, 1992). Such cooperative effort could result in a new shared social identity for the groups (Gaertner, Mann, Murrell, & Dovidio, 1989).

A successful contact in reducing prejudice should also be based on an egalitarian structure (Singh, 1992). In normal group interaction, group members usually behave as if status characteristics (age, color, sex, and ethnicity) were relevant to the skills involved in the task (Cohen, 1984). Because race is considered as a status characteristic, it was found that in situations where blacks and whites participate, whites were both given and took more opportunities to perform and their performance was evaluated as better. Whites were also more active and influential in these situations and ranked higher on the number of initiated acts than blacks (Singh, 1992). Similarly, suggestions by whites more often became the group's decision than suggestions by blacks. It seems that "When a racial status characteristic becomes salient in the situation, the prestige and power order of the small group working on a collective task comes to reflect the broader social status ranking of the races in a kind of self-fulfilling hypothesis" (Cohen, 1982, p. 213). It is therefore important that expectations regarding competence based on external status should be changed prior to contact between groups in addition to giving equal opportunity to all members to participate and contribute to the team product (Cook, 1969).

Having the opportunity to know members of other groups and interact with them as individuals may reduce prejudice and discrimination (Cook, 1978; Harrington & Miller, 1992). Harrington and Miller (1992) suggested that the differentiation of an out-group and discovering the uniqueness of its individual members may increase positive responses to them. Contacts with individual members of the group may also be less stressful or anxiety provoking than with a large number of the same group, and thus will have more positive effect (Harrington & Miller, 1992). The role of anxiety in prejudice may explain how intergroup contact under specific conditions (equal status, pleasant, intimate, cooperative, and supported by social norms) reduces prejudice by desensitizing subjects to anxiety (Stephan, 1992). Desensitization aimed at reducing anxiety was shown to reduce prejudice (Sappington, 1976).

Positive contact must meet with normative support from authority figures.

In addition to social, cultural, and familial norms regarding intergroup contact, individuals are influenced at an early age by the attitudes of teachers, administrators, and their peers (Harrington & Miller, 1992; Allen & Wilder, 1975). It is more difficult to deal with discrimination when it is institutionalized and prejudice has become part of the entire social system than when it lies within the prejudiced individual. Hence, there should be a change in the whole system that provides privileges and power to certain groups (Pettigrew, 1986).

One function of positive contact is to provide members of different groups the opportunity to disconfirm existing stereotypes. Knowledge of similarity between the person and the out-group through direct contact should lead to reducing intergroup anxiety and result in a positive change that may disconfirm negative stereotypes (Stephan & Stephan, 1985). One must be cautious, however, about the resulting effects of positive contact with individuals from a minority group. Out-group members who disconfirm stereotypes during the contact will often be discounted as the exception and generalization to the whole group may not take place (Harrington & Miller, 1992).

SUMMARY AND CONCLUSION

There has been an increasing interest in the study of prejudice, racism, and discrimination by social psychologists during the second half of this century. These areas of research have become more important because of many factors such as the Nazi atrocities during World War II, the recent rise of right-wing ideologies in Europe and North America, population movements throughout the globe, and the emergence of multicultural societies. Like other human psychopathologies, the origin of prejudice is multifactorial. Some of the early theories of prejudice are the scapegoat theory, the realistic conflict theory, and the social identity theory. These theories suggest certain precipitating factors related to prejudice and discrimination such as frustration, conflicts of interest, and competition for a positive social identity. On the other hand, the authoritarian personality, and social learning and cognitive theories suggest certain vulnerability factors that predispose individuals toward prejudice and discrimination. For example, cognitive theory emphasizes categorization, which is the basis for prejudice.

In the West, the history of colonization and slavery has created a domination complex in white Europeans in relation to other races and nations, using science and Christian religion to support the belief in their own superiority as well as the inferiority of other cultures (Noël, 1994). The influence of this historical background of Western ethnocentrism (Noël, 1994) has been perpetuated from one generation to another through social learning in the family or through the media, schools, and institutions. This cultural bias toward "whites" is so pervasive in the West that it is seen even among minorities such as Asians, blacks, and Native Indians, who identify with whites in early childhood, demonstrating a positive white and a negative black color bias (Fishbein, 1992; Chapter 13, this volume). One disturbing aspect of prejudice and discrimination is that its effects are not limited to its victims but touch the whole fabric of society as demonstrated in the devastating effects of Nazi ideology during World War II. Unfortunately, recent human rights legislation in some Western countries has not eliminated prejudice and discrimination, but has given rise to more subtle and indirect aversive racism, which is more difficult to confront and combat. This "new racism" tends to hide behind the legal system or is rationalized by some cherished Western democratic or Christian principles. Unless attention is given to the multiplicity of factors associated with prejudice, discrimination, and aversive racism, contact between ethnic groups to create social and racial harmony in Western multicultural society would be doomed to failure.

REFERENCES

Adorno, T. W., Frenkel-Brunswik, E., Levinson, D. J., & Sanford, R. N. (1950). *The authoritarian personality.* New York: Harper & Row.

Albert, M., & Darby, B. (1992). The development of racial attitudes in children. In J. Lynch, C. Modgil, & S. Modgil (Eds.), *Cultural diversity and the schools* (Vol. 2). *Prejudice, polemic or progress?* (pp. 93–106). London: Falmer Press.

Al-Issa, I. (1980). *The psychopathology of women.* Englewood Cliffs, NJ: Prentice-Hall.

Allen, V. L., & Wilder, D. A. (1975). Categorization, beliefs, similarity, and intergroup discrimination. *Journal of Personality and Social Psychology, 32,* 971–977.

Allport, G. W. (1954). *The nature of prejudice.* Reading, MA: Addison-Wesley.

Altemeyer, B. (1988). *Enemies of freedom: Understanding right-wing authoritariansism.* San Francisco: Jossey-Bass.

Altemeyer, B. (1994). Reducing prejudice in right-wing authoritarians. In M. P. Zanna & J. M. Olson (Eds.), *The psychology of prejudice: The Ontario symposium* (Vol. 7, pp. 131–148). Hillsdale, NJ: Lawrence Erlbaum.

Ashmore, R. D. (1970). The problem of intergroup prejudice. In B. E. Collins (Ed.), *Social psychology* (pp. 246–296). Reading, MA: Addison-Wesley.

Barna, L. M. (1983). The stress factor in intercultural relations. In D. Landis & R. W. Brislin (Eds.), *Handbook of intercultural training* (Vol. 2, pp. 19–49). New York: Pergamon Press.

Bothwell, R. K., Brigham, J. C., & Malpass, R. S. (1989). Cross-racial identification. *Personality and Social Psychology Bulletin, 15,* 19–25.

Brigham, J. C. (1971). Ethnic stereotypes. *Psychological Bulletin, 76,* 15–38.

Brigham, J. C., & Malpass, R. S. (1985). The role of experience and contact in the recognition of faces of own- and other-race persons. *Journal of Social Issues, 41,* 139–155.

Brigham, J. C., & Williamson, N. L. (1979). Cross-racial recognition and age: When you're over 60, do they still all look alike? *Personality and Social Psychology Bulletin, 5,* 218–222.

Chance, J. E., & Goldstein, A. G. (1981). Depth of processing in response to own- and other-race faces. *Personality and Social Psychology Bulletin, 7,* 475–480.

Cohen, E. G. (1982). Expectation status and interracial interaction in school settings. *Annual Review of Sociology, 8,* 209–235.

Cohen, E. G. (1984). The desegregated school: Problems in status power and interethnic climate. In N. Miller & M. B. Brewer (Eds.), *Groups in contact: The psychology of desegregation* (pp. 77–96). New York: Academic Press.

Cook, S. W. (1969). Motives in a conceptual analysis of attitude-related behavior. In W. J. Arnold & D. Levine (Eds.), *Nebraska symposium on motivation* (Vol. 17, pp. 179–231). Lincoln: University of Nebraska Press.

Cook, S. W. (1978). Interpersonal and attitudinal outcomes in co-operating interracial goups. *Journal of Research and Development in Education, 12,* 97–113.

Crocker, J., & Major, B. (1994). Reaction to stigma: A moderating role to justification. In M. P. Zanna & J. M. Olson (Eds.), *The psychology of prejudice: The Ontario symposium* (pp. 289–314). Hillside, NJ: Lawrence Erlbaum.

Devine, P. G., Monteith, M. J., Zuwerink, J. R., & Elliot, A. J. (1991). Prejudice with and without compunction. *Journal of Personality and Social Psychology, 60,* 817–830.

Dijker, A. J. M. (1987). Emotional reactions to ethnic minorities. *European Journal of Social Psychology, 17,* 305–325.

Dion, K. L. (1979). Intergroup conflict and intragroup cohesiveness. In W. G. Austin & S. Worchel (Eds.), *The social psychology of intergroup relations* (pp. 211–224). Belmont, CA: Brooks/Cole.

Dion, K. L. (1986). Responses to perceived discrimination and relative deprivation. In J. M. Olson, C. P. Herman, & M. P. Zanna (Eds.) *Relative deprivation and social comparison: The Ontario symposium* (Vol. 4, pp. 159–179). Hillsdale, NJ: Lawrence Erlbaum.

Dion, K. L., Dion, K. K., & Pak, A. W.-P. (1992). Personality-based hardiness as a buffer for discrimination-related stress in members of Toronto's Chinese community. *Canadian Journal of Behavioural Science, 24,* 517–536.

Dion, K. L., & Earn, B. M. (1975). The phenomenology of being a target of prejudice. *Journal of Personality and Social Psychology, 32,* 944–950.

Dion, K. L., & Giordano, C. (1990). Ethnicity and sex as correlates of depression symptoms in a Canadian university sample. *The International Journal of Social Psychiatry, 36,* 30–41.

Dollard, J., Doob, L. W., Miller, N. E., Mowrer, O. H., & Sears, R. R. (1939). *Frustration and aggression.* New Haven: Yale University Press.

Dovidio, J. F., & Gaertner, S. L. (1986). Prejudice, discrimination, and racism: Historical trends and contemporary approaches. In J. F. Dovidio & S. L. Gaertner (Eds.), *Prejudice, discrimination, and racism* (pp. 1–34). London: Academic Press.

Duncan, B. L. (1976). Differential social perception and attribution of intergroup violence: Testing the lower limits of stereotyping of blacks. *Journal of Personality and Social Psychology, 34,* 590–598.

Eagly, A. H. (1987). *Sex differences in social behavior: A social-role interpretation.* Hillsdale, NJ: Lawrence Erlbaum.

Ellis, H. D. (1981). Theoretical aspects of face recognition. In G. H. Davies, H. D. Ellis, & J. Shepherd (Eds.), *Perceiving and remembering faces* (pp. 171–197). London: Academic Press.

Esses, V. M., Haddock, G., & Zanna, M. P. (1993). Values, stereotypes, and emotions as determinants of intergroup attitudes. In D. M. Mackie & D. L. Hamilton (Eds.), *Affect, cognition, and stereotyping: Interactive processes in group perception* (pp. 137–166). San Diego, CA: Academic Press.

Farina, A. (1982). The stigma of mental disorders. In A. G. Miller (Ed.), *In the eye of the beholder: Contemporary issues in stereotyping* (pp. 305–363). New York: Praeger.

Fishbein, H. D. (1992). The development of peer prejudice and discrimination in children. In J. Lynch, C. Modgil, & S. Modgil (Eds.), *Cultural diversity and the schools* (Vol. 2). *Prejudice, polemic or progress?* (pp. 43–74). London: Falmer Press.

Gaertner, S. L. (1973). Helping behavior and racial discrimination among liberals and conservatives. *Journal of Personality and Social Psychology, 25,* 335–341.

Gaertner, S. L., & Dovidio, J. F. (1986). The aversive form of racism. In J. F. Dovidio & S. L. Gaertner (Eds.), *Prejudice, discrimination, and racism* (pp. 61–89). London: Academic Press.

Gaertner, S. L., Mann, J., Murrell, A., & Dovidio, J. F. (1989). Reducing intergroup bias: The benefits of recategorization. *Journal of Personality and Social Psychology, 57,* 239–249.

Gaertner, S. L., & McLaughlin, J. P. (1983). Racial stereotypes: Associations and ascriptions of positive and negative characteristics. *Social Psychology Quarterly, 46,* 23–30.

Goffman, E. (1963). *Stigma: Notes on the management of spoiled identity.* Englewood Cliffs, NJ: Prentice-Hall.

Greeley, A. M., & Sheatsley, P. B. (1971). Attitudes toward racial integration. *Scientific American, 225,* 13–19.

Gudykunst, W. B. (1988). Culture and intergroup processes. In M. H. Bond (Ed.), *The cross-cultural challenge to social psychology* (pp. 165–195). Newbury Park, CA: Sage.

Hamilton, D. L., & Gifford, R. K. (1976). Illusory correlation in interpersonal perception: A cognitive basis of stereotypic judgments. *Journal of Experimental Social Psychology, 12,* 392–407.

Hamilton, D. L., & Rose, T. L. (1980). Illusory correlation and the maintenance of stereotypic beliefs. *Journal of Personality and Social Psychology, 39,* 832–845.

Hamilton, D. L., & Sherman, S. J. (1989). Illusory correlations: Implications for stereotype theory and research. In D. Bar-Tal, C. F. Graumann, A. W. Kruglanski, & W. Stroebe (Eds.), *Stereotyping and prejudice* (pp. 59–82). New York: Springer-Verlag.

Hamilton, D. L., & Trolier, I. K. (1986). Stereotypes and stereotyping: An overview of the cognitive approach. In J. F. Dovidio & S. L. Gaertner (Eds.), *Prejudice, discrimination, and racism* (pp. 127–163). London: Academic Press.

Harrington, H. J., & Miller, N. (1992). Research and theory in intergroup relations: Issues of consensus and controversy. In J. Lynch, C. Modgil, & S. Modgil (Eds.), *Cultural diversity and the schools* (Vol. 2). *Prejudice, polemic or progress?* (pp. 159–178). London: Falmer Press.

Jones, J. M. (1972). *Prejudice and racism.* Reading, MA: Addison-Wesley.

Kleck, R. E., & Strenta, A. (1980). Perception of the impact of negatively valued physical characteristics on social interaction. *Journal of Personality and Social Psychology, 39,* 861–873.

Kuo, W. H., & Tsai, Y.-M. (1986). Social networking, hardiness, and immigrant's mental health. *Journal of Health and Social Behavior, 27,* 133–149.

Langer, E. J., & Abelson, R. P. (1974). A patient by any other name ...: Clinician group difference in labeling bias. *Journal of Consulting and Clinical Psychology, 42,* 4–9.

Langer, E. J., & Imber, L. (1980). The role of mindlessness in the perception of deviance. *Journal of Personality and Social Psychology, 39,* 360–367.

LaPierre, R. T. C. (1934). Attitudes versus actions. *Social Forces, 13,* 230–237.

Lemyre, L., & Smith, P. M. (1985). Intergroup discrimination and self-esteem in the minimal group paradigm. *Journal of Personality and Social Psychology, 49,* 660–670.

McConahay, J. B. (1986). Modern racism, ambivalence, and the modern racism scale. In J. F. Dovidio & S. L. Gaertner (Eds.), *Prejudice, discrimination, and racism* (pp. 91–125). London: Academic Press.

Minard, R. D. (1952). Race relationships in the Pocahontas coal field. *Journal of Social Issues, 8,* 29–44.

Moritsugu, J., & Sue, S. (1983). Minority status as a stressor. In R. D. Felner, L. A. Jason, J. N. Moritsugu, & S. S. Farber (Eds.), *Preventive psychology: Theory, research, and practice* (pp. 162–174). New York: Pergamon.

Noël, L. (1994). *Intolerance: A general survey.* Montreal and Kingston: McGill-Queen's University Press.

Oakes, P. J., & Turner, J. C. (1980). Social categorization and intergroup behaviour: Does the minimal intergroup discrimination make social identity more positive? *European Journal of Social Psychology, 10,* 295–301.

Pak, A. W.-P., Dion, K. L., & Dion, K. K. (1991). Social–psychological correlates of experienced discrimination: Test of the double jeopardy hypothesis. *International Journal of Intercultural Relations, 15,* 243–254.

Pettigrew, T. F. (1958). Personality and sociocultural factors in intergroup attitudes: A cross-national comparison. *Journal of Conflict Resolution, 2,* 29–42.

Pettigrew, T. F. (1964). *A profile of the American Negro.* Princeton, NJ: D. Van Nostrand.

Pettigrew, T. F. (1986). The intergroup contact hypothesis reconsidered. In M. Hewstone & R. Brown (Eds.), *Contact, conflict, and intergroup relations* (pp. 169–195). Oxford: Blackwell.
Pettigrew, T., & Meertens, R. (1991). *Relative deprivation and intergroup prejudice.* Unpublished manuscript, University of Amsterdam.
Quattrone, G. A., & Jones, E. E. (1980). The perception of variability within ingroups and outgroups: Implications for the law of small numbers. *Journal of Personality and Social Psychology, 38,* 141–152.
Reitzes, D. C. (1953). The role of organizational structures: Union versus neighborhood in a tension situation. *Journal of Social Issues, 9*(1), 37–44.
Sagar, H. A., & Schofield, J. W. (1980). Racial and behavioral cues in black and white children's perceptions of ambiguously aggressive acts. *Journal of Personality and Social Psychology, 39,* 590–598.
Sappington, A. A. (1976). Effects of desensitization of prejudiced whites to blacks upon subjects' stereotypes of blacks. *Perceptual and Motor Skills, 43,* 311–411.
Sherif, M. (1967). *Group conflict and cooperation.* London: Routledge & Kegan Paul.
Singh, B. R. (1992). Teaching methods that enhance human dignity, self-respect and academic achievement. In J. Lynch, C. Modgil, & S. Modgil (Eds.), *Cultural diversity and the schools* (Vol. 2). *Prejudice, polemic or progress?* (pp. 207–229). London: Falmer Press.
Sniderman, P. M., Piazza, T., Tetlock, P. E., & Kendrick, A. (1991). The new racism. *American Journal of Political Science, 35,* 423–447.
Stephan, C. W. (1992). Intergroup anxiety and intergroup interaction. In J. Lynch, C. Modgil, & S. Modgil (Eds.), *Cultural diversity and the schools* (Vol. 2). *Prejudice, polemic or progress?* (pp. 145–158). London: Falmer Press.
Stephan, W. G., & Rosenfield, D. (1982). Racial and ethnic attitudes. In A. G. Miller (Ed.), *In the eye of the beholder: Contemporary issues in stereotyping* (pp. 92–136). New York: Praeger.
Stephan, W. G., & Stephan, C. W. (1985). Intergroup anxiety. *Journal of Social Issues, 41,* 157–175.
Tajfel, H. (1969). Cognitive aspects of prejudice. *Journal of Social Issues, 25,* 79–97.
Tajfel, H. (1981). *Human groups and social categories.* Cambridge, England: Cambridge University Press.
Tajfel, H., & Billig, M. (1974). Familiarity and categorization in intergroup behavior. *Journal of Experimental Social Psychology, 10,* 159–170.
Tajfel, H., & Turner, J. (1985). The social identity theory of intergroup behavior. In S. Worchel & W. G. Austin (Eds.), *Psychology of intergroup relations* (pp. 7–24). Chicago: Nelson-Hall.
Vidulich, R. N., & Krevanick, F. W. (1966). Racial attitudes and emotional response to visual representation of the Negro. *Journal of Social Psychology, 68,* 82–93.
Weitz, S. (1972). Attitude, voice, and behavior: A repressed affect model of interracial interaction. *Journal of Personality and Social Psychology, 24,* 14–21.
Wirtenberg, J. (1978). *Cultural fairness in materials development.* [Abstract]. Paper presented at the skills workshop of the Women's Educational Equity Act program, Washington, DC.
Word, C. O., Zanna, M. P., & Cooper, J. (1974). The nonverbal mediation of self-fulfilling prophecies in interracial interaction. *Journal of Experimental Social Psychology, 10,* 109–120.
Zanna, M. P. (1994). On the nature of prejudice. *Canadian Psychology, 35,* 11–23.
Zuckerman, D., Singer, D., & Singer, J. (1980). Children's television viewing, racial and sex-role attitudes. *Journal of Applied Social Psychology, 10,* 281–294.

II

Ethnic Groups and Immigrants in North America

3

Southeast Asian Refugees in Canada

MORTON BEISER and ILENE HYMAN

The so-called "Vietnamese boat people crisis" erupted in 1978. During the next few years, the electronic and print media startled the world with pictures of and reports about Southeast Asians who fled their homes and then endured pirate attacks and hazardous seas in ill-equipped boats only to be turned away by countries who could have offered them refuge. During the height of the crisis, Canada provided haven to 60,000 Southeast Asians, the largest number of refugees ever admitted to the country during such a short time. This response to the crisis marked a high point in the country's evolution from an insular, indifferent nation to one now widely admired for her compassion. In 1986, the United Nations acknowledged Canada's international leadership in refugee affairs by its award of the Nansen medal for humanitarianism.

The Clarke Institute and University of Toronto Department of Psychiatry Refugee Resettlement Project (RRP), initiated in 1981, is a study of 1348 Southeast Asian refugees admitted to Canada during the "boat people" crisis, who resettled in and around Vancouver, British Columbia. This decade-long investigation documents the adaptation of the Southeast Asians in their new home, the factors that facilitated their success, and the social and psychological forces that created mental health risk.

MORTON BEISER • Department of Psychiatry, University of Toronto, and Department of Culture, Community, and Health Studies, Clarke Institute of Psychiatry, Toronto, Ontario, Canada M5T 1R8. **ILENE HYMAN** • Department of Culture, Community, and Health Studies, Clarke Institute of Psychiatry, Toronto, Ontario, Canada M5T 1R8.

Ethnicity, Immigration, and Psychopathology, edited by Ihsan Al-Issa and Michel Tousignant. Plenum Press, New York, 1997.

SOCIAL AND CULTURAL BACKGROUND

The term, "Vietnamese boat people," is misleading on two counts. First, many Southeast Asian refugees were not Vietnamese. Second, most escaped their home countries over land, not by boat.

Saigon fell to North Vietnam in 1975. Before Hanoi's armies took control of the South, 135,000 Vietnamese fled as refugees. Although the vast majority of this predominantly urban, middle-class, well-educated group were relocated to the United States, about 9000 resettled in Canada, primarily in Montreal and Quebec City.

Shortly after this wave of refugee exodus, Hanoi sealed the borders of a country that was plunging into economic crisis. The Sino-Vietnamese war had emptied the country's treasury, and the US military's jungle defoliation offensive had stripped it of one fifth of its fruit and lumber-producing forests. Added to these problems, floods and droughts in the late 1970s seriously affected rice production. The crisis prompted the government to send the merchant class (many of whom were ethnic Chinese) from the cities to be "reeducated" as pioneer agricultural workers in "new economic zones."

Resorting to conquest of its neighbors in order to deal with its internal problems, Vietnam invaded Cambodia in 1978. When China retaliated with military action along its border with North Vietnam, Hanoi began to persecute and expel ethnic Chinese residents, many of whom could trace hundreds of years of ancestry in Vietnam.

The forced expulsion of Chinese, together with the escape of many Vietnamese who felt they could no longer live in their country, set the so-called boat people crisis in motion. More people escaped from Vietnam over land routes through Cambodia to Thailand than by sea. Nevertheless, the image of people on boats trying to reach safe harbor in Hong Kong, the Philippines, Malaysia, and Indonesia remains the most potent icon of the Southeast Asian exodus.

Sandwiched between Vietnam, Thailand, and China, and officially neutral, Laos could not escape international politics. Within its borders, battles for control of the country flared between the communist Pathet Lao, backed by China, and rightist-dominated government forces, backed by the United States and the Philippines. From the early 1960s, Laos's fate became increasingly tied to Vietnam. In return for Pathet Lao support of North Vietnamese guerrilla movements along the Ho Chi Minh Trail and from there into South Vietnam, Hanoi helped the Lao Communists gain control of Vientiane, the capital of Laos. The fall of Saigon in 1975 finally broke the deadlock between government-led military and the Pathet Lao. Their morale in collapse, rightist politicians and soldiers fled to Thailand, to be quickly followed by other citizens, fearful of what communist domination might mean and of how the Pathet Lao might retaliate against former supporters of the West.

Meanwhile, in Cambodia, Vietnam's armies ultimately defeated the notorious warlord, Pol Pot. During the confusion of the war, the wealthy, the entrepreneurs, and the intellectuals—all of whom Pol Pot had marked for his genocidal programs—escaped their prisons in the forests of Cambodia to become part of the refugee torrent gushing out of Southeast Asia.

Refugees who managed to find asylum in Hong Kong, Thailand, Indonesia, Malaysia, the Philippines, or Singapore were placed in holding camps administered by the respective countries. Although supported by the United Nations High Commission for Refugees, as well as nongovernmental, voluntary, international agencies (often referred to as NGOs or VOLAGs) such as the International Red Cross, the Mennonite Central Committee, and Save the Children, the refugees had to face harsh camp conditions and endure enforced idleness—sometimes for weeks, but often for years—until selected by a resettlement country. On the basis of the ratio of refugee admissions to indigenous population, Canada and Australia became the era's most generous countries of permanent asylum. Between 1979 and 1981, Canada admitted 60,000 "second-wave" Southeast Asian refugees. Compared with the first-wave group, second-wave refugees came from a wider socioeconomic spectrum, were less well-educated, and had less previous exposure to the west. More than 90% spoke neither English nor French. Following government policy, the second-wave refugees were scattered across Canada, in rural areas as well as in cities (Nguyen, 1982b).

REFUGEES AND MENTAL ILLNESS

Common sense together with behavioral science theory suggest that the survivors of prolonged wars, of persecution, of hazardous escapes from their homelands, and of internment in refugee camps, forced to adjust to resettlement countries dominated by unfamiliar customs and languages, must be people at risk for mental disorder. In Canada, concerns about the mental health of refugees, and of immigrants in general, prompted the creation of a federal task force to investigate the situation and to formulate recommendations. After a comprehensive literature review, the task force concluded that about half the available literature supported theory and common sense by demonstrating that migrants experience more mental health risk than host country indigens. The other half, however, revealed either no differences or, in some cases, a mental health advantage for newcomers.

The task force findings underline the need for theory that permits more complex formulations than a simple stress = distress model (Canadian Task Force on Mental Health Issues Affecting Immigrants and Refugees, 1988). Although persecution, flight, and resettlement create mental health risk, their effects are modified by a context of psychological and social resources. For example, the availability of a close and confiding relationship during resettle-

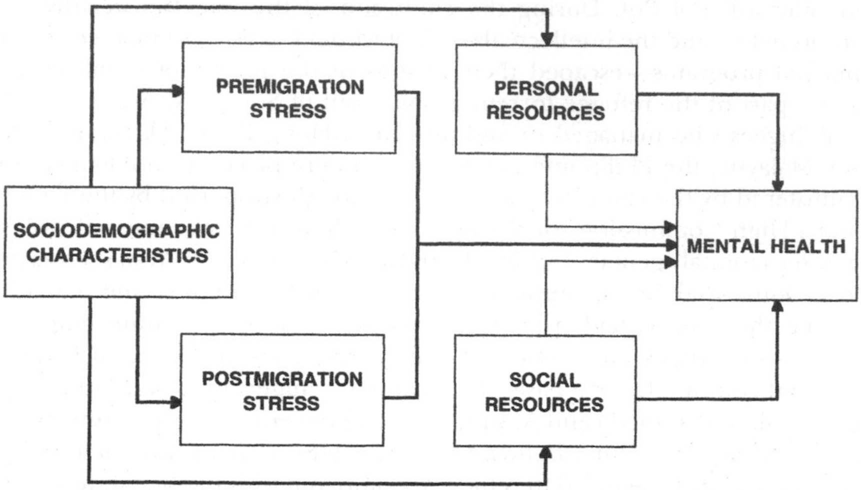

Figure 1. Refugee resettlement and mental health.

ment is a microlevel social resource that modifies risk and contributes to mental health. At a macrolevel, a supportive social network (typically available to newcomers through their like-ethnic community) can also protect and support mental health. Drawing on stress process theory, Fig. 1 presents a model of the relationship between risk, protective factors, and mental health that has guided the RRP investigations.

The model posits that pre- and postmigration stressors are independent variables that exert a direct effect on mental health. Social and psychological resources affect mental health directly (thus acting as independent variables) or, by affecting the experience of stress, influence mental health indirectly (thereby acting as moderating variables).

PSYCHIATRIC DISORDER

Since categories such as depressive disorder denote concepts of mental disorder whose origins are largely North American and European, their cross-cultural applicability is subject to continuing challenge. On the grounds that cultural differences in idioms of distress, in the experience of illness, and in the construction of illness categories make such comparisons impossible, cultural relativists (Kleinman, 1987; Littlewood, 1992; Obeyesekere, 1985; Lutz, 1985) decry the use of traditional psychiatric categories to compare the mental health of groups like Southeast Asian refugees with native-born residents of host countries like Canada. The argument that Eastern expressions and experiences of illness differ from Western is summarized in a popular apothegm: "Asians somatize and North Americans psychologize" (see Kleinman, 1980; Tseng, 1975; Yap, 1965).

RRP data refute the apothegm and its chain of related assumptions. Factor analyses of symptoms reported by the Southeast Asian refugees and a comparison sample of longtime residents of Canada have yielded remarkably similar results. Confirmatory factor analyses of data from community samples of Southeast Asian refugees and Canadian residents revealed that depressive affect, somatic distress, panic, and feelings of well-being accounted for most of the symptoms variance in each of these "Western" and "Eastern" groups, and that their structure was cross-culturally invariant. These results strongly suggest the universality of common forms of distress and of positive affect (Beiser, 1985; Beiser & Fleming, 1986; Devins, Beiser, Dion, Pelletier, & Edwards, in press). Since factors are orthogonal structures, the data also challenge the assertion that Asians somatize depression. Rather than being a cultural equivalent for depression, somatization is probably a unique and independent dimension of distress.

Critics of attempts to create cross-culturally stable measures of distress and disorder have pointed out that the reliance of symptom inventories such as the Present State Examination (PSE) or the Diagnostic Interview Schedule (DIS) on Euroamerican expressions of distress virtually ensures that the resultant categories will mirror the constructs from which they were derived. These critics argue that symptom inventories should include culture-specific idioms of distress, an innovation that would permit the emergence of culture-specific aggregations of symptoms (Lin, 1983). However, the RRP inventory did include culture-specific items, some derived from other instruments (Kinzie et al., 1982) and some from key-informant interviews. Rather than producing new categories, the culture-specific items clustered with the "universal" expressions of depressive affect and of somatization derived from symptom inventories in popular use (Beiser & Fleming, 1986).

Dimensions of distress seem remarkably stable across groups. Culture, however, may play a role in shaping the metric of intensity. Although it seems counterintuitive, resident Canadians taking part in the RRP endorsed more intense expressions of depressive affect than did the refugees. There were no differences in endorsement patterns on the somatization items, and refugees tended to score lower on positive affect (Beiser & Fleming, 1986; Devins et al., in press). The findings suggest that, although the same spectrum of emotional expression is available to Southeast Asians and to North Americans, the latter may communicate in bolder colors, the former with a more muted palette.

A related set of investigations has centered on psychiatric diagnosis, rather than dimensions of distress. The application of grade of membership (GOM) analysis (a multivariate clustering technique appropriate for testing the validity of clinical constructs) to the Southeast Asian and resident Canadian data

University of Toronto investigative team is addressing the apparent paradox of increased risk for psychopathology together with exceptional achievement.

STRESSORS

Figure 1 calls attention to the influence of both pre- and postmigration stressors on mental health. Consistent with reports by others (Westermeyer, Vang, & Neider, 1983a,b; Westmeyer, Neider, & Vang, 1984), RRP data suggest that, in the early phases of resettlement, premigration traumata affect mental health less profoundly than postmigration stressors. For example, although harsh conditions prevailed in all the refugee camps in Southeast Asia, it was possible to array them on a scale, with Thai camps rating the worst, Hong Kong camps the best, and the others in between. RRP respondents who had been in Thai camps showed the highest distress and those from Hong Kong camps the lowest. However, the relationship between this premigration stressor and mental health proved evanescent. After the refugees had been in Canada more than 6 months, the relationship between refugee camp stress and depression disappeared (Beiser, Turner, & Ganesan, 1989).

Unemployment creates mental health risk for refugees (Beiser, Johnson, & Turner, 1993b; Westermeyer et al., 1983a,b; Westermeyer, Callies, & Neider, 1990; Lin, 1986) as it does for everyone (Kessler, Houser, & Turner, 1987a; Kessler, Turner, & House, 1987b; Bland, Stebelsky, Orn, & Newman, 1988). Parallel statistical associations in different population groups do not, however, necessarily imply parallel dynamics. Context determines the experience of unemployment. Personal and household financial strain created by unemployment proved to be salient stressors for refugees as well as host country residents. However, unemployment also created a unique and additional mental health risk for refugees. Not working undermined more than self-support and the support of family present in Canada. It also meant a failure in the obligation to family left behind in refugee camps or in the home country. This finding, highlighting differences between the individually centered ethos of North American society and the more sociocentric, familistic orientation of Southeast Asians (Haines & Rutherford, 1981), illustrates the role of cultural and situational context in the definition of stress. The role of occupationally derived status is another illustration of how situation shapes the meaning of stress. Under ordinary circumstances, work is an index of social status. As a consequence, unemployment threatens both self-esteem and the maintenance of social contacts (Warr, 1982). However, assaults to status and restriction of social contact were not the salient factors linking unemployment to refugee mental health. Instead, individual deprivation and failed familial obligation consequent on unemployment constituted accounted for mental distress among the refugees (Beiser et al., 1993b).

RRP data demonstrated a reciprocal relationship between unemployment and depression. Unemployed people were more likely to be depressed than their employed counterparts. Job loss predicted later depression; finding a job led to improved mental health (Beiser et al., 1993b). On the other hand, depressed refugees were more likely than the nondepressed to lose their jobs. Untreated depression may thus create social difficulties, leading to the stabilization of symptoms and to increasing social maladaptation (Beiser et al., 1993b).

During the early years of resettlement, refugees typically suffer high rates of unemployment. Initial trends frequently register in public consciousness, giving rise to an erroneous belief that refugees are an inevitable drain on a host country's economy. Long-term trends refute this idea. The longer refugees live in resettlement countries, the higher their rate of employment (Caplan et al., 1989). In 1991, 10 to 12 years after the refugees in the RRP cohort arrived in Canada, their unemployment rate was lower than the national average (8% for former refugees versus a 10.3% national average). Refugees experience difficulty in finding jobs at the level their training and former experience might lead them to expect (Canadian Task Force on Mental Health Issues Affecting Immigrants and Refugees, 1988). During their early years in Canada, both men and women experienced a drop in occupational status relative to their positions in Vietnam. Teachers became domestics and electricians worked as farmhands. As might be expected, the most highly educated experienced the sharpest declines in occupational prestige. The drop in occupational status was even more severe for men than for women. Underemployment has been posited to be a mental health risk (Canadian Task Force on Mental Health Issues Affecting Immigrants and Refugees, 1988). However, according to RRP data, although underemployed resident Canadians were at risk for depression, the Southeast Asian refugees were not (Beiser et al., 1993b; Edwards, 1994). Qualitative RRP data suggest that the refugees' hopes for their children helped ease and rationalize personal deprivations (Beiser et al., 1993b).

Ten to twelve years postarrival, the picture had brightened. Most refugees were not only working, but were no longer underemployed. Occupational status for males improved to the point where men were working at jobs equal to or even slightly higher in prestige than those they had held in Vietnam. Female occupational status gains were even more dramatic. Having begun at prearrival occupational levels considerably lower than their male counterparts, women had achieved virtual parity in employment prestige after their first decade in Canada (Edwards, 1994).

An emerging Southeast Asian entrepreneurial presence is helping to revitalize the "Chinatowns" of Montreal, Toronto, and Vancouver. Given Canada's increasing interest in cultivating economic ties with the "Little Economic Tigers" of Southeast Asia, the former refugees seem well positioned to help create important links and to provide much needed cross-cultural understanding. The contributions of refugees to their adopted country remain more a matter of conjecture than the subject of study (Bun & Christie, 1995).

Although underemployment had no apparent effect on rates of mental disorder, it did affect well-being. Refugees who experienced gains in occupational prestige over the years also achieved higher levels of positive affect than others who remained at the same levels or experienced decline. The finding that although underemployment does not create mental health risk, it does jeopardize well-being, highlights the importance of maintaining a conceptual distinction between positive and negative affects. These dimensions of mental health are not only factorially separable, but etiologically distinct (Devins et al., in press; Beiser & Fleming, 1986; Bradburn, 1969).

Family separation creates emotional distress. Although Part I.3.(c) of Canada's Immigration Act of 1976 defines family reunification as one of its cornerstones (also see Minister of Supply and Services, 1994, p. xi), administrative policy and bureaucratic process often stand in the way (Canadian Council for Refugees Task Force on Family Reunification, 1995). Many of the Southeast Asian refugees arriving in Canada between 1979 and 1981 reported that they had at least two important family members either in refugee camps or still living in the homeland with whom they wished to be reunited.

Based on a study of Vietnamese refugees in mental health care, Nguyen (1982a) identified separation from immediate family members as a major mental health risk. According to RRP results, people separated from important family members had higher levels of depressive affect than individuals reporting no separation. Family relationship affected mental health risk: separation from spouse had the greatest psychological impact, separation from siblings the least, with that from parents in between. Refugees who were eventually able to bring their relatives to Canada experienced an improvement in mental health (Beiser et al., 1993b).

TIMING AND MENTAL HEALTH RISK

According to a popular model, the risk for developing mental disorders is not particularly high immediately after resettling in a foreign country. Instead, mental disorders begin to emerge only after an initial "incubation" period, weeks or even months after initial arrival. The appeal of predictable simplicity probably accounts for the widespread acceptance of this model of phase-related risk, despite the fact that its initial formulation was based on a surprisingly small number of clinical, and therefore methodologically limited studies (Tyhurst, 1951; Holmes & Masuda, 1973; Mathers, 1974; Grinberg, 1984). Generalizing from clinical samples to a population at large is perilous and always questionable.

Rumbaut's (1985) community-based study of Southeast Asian refugees in

San Diego offered a methodological advance over clinical investigations. His findings suggested a period of maximum risk of 12 to 18 months postarrival. In a study of immigrant and refugee women, Franks and Faux (1990) reported that the most recent arrivals had lower depressions scores than people resident in Canada for 8.5 to 15.5 years. These authors suggested that a group's past hardships may make current conditions seem more tolerable, at least in the short run. The validity of Rumbaut's and of Franks and Faux's conclusions, however, is jeopardized because both studies are cross-sectional rather than longitudinal. Comparing the mental health of refugees present in a resettlement country for varying lengths of time rather than following one group over time risks the confounding of time with cohort effects.

Longitudinal data from the RRP confirm but also qualify the concept of phase-related mental health risk. Ten to twelve months after arrival, levels of depressive affect among the refugees were higher than in previous or subsequent periods. However, the experience of increased risk was not universal. Instead, it appeared only among refugees bereft of family and limited or no access to a like-ethnic community (Beiser, 1988).

According to a study by Nguyen (1982b), it takes a refugee 3 to 5 years after initial resettlement to regain a sense of equilibrium and to develop confidence in his or her future. Among the factors facilitating restabilization, Nguyen concurs with the Canadian Task Force report (1988) in identifying employment, reunification with family, and language competence as the most important.

The longer that refugees in the RRP study remained in Canada, the more their levels of depressive affect fell. These findings, however, do not offer grounds for complacency. Consistent with other research (Westermeyer et al., 1984), RRP data demonstrate that depression in a vulnerable population is not a transient problem. Intense distress tends to persist and probably creates a condition of risk for full-blown, potentially chronic, clinical depressive disorder (Keller, Lavori, Rice, Coryell, & Herschfeld, 1986; Weissman, Myers, & Thompson, 1986).

PROTECTIVE FACTORS AND MENTAL HEALTH

Mental health depends on a complex interaction between risk factors that jeopardize mental health and social and psychological factors that protect it.

Social Resources

H.B.M. Murphy (1977) was probably the first psychiatrist to direct attention to the psychologically protective influence of the like-ethnic community. Although subsequent research consistently supports the cogency of Murphy's observations (Beiser, 1982, 1988; Beiser et al., 1989; Berry & Blondel, 1982), it has done little to elucidate how a "critical mass" of like-ethnics supports individual mental health.

Chinese refugees in the RRP study enjoyed an initial mental health advantage over the non-Chinese. Instrumental support available through the Chinese community offers, at best, only a partial explanation for the Chinese refugees' mental health advantage. For example, although marginally employable persons, such as elderly, Chinese, non-English-speaking females had an easier time finding work than their non-Chinese peers, the employment advantages for the Chinese as a whole were less than overwhelming (Johnson, 1988).

Symbolic interaction theory provides a more promising interpretive possibility. According to symbolic interactionists such as C. H. Cooley (1902) and G. H. Mead (1934), self-evaluation and social identity—both important determinants of mental health—originate in social interaction. By providing opportunities for friendship and by reaffirming ethnic and social identity, a like-ethnic community of significant size supports feelings of self-worth.

Alternative explanations for the Chinese refugees' mental health advantage are possible. Although their ancestors had been in Vietnam for generations, the Chinese were an identifiable ethnocultural minority, whereas the Vietnamese and Laotians were members of the dominant culture in their respective countries. Historical differences may have prepared the Chinese refugees better than their non-Chinese counterparts for life in a new country in which all were relegated to minority status. Another possibility is that the Vietnamese, Laotians, and Cambodians who were uprooted from their respective homelands had more to mourn than the Chinese, who were sojourners in a foreign country.

Longitudinal data from the RRP throw some light on competing hypotheses. If the Chinese were more adaptable than the non-Chinese rather than better supported, one might expect their initial advantage to continue over time. Instead, the powerful ethnic effect on mental health observed during the initial period of resettlement disappeared several years later (Beiser et al., 1989). It seems plausible that during the intervening years, the non-Chinese refugees began to create new ethnocultural communities or to cultivate relationships with the majority culture that provided new resources for self-affirmation, thereby enabling them to "catch up" with the Chinese. The RRP longitudinal data not only suggested eventual dissipation of the initial Chinese mental health advantage, but, in addition, some long-term gains for the non-Chinese. In comparison with Chinese refugees, Laotians, Vietnamese, and Cambodians seemed to be integrating more quickly with the larger society, learning English faster, and including more nonethnics in their friendship networks.

Resettlement theory suggests that the degree of openness of the host society affects the mental health of newcomers (Aylesworth, Ossario, & Osaki,

1977; Beiser & Collomb, 1981; Beiser, 1982). An intuitively appealing construct, "host country receptivity," is difficult to operationalize. A Canadian government program, expanded during the refugee crisis of the late 1970s, provided a natural experiment to test the proposition. Most refugees entering Canada come under government sponsorship, under which terms they receive income and housing support for 1 year and, for those deemed likely to enter the paid workforce, English language training. Families, organizations such as churches, and groups of private citizens can and do act as private sponsors by guaranteeing income support for 1 year or until a sponsored refugee becomes self-sufficient.

Canada's Conservative government of the day tried to fulfill its commitment to resettle Southeast Asian refugees without compromising its philosophy that private citizens should do more and government less. To achieve these ends, the Department of Immigration and Employment initiated a private sponsorship campaign under the terms of which it pledged to match each refugee brought in under private auspices with one sponsored by the government. Hypothesized program benefits included: (1) by bearing part of the material cost for the refugees' first year in Canada, the private sector would reduce the government's financial burden, and (2) advocates would have the opportunity to increase overall refugee levels by assuming individual responsibility. The third aim of the program—to facilitate refugee integration and reduce racial backlash through community participation (Adelman, 1980)—suggested the hypothesis that in comparison with government agencies, private individuals would devote more attention to and likely have more time for the people they sponsored. As a result of this advantage in hospitality, privately sponsored refugees would experience better mental health than government sponsored.

RRP data do not support the last hypothesis. In retrospect, government and academics may have been more impressed with the virtues of private sponsorship than the refugees themselves. Adelman (1984), for example, reports that private sponsors tended to find housing for their charges that, on termination of the sponsorship, the refugees could no longer afford. In addition, sponsors looked for housing accessible to them rather than, as the refugees might have preferred, close to ethnic communities or to potential workplaces. Despite the fact that at the end of their first year in Canada, privately sponsored refugees were financially better off and had learned more English than their government-sponsored counterparts, 50% said they would have preferred government sponsorship (Woon, 1987). Many complained that their sponsors were overly intrusive. The privately sponsored group also felt disadvantaged by inequity. Some sponsor groups provided treatment of almost opulent proportions. Other sponsors, disillusioned after a first flush of enthusiasm, became indifferent (Woon, 1987).

Power asymmetries created vulnerability. Refugees in the RRP sample whose religions were incongruent with their sponsors (for example, Buddhist refugees sponsored by a Christian church group) were at higher risk for depression than those whose religions matched (Beiser et al., 1989). Interpreting similar findings, other investigators (Westermeyer et al., 1983a,b) have described refugee distress attendant on sexual exploitation or proselytization. RRP observations suggest that, if some private sponsors consciously or unconsciously may have considered the religious conversion of the refugees a good idea, most were not overtly coercive. Nevertheless, many refugees felt pressured. Unable to understand why strangers would be willing to help them and trying to comprehend what was expected of them in return, some refugees stumbled on the idea that they could please their sponsors by adopting their religion (Beiser et al., 1989).

The RRP findings should act as a caution to rather than an indictment of churches, institutions that have been major advocates for refugees and that have assumed major responsibility for refugee welfare in resettlement countries. Neuwirth and Clark (1981) have described the conundrum of beneficence versus undue influence. Religious sponsors tend to provide assistance predicated on an assumption—perhaps misguided—that refugees will eventually assimilate to the dominant culture and that religious conversion will be a natural concomitant of assimilation. The assumption sometimes creates stress for sponsored refugees. It also helps to account for the devotion of church-affiliated sponsors, whose commitment tends to be more sustained than that of others who become sponsors out of a sometimes evanescent sense of compassion or in order to foster their own personal growth.

Like-ethnic community support and the host society's receptivity are macrosocial variables affecting mental health. At a more microlevel, marriage can be a potent protective factor. Married refugees whose spouses were with them in Canada had lower levels of depression than single, divorced, or widowed adults or those involuntarily separated by circumstance. Over time, singles who married experienced an improvement in mental health and people who separated, divorced, or were widowed experienced a decline (Beiser et al., 1993b). Family and community relations also affect self-concept. In a study of Vietnamese and Sino-Vietnamese resettling in Alberta, Indra (1988) found a positive association between self-esteem on the one hand and family and community involvement on the other.

Personal Resources

Keeping the past out of awareness seems an effective way to ward off depression. RRP qualitative interviews suggested that in the camps the refugees concentrated on day-to-day survival. The most successful neither ruminated about the past nor allowed expectations for the future to occupy much of their attention. Concentrating on the present and to a limited extent the future also proved the most successful strategy during the early years of resettlement. Data from a quantitative method developed for the RRP confirmed the impression that individuals who fixated on the past were likely to fall prey to depression. Splitting the past from the present and future not only seemed to protect individual mental health, but to offer a psychological buffer against the memory of past deprivations. Compared with resident Canadians, refugees were more likely to avoid focusing on the past (referred to as "nostalgia" in the RRP investigations) and to split the present from future and past (referred to as an "atomistic" approach to handling time).

Although "time-bindedness," the integration of past, present, and future, is, according to Mowrer (cited in May, 1958), probably the natural human state, the reemergence of the past and its reconnection with present and future are mental processes that create a risk for depression (Beiser, 1987; Beiser et al., 1989; Beiser & Hyman, in press).

Avoidance of the past is related to Freud's concept of *Unterdruckung*, or "pressing under." Later elaborated by others as *suppression*, the concept describes a psychological defense involving the temporary setting aside of painful percepts. Many psychiatrists draw a distinction between suppression (more or less a conscious act of inattention) and the psychopathology-inducing mechanism of repression (or motivated forgetting) through which unwanted memories are forced into the unconscious. Basing his conclusions on a study of successful people, George Vaillant (1977) suggests that suppression is the most common and perhaps the most effective defense against internal conflict. Commenting on the role of repression in her study of victims of catastrophic stress, Terr (1994) argues that the return of painful, repressed memory invariably invokes symptoms: the presence of symptoms helps distinguish between genuine remembering and the so-called "false memory" syndrome (for further discussion of these psychodynamic concepts, see Moore & Fine, 1990).

The refugees' avoidance of past percepts and their proclivity to split time spheres apart are probably adaptive mechanisms, akin to suppression, rather than indicators of psychopathology. The psychophysiological mechanisms underlying and sustaining these phenomena are poorly understood and require further study. It is probably even more important to study the process that makes recovery of the past and its reintegration with present and future possible without jeopardizing mental health. An understanding of constructive ways to respond to what some have called the migrant's "impulse to restore the past" (Baskaukos, 1981) has important treatment implications. For example, does the availability of a community of survivors of a shared experience not only facilitate the recapture of memory but make it easier to deal with inevitable feelings of loss, since loss will have been a common experience (Portes & Bach, 1985)? Alternatively, could small-group techniques to instill future orientation (Kandel, Langrod, & Ruiz, 1981) prove helpful to refugees?

TREATMENT ISSUES

Although most refugees do not become mental health casualties, there will always be a minority who develop psychiatric problems. On the whole, immigrants and refugees either avoid or tend to be ill-served by the formal mental health care system (Munroe-Blum, Boyle, Offord, & Kates, 1989; Beiser, Gill, & Edwards, 1993a). However, when culturally sensitive service is available, refugees and immigrants from cultures popularly perceived as resistant to psychiatric help do not conform to stereotype. Instead, they make use of services and evidently benefit from them (Kinzie, 1985).

Approximately half of all persons in the general population suffering from a major mental disorder consult the general medical sector (Narrow, Regier, Rae, & Manderscheid, 1993), a pattern that has prompted the conceptualization of primary health care as a "de facto mental health care system" (Regier, Goldberg, & Taube, 1978). Many people, however, either define their problems in physical terms or emphasize physical complaints, while downplaying the psychological (Schurman, Kramer, & Mitchell, 1985). Physician propensity to emphasize the physical aspects of health compounds patient reticence to volunteer emotional symptoms, resulting in a 25 to 50% underrecording of mental health problems in primary care practice (Hoeper et al., 1980; Hankin et al., 1982).

Given the Southeast Asian reluctance to divulge symptoms of emotional distress unless appropriately questioned (Cheung & Dobkin de Rios, 1982; Kinzie & Manson, 1983), one might hypothesize that the proportion of "missed cases" of mental disorder among the refugees would be even higher than among the general population. However, RRP data (Beiser, 1994) are inconsistent with the hypothesis: The association between psychiatric disorder and propensity to seek help in the primary health care sector is weaker among refugees than in the general population.

The answer to this seeming paradox may be that Asians have no difficulty identifying mental health problems but avoid consulting physicians for help. For example, Ying (1990) asked 40 female Chinese immigrants living in the United States to explain what was wrong with a woman described in a vignette designed to cover the syndrome described as major depression in the DSM-III-R (American Psychiatric Association, 1987). Although 60% identified the problem as psychological distress, the majority felt it would be inappropriate to consult a doctor. Asked what the woman in the vignette should do, the majority of the interviewees responded that people with such problems should rely on themselves, on family, or on friends. Only those respondents who conceptualized the distress as physical disorder recommended that the subject of the vignette consult a doctor. Pham's (1986) exploration of concepts of mental health among Vietnamese in Calgary is consistent with Ying's work. Most of the 29 refugees participating in Pham's inquiry had a rich concept of mental health that involved concepts of simplicity, equilibrium, and harmony between mind and body derived from Tao philosophy. Perceived threats to mental health involved concerns for survival and difficulties in adapting to a new environment. Asked about methods for dealing with mental breakdown, the Calgary cohort emphasized self-reliance, religious solace, and avoiding stressful situations.

Refugees use the health care system about as often as people in the general population. Responding to a question about physician utilization included in the RRP survey, 16.5% of the refugees reported having seen a doctor in the few weeks prior to interview. The corresponding figures for resident Canadians was about 17.0%. Patterns of use varied, however. Non-Chinese refugees were more likely than either Chinese refugees or resident Canadians to see doctors for apparently trivial symptoms like mild headaches (Beiser, 1994).

What might account for this pattern of apparently inappropriate use of the health care system? In Southeast Asia, the family, a community authority, or a religiotraditional healer constitute the usual first line of resort in the struggle against illness; the biomedical system is consulted only after other resources have been consulted and found wanting (Kleinman, 1980; Tung, 1980). In comparison with the ethnic Vietnamese and Laotian refugees making up the current study sample, ethnic Chinese refugees were more likely to have migrated in family units rather than as individuals. On arrival in Vancouver, the refugees encountered a city boasting one of the largest Chinese communities in North America, but no preexisting Vietnamese or Laotian counterparts. These community characteristics probably helped shape Vietnamese and Laotian recourse to the primary health system. Compared to the Chinese refugees, the Vietnamese and Laotians were less likely to have access to trusted family members to help interpret symptoms, to give them meaning, to prescribe time-tested home remedies, and to provide authoritative wisdom. Although there were persons selling Chinese-derived herbs and medicines in Vancouver, the site of the RRP, there were no traditional healers from other cultural traditions, such as the Laotian *mo* (traditional healers) or *moyaa* (herbal specialists) to act as first-line health care providers. It seems a reasonable conjecture that the refugees sometimes turned to the health care system for what seem to be inappropriate reasons because they had nowhere else to go. In support of this conjecture, other studies have demonstrated that when they have alternatives, Southeast Asian refugees avoid taking minor medical complaints to physicians (Cheon-Klessig, Camilleri, McElmurry, & Ohlson, 1988; Deuschle & Diaz, 1981).

CONCLUSIONS

The Southeast Asian exodus to North America stimulated Canadian and US research in refugee mental health on an unprecedented scale. Although the information from these efforts is undeniably valuable, it is difficult to judge the extent to which it can be extrapolated to other refugees during other historical periods. There is a need to test models derived from the Southeast Asian experience in other groups. Longitudinal studies of adaptation and mental health should be encouraged. Changing contexts change the salience of mental health stressors and call on changing patterns of social and psychological resources for their amelioration.

Countries like Canada admit refugees out of a sense of compassion. Too often, resettlement countries behave as if their responsibility for the welfare of newcomers ends at the point of entry. However, ensuring the mental health of migrants—and in particular of refugees who come to a new country having endured much—is important, both in order to achieve compassionate goals and to realize the eventual contribution refugees can make to their adopted homes.

Acknowledgments. This study was made possible by grants from Canada Health and Welfare NHRDP 6610-1249, the Secretary of State's Multiculturalism Directorate, the United Way and Woodward Foundations of Vancouver, as well as by a National Health Scientist Award from NHRDP, and a Rockefeller Foundation Resident Scholar Award, both to Dr. Beiser, and a postdoctoral fellowship from NHRDP to Dr. Hyman. Principal investigators for the Refugee Resettlement project were Morton Beiser, Clarke Institute and Department of Psychiatry, University of Toronto; and Phyllis J. Johnson, Family and Nutritional Sciences, and Richard C. Nann, Social Work, both at the University of British Columbia.

REFERENCES

Adelman, H. (1980). *The Indochinese refugee movement.* Toronto: Operation Lifeline and Copp Clark.

Adelman, H. (1984). Support systems for refugee resettlement. In R. C. Nann, P. J. Johnson, & M. Beiser (Eds.), *Refugee resettlement: Southeast Asians in transition* (pp. 114–118). Vancouver: University of British Columbia Refugee Resettlement Project.

Amaral-Dias, C. A., Vicente, T. N., Cabrita, M. F., & de Mendon, A. R. (1981). Transplantation, identity and drug addiction. *Bulletin of Narcotics, 33,* 21–26.

American Psychiatric Association. (1987). *Diagnostic and statistical manual of mental disorders* (3rd ed., rev.). Washington, DC: Author.

American Psychiatric Association. (1994). *Diagnostic and statistical manual of mental disorders* (4th ed.). Washington, DC: Author.

Aylesworth, L. S., Ossario, P. G., & Osaki, L. T. (1977). *Stress and mental health among Vietnamese in the United States: Preliminary findings of a mental health needs assessment among Vietnamese refugees in Colorado.* Paper presented at the Health, Education and Welfare Conference on Mental Health Needs of Indochinese Refugees, Denver, Colorado.

Baskaukos, L. (1981). The Lithuanian refugee experience and grief. *International Migration Review, 15,* 276–291.

Beiser, M. (1982). Migration in a developing country: Risk and opportunity. In R. C. Nann (Ed.), *Uprooting and surviving: Adaptation and resettlement of migrant families and children* (pp. 119–146). Dordrecht, Holland: D. Reidel.

Beiser, M. (1985). The grieving witch: A framework for applying principles of cultural psychiatry to clinical practice. *Canadian Journal of Psychiatry, 30*, 130–141.

Beiser, M. (1987). Changing time perspective and mental health among Southeast Asian refugees. *Culture, Medicine and Psychiatry, 11*, 437–464.

Beiser, M. (1988). Influences of time, ethnicity, and attachment on depression in Southeast Asian refugees. *American Journal of Psychiatry, 145*, 46–51.

Beiser, M. (1994). *The use of primary health care by Southeast Asian refugees and resident Canadians.* Unpublished manuscript.

Beiser, M., Cargo, M., & Woodbury, M. A. (1994). A comparison of psychiatric disorder in different cultures: Depressive typologies in Southeast Asian refugees and resident Canadians. *International Journal of Methods in Psychiatric Research, 4*, 157–172.

Beiser, M., & Collomb, H. (1981). Mastering change: Epidemiological and case studies in Senegal, West Africa. *American Journal of Psychiatry, 138*, 455–459.

Beiser, M., & Fleming, J. A. (1986). Measuring psychiatric disorder among Southeast Asian refugees. *Psychological Medicine, 16*, 627–639.

Beiser, M., Gill, K., & Edwards, R. G. (1993a). Mental health care in Canada: Is it accessible and equal? *Canada's Mental Health, 41*, 2–7.

Beiser, M., & Hyman, I. (in press). Refugee time perspective and mental health. *American Journal of Psychiatry.*

Beiser, M., Johnson, P., & Turner, R. J. (1993b). Unemployment, underemployment and depressive affect among Southeast Asian refugees. *Psychological Medicine, 23*, 731–743.

Beiser, M., Turner, R. J., & Ganesan, S. (1989). Catastrophic stress and factors affecting its consequences among Southeast Asian refugees. *Social Science and Medicine, 28*, 183–195.

Berry, J. W., & Blondel, T. (1982). Psychological adaptation of Vietnamese refugees in Canada. *Canadian Journal of Community Mental Health, 1*, 81–88.

Bland, R. C., Stebelsky, G., Orn, H., & Newman, S. C. (1988). Psychiatric disorders and unemployment in Edmonton. *Acta Psychiatrica Scandinavica Supplementum, 77*, 72–80.

Bradburn, N. M. (1969). *The structure of psychological well-being.* Chicago: Aldine.

Bun, C. K., & Christie, K. (1995). Past, present and future: The Indochinese refugee experience twenty years later. *Journal of Refugee Studies, 8*, 75–94.

Burke, A. W. (1982). Determinants of delinquency in female West Indian migrants. *International Journal of Social Psychiatry, 28*, 28–34.

Canadian Council for Refugees Task Force on Family Reunification. (1995). *Refugee family reunification.* Montreal: Canadian Council for Refugees.

Canadian Task Force on Mental Health Issues Affecting Immigrants and Refugees. (1988). *Review of the literature on migrant mental health.* Cat. No. Ci96-37/1988E. Ottawa: Ministry of Supply and Services.

Caplan, N., Whitmore, J. K., & Choy, M. H. (1989). *The boat people and achievement in America: A study of family life, hard work and cultural values.* Ann Arbor: University of Michigan Press.

Chan, D. W. (1985). The Chinese version of the General Health Questionnaire: Does language make a difference? *Psychological Medicine, 15*, 147–155.

Cheng, T. A. (1989). Sex difference in prevalence of minor psychiatric morbidity: A social epidemiological study in Taiwan. *Acta Psychiatrica Scandinavica, 80*, 395–407.

Cheon-Klessig, Y., Camilleri, D. D., McElmurry, B. J., & Ohlson, V. M. (1988). Folk medicine in the health practice of Hmong refugees. *Western Journal of Nursing Research, 10*, 647–660.

Cheung, F., & Dobkin de Rios, M. F. (1982). Recent trends in the study of the mental health of Chinese immigrants to the United States. *Research in Race and Ethnic Relations, 3*, 145–163.

Cooley, C. H. (1902). *Human nature and the social order.* Glencoe, IL: Free Press.

Deuschle, K. W., & Diaz, M. (1981). The shortfall in Hispanic health manpower: The national and Mount Sinai–East Harlem picture. *Mount Sinai Journal of Medicine, 48,* 339–344.

Devins, G. M., Beiser, M., Dion, R., Pelletier, L. G., & Edwards, R. G. (in press). Cross-cultural measurement of psychological well-being: Psychometric equivalence of Cantonese, Vietnamese, and Laotian translation of the affect balance scale. *American Journal of Public Health.*

Edwards, R. G. (1994). *Southeast Asian refugees in Canada: Gender differences in adaptation and mental health.* Waterloo: Wilfred Laurier University (unpublished thesis).

Franks, F., & Faux, S. A. (1990). Depression, stress, mastery, and social resources in four ethnocultural women's groups. *Research in Nursing and Health, 13,* 283–292.

Grinberg, L. (1984). A psychoanalytic study of migration: Its normal and pathological aspects. *Journal of American Psychoanalytic Association, 32,* 13–38.

Haines, D. W., & Rutherford, P. T. (1981). Family and community among Vietnamese refugees. *International Migration Review, 15,* 310–319.

Hall, B. L. (1993). Elderly Vietnamese immigrants: Family and community connections. *Community Alternatives: International Journal of Family Care, 5,* 81–96.

Hankin, J. R., Steinwachs, D. M., Regier, D. A., Burns, B. J., Goldberg, I. D., Hoeper, & E. W. (1982). Use of general medical care services by persons with mental disorders. *Archives of General Psychiatry, 39,* 225–231.

Hirschfield, R., & Cross, C. K. (1982). Epidemiology of affective disorders. *Archives of General Psychiatry, 39,* 35–46.

Hoeper, E. W., Nycz, G. R., Regier, D. A., Goldberg, I. D., Jacobson, A., & Hankin, J. (1980). Diagnosis of mental disorder in adults and increased use of health services in four outpatient settings. *American Journal of Psychiatry, 137,* 207–210.

Holmes, T. H., & Masuda, M. (1973). Life change and illness susceptibility. In J. P. Scott & E. C. Senay (Eds.), *Separation and depression: Clinical and research aspects* (pp. 161–186). Washington, DC: American Association for the Advancement of Science.

Indra, D. M. (1988). Self-concept and resettlement: Vietnamese and Sino-Vietnamese in a small prairie city. In L. J. Dorais, K. B. Chan, & D. M. Indra (Eds.), *Ten years later: Indochinese communities in Canada* (pp. 69–93). Montreal: Canadian Asian Studies Association.

Johnson, P. J. (1988). The impact of ethnic communities on the employment of Southeast Asian refugees. *Amerasia, 14*(1), 1–22.

Kandel, A., Langrod, J., & Ruiz, P. (1981). Change in future time perception of day hospital psychiatric patients in response to small group treatment approaches. *Journal of Clinical Psychology, 37,* 769–775.

Keller, M. B., Lavori, P. W., Rice, J., Coryell, W., & Herschfeld, R. M. A. (1986). The persistent risk of chronicity in recurrent episodes of nonbipolar major depressive disorder: A prospective follow-up. *American Journal of Psychiatry, 143,* 24–28.

Kessler, R. C., House, J. S., & Turner, J. B. (1987a). Unemployment and health in a community sample. *Journal of Health & Social Behavior, 28,* 51–59.

Kessler, R. C., Turner, J. B., & House, J. S. (1987b). Intervening processes in the relationship between unemployment and health. *Psychological Medicine, 17,* 949–961.

Kinzie, J. D. (1985). Cultural aspects of psychiatric treatment with Indochinese refugees. 137th Annual Meeting of the American Psychiatric Association (1984, Los Angeles, California). *American Journal of Social Psychiatry, 5,* 47–53.

Kinzie, J. D., & Manson, S. M. (1983). Five years' experience with Indochinese refugee psychiatric patients. *Journal of Operational Psychiatry, 14,* 105–111.

Kinzie, J. D., Manson, S. M., Vinh, D. T., Nolan, N. T., Anh, B., & Pho, T. N. (1982). Development and validation of a Vietnamese language depression rating scale. *American Journal of Psychiatry, 139,* 1276–1281.

Kleinman, A. (1980). *Patients and healers in the context of culture.* Berkeley: University of California Press.

Kleinman, A. (1987). Anthropology and psychiatry: The role of culture in cross-cultural research on illness. *British Journal of Psychiatry, 151,* 447–454.

Lin, K. M. (1986). Psychopathology and social disruption in refugees. In C. C. Williams & J. Westermeyer (Eds.), *Refugee mental health in resettlement countries* (pp. 61–73). Washington, DC: Hemisphere.

Lin, T. Y. (1983). Psychiatry and Western culture. *Western Journal of Medicine, 139*, 862–867.

Littlewood, R. (1992). Psychiatric diagnosis and racial bias: Empirical and interpretative approaches. *Social Science and Medicine, 34*, 141–149.

Lutz, C. (1985). Depression and the translation of emotional worlds. In A. Kleinman & B. Good (Eds.) *Culture and depression* (pp. 63–100). Berkeley: University of California Press.

Mathers, J. (1974). The gestation period of identity change. *British Journal of Psychiatry, 125*, 472–474.

May, R. (1958). Contributions of existential psychotherapy. In R. May, E. Angel, & H. F. Ellenberger (Eds.), *Existence: A new dimension in psychiatry and psychology* (pp. 37–91). New York: Basic Books.

Mead, G. H. (1934). *Mind, self and society*. Chicago: University of Chicago Press.

Minister of Supply and Services. (1994). *Into the 21st century: A strategy for immigration and citizenship*. Ottawa: Author.

Moore, B. E., & Fine, B. D. (1990). *Psychoanalytic terms and concepts*. New York: American Psychoanalytic Association.

Morgan, M. C., Wingard, D. L., & Felice, M. E. (1984). Subcultural differences in alcohol use among youth. *American Journal of Psychiatry, 5*, 191–195.

Munroe-Blum, H., Boyle, M. G., Offord, D. R., & Kates, N. (1989). Immigrant children: Psychiatric disorder, school performance, and service utilization. *American Journal of Orthopsychiatry, 59*, 510–519.

Murphy, H. B. (1977). Migration, culture and mental health. *Psychological Medicine, 7*, 677–684.

Murphy, H. B. M. (1979). Migration and the major mental disorders. In C. Zwingman & M. Pfister-Ammende (Eds.), *Uprooting and after* (pp. 204–220). Heidelberg: Springer.

Narrow, W. E., Regier, D. A., Rae, D. S., & Manderscheid, R. W. (1993). Use of services by persons with mental and addictive disorders: Findings from the National Institute of Mental Health Epidemiologic Catchment Area Program. *Archives of General Psychiatry, 50*, 95–107.

Neuwirth, G., & Clarke, L. (1981). Indochinese refugees in Canada: Sponsorship and adjustment. *International Migration Review, 15*, 131–140.

Nguyen, S. D.(1982a). Psychiatric and psychosomatic problems among Southeast Asian refugees. *The Psychiatric Journal of the University of Ottawa, 7*, 163–172.

Nguyen, S. D. (1982b). The psycho-social adjustment and the mental health needs of Southeast Asian refugees. *The Psychiatric Journal of the University of Ottawa, 7*, 26–35.

Obeyesekere, G. (1985). Depression, Buddhism, and the work of culture in Sri Lanka. In A. Kleinman & B. Good (Eds.), *Culture and depression* (pp. 134–152). Berkeley: University of California Press.

Pham, T. N. (1986). The mental health problems of the Vietnamese in Calgary: Major aspects and implications for service. *Canada's Mental Health, 34*, 5–9.

Portes, A., & Bach, R. (1985). *Latin journey: Cuban and Mexican immigrant in the US*. Berkeley: University of California Press.

Regier, D. A., Goldberg, I. D., & Taube, C. A. (1978). The de facto US mental health services system: A public health perspective. *Archives of General Psychiatry, 35*, 685–693.

Robins, L. N., & Regier, D. A. (1991). *The validity of psychiatric disorders in America: The Epidemiologic Catchment Area Study*. New York: Free Press.

Rumbaut, R. G. (1985). Mental health and refugee experience: A comparative study of Southeast Asian refugees. In T. C. Owan (Ed.), *Southeast Asian mental health, treatment, prevention, services, training and research* (pp. 433–486). Rockville, MD: National Institute of Mental Health.

Rumbaut, R. G. (1991). The agony of exile: A study of the migration and adaptation of Indochinese refugee adults and children. In F. L. J. Ahearn & J. L. Athey (Eds.), *Refugee children: Theory, research, and services* (pp. 53–91). Baltimore: The Johns Hopkins University Press.

Rumbaut, R. G., & Ima, K. (1988). *The adaptation of Southeast Asian refugee youth: A comparative study.* Washington, DC: US Office of Refugee Resettlement.

Sack, W. H. (1985). Post-traumatic stress disorders in children. *Integrative Psychiatry, 3,* 162–164.

Schurman, R. A., Kramer, P. D., & Mitchell, J. B. (1985). The hidden mental health network: Treatment of mental illness by nonpsychiatrist physicians. *Archives of General Psychiatry, 42,* 89–94.

Skhiri, Annabi, & Allani. (1982). Enfants d'immigres: Facteurs de liens ou de rupture? *Annales Medico Psychologiques, 140,* 597–602.

Terr, L. (1994). *Unchained memories: True stories of traumatic memories, lost and found.* New York: Basic Books.

Tseng, W. S. (1975). The nature of somatic complaints among psychiatric patients: The Chinese case. *Comparative Psychiatry, 16,* 237–245.

Tung, T. M. (1980). *Indochinese patients: Cultural aspects of the medical and psychiatric care of Indochinese refugees.* Fall Church, VA: Action for Southeast Asians.

Tyhurst, L. (1951). Displacement and migration: A study in social psychiatry. *American Journal of Psychiatry, 107,* 561–568.

Vaillant, G. (1977). *Adaptations to life.* Boston: Little, Brown.

Warr, P. (1982). Psychological aspects of employment and unemployment. *Psychological Medicine, 12,* 7–11.

Weissman, M. M., Myers, J. K., & Thompson, W. D. (1986). Depressive symptoms as a risk factor for mortality and for major depression. In L. Erlenmeyer-Kimling & N. Miller (Eds.), *Life span research on the prediction of psychopathology* (pp. 251–260). Hillsdale, NJ: Lawrence Erlbaum.

Westermeyer, J., Callies, A., & Neider, J. (1990). Welfare status and psychosocial adjustment among 100 Hmong refugees. *Journal of Nervous and Mental Disease, 178,* 300–306.

Westermeyer, J., Neider, J., Vang, T. F. (1983a). Migration and mental health among Hmong refugees: Association of pre- and postmigration with self-rating scales. *Journal of Nervous and Mental Disease, 171,* 92–96.

Westermeyer, J., Vang, T. F., & Neider, J. (1983b). Refugees who do and do not seek psychiatric care: An analysis of premigratory and postmigratory characteristics. *Journal of Nervous and Mental Disease, 171,* 86–91.

Westermeyer, J., Vang, T. F., & Neider, J. (1984). Acculturation and mental health: A study of Hmong refugees at 15 and 35 years post-migration. *Social Science and Medicine, 18,* 87–93.

Woon, Y. F. (1987). The mode of refugee sponsorship and the socio-economic adaptation of Vietnamese in Victoria: A three-year perspective. In K. B. Chan & D. M. Indra (Eds.), *Uprooting, loss and adaptation: The resettlement of Indochinese in Canada* (pp. 132–146). Ottawa: Canadian Public Health Association.

Yap, P. M. (1965). Phenomenology of affective disorders in Chinese and other cultures. In A. V. S. de Reuck & R. Porter (Eds.), *Transcultural psychiatry* (pp. 84–108). London: Churchill.

Ying, Y. W. (1990). Explanatory models of major depression and implications for help-seeking among immigrant Chinese-American women. International Symposium on Mental Health (1989, Taipei, Taiwan). *Culture, Medicine and Psychiatry, 14,* 393–408.

4

Refugees and Immigrants in Quebec

MICHEL TOUSIGNANT

HISTORY OF IMMIGRATION IN QUEBEC

Nearly 85% of the immigrants settling in Quebec chose to reside in Montreal. This metropolitan area receives 16% of Canadian immigrants and, by the turn of the century, half of its school population will have foreign-born parents. Two thirds of the residents speak French and one third English. A law now obliges immigrants' children to attend French-speaking schools unless one of their parents has been previously attending a Quebec English-speaking school. This policy has radically transformed the social portrait of immigration during the last 20 years. For this reason, Montreal and the province of Quebec offer unique features to study the adaptation of immigrants to a new environment.

After the English conquest in 1760 and up to 1950, the history of immigration in Quebec has followed the trends witnessed in the rest of Eastern Canada and North America. Large groups from European descent, the most representative being from Britain, Ireland, and the Jewish diaspora, assimilated into the English group and threatened the survival of the French population. Deeply concerned for its cultural and Catholic identity, the native population survived by retreating into an isolationist attitude reinforced by the arrival of conservative priests exiled from France in the aftermath of the Revolution. The church attempted to stifle the movement of European and American liberalism

MICHEL TOUSIGNANT • Laboratory for Research in Human and Social Ecology, University of Quebec at Montreal, Montreal, Quebec, Canada H3C 3P8.

Ethnicity, Immigration, and Psychopathology, edited by Ihsan Al-Issa and Michel Tousignant. Plenum Press, New York, 1997.

and promoted a high birthrate appropriately named the "revenge of the cradles" to counteract the demographic imbalance.

After 1950, immigrants came predominantly from Italy first, and then from Portugal and Greece. The French institutions were still unprepared to integrate them, though many were Latin and Catholic. The cultural and economic attraction of English North America weighed very much against a reversal. After 1965, this trend was tempered by the entrance of French-speaking groups, the Sephardic Jews from Morocco, and the middle-class intellectuals from Haiti. With an elected government in 1976 advocating sovereignty, the balance swiftly switched over and new immigrants, with a majority non-European, were increasingly pressured to join the French community. Paradoxically, the French-Canadians who until then had sent their missionaries all the world over were only then starting to pay serious attention to their foreign-born citizens.

Montreal has no real monocultural immigrant ghettos as we find them in Toronto, for instance. A cultural group may occupy several contiguous apartment buildings or a couple of streets, but most groups are generally spread over a large territory and many have a density barely sufficient to ensure cultural survival. The "immigrant" districts host a heterogeneous community where the dominant group seldom exceeds a quarter of the local population. In the district of Park Extension, for instance, as many as 80 languages are spoken within a single square mile. Moreover, there are large mixed sectors surrounding this core immigrant population. Starting with the Jewish immigration at the beginning of the century, new immigrants have traditionally occupied a north–south corridor, sometimes referred to as a "no-man's land" between the French area to the east and the English area to the west. This relative isolation as well as the competition between two dominant cultures have certainly slowed the pace of integration and helped to reinforce the culture of origin. The large English Jewish community of Montreal is perceived by some as more conservative than the other North American Jewish communities. Many groups, including the Creole- and French-speaking Haitians, are divided between their allegiance to the host culture and their narrow contacts with a North American diaspora. With a high unemployment rate chronically in the two digits, immigrants have regularly traveled outside of the province for job opportunities or to find specialized folk-medicine centers. As a consequence, the interprovincial mobility is quite high.

Research has focused more on refugees than on immigrants during the last decade. In the last 20 years, refugees have enjoyed a positive attitude from the host population, even to the point where pressures have occasionally been brought to bear to nullify deportation orders when claims had been refused. A large number of the refugees entered the country through the international airport of Mirabel, for a long time known around the world to be a soft point of entry, a factor contributing to a high load of individual applicants. Consequently, the largest group of refugees barely exceeds 20,000 and most of them do not include more than a few hundred.

Despite the cultural specificity of French Quebec, there are many other factors besides the bilingual context to explain the findings reported in this chapter. Only a large comparative analysis would eventually demonstrate the contribution of the specific Quebec context. Other general factors proposed by theories of immigration evidently also play a role. Because of the diversity of the groups surveyed, in contrast to other chapters in this volume, we structured the presentation around the theme of integration. The fact that the recent contributions in Quebec have been mainly on children and adolescents, this topic will provide a unifying theme and highlight the developmental perspective in discussing immigrant adaptation.

REFUGEES

Inspired by the Beiser report (Task Force on the Mental Health of Immigrants and Refugees, 1989), which had shown the difficulties of Canadian adolescent immigrants, a study was conducted between 1991 and 1993 on a sample of 204 male and female adolescents from refugee families (Tousignant, Habimana, Brault, Bendris, & Sidoli-Leblanc, 1993). The age range was between 14 and 19 years old. More than 35 nations were included. Salvador had the largest number but with no more than 15% of the total sample. All of the main regions of the world were represented: Southeast Asia (29%), Central America (27%), the Middle East (12%), Eastern Europe (11%), sub-Saharan Africa (7%), South America (7%), and other Asian countries (6%). Two thirds of the sample lived in the Montreal area and the other third in small industrial centers (Quebec City, Sherbrooke, Trois Rivières). Only 15 adolescents were born in Canada and 69% had entered the country after their sixth birthday. The range of parental education was quite spread out: 55% of the fathers and 40% of the mothers had reached postsecondary level. The percentage of two-parent families was 69%. Only 62% of the fathers were employed with two thirds showing downward mobility.

The sample was selected from volunteering schools in immigrant neighborhoods. Letters were sent to all adolescents whose parents were born in countries with a recent civil strife. A phone call later confirmed if the family had obtained a refugee status or had come to Canada mainly for political motives. All the families had been in Canada for more than 3 years and all the interviews were done in French by interviewers from five nationalities. The goal of the project was the assessment of family vulnerability and resilience. A 3-hour interview included, among other instruments, the Child Experiences of Care and Abuse (Bifulco, Brown, & Harris, 1994) and the family history of exile. The psychiatric status was assessed with the Diagnostic Interview Schedule for Children-II, based on the *Diagnostic and Statistical Manual of Mental Disorders*, 3rd edition, revised (DSM-III-R) (American Psychiatric Association, 1987) criteria.

The rate of simple phobia was very high (18.2%), especially among girls

(27.6%). This result could either be the outcome of a high prevalence of posttraumatic syndromes or could reflect some cultural bias. Because all cases of simple phobia did not result in social impairment in daily roles, it was finally decided to omit this diagnosis from the assessment of prevalence.

A parallel provincial Santé Québec survey, which included a 13- to 14-year-old group, had been completed shortly before this survey and had used the same diagnostic instrument (Bergeron, Valla, & Breton, 1992). This younger age group could be used for comparison with the refugee group because there was no significant age differences in the latter. The refugee rate (21.2%) was twice that of the Santé Québec sample (11.4%). Major depression, dysthymia, and conduct disorders were from one and a half to two times higher in the refugee group than in adolescents in the general population, while the anxiety rate was seven times higher in the refugee group. The boy : girl ratio was similar in both samples, 0.57 in the refugee group and 0.63 in the Quebec sample. Six girls and one boy had attempted suicide during the last year in the refugee group, which amounts to the rate found among Quebec high schools for the same grades (Tousignant, Bastien, & Hamel, 1993).

The high rate of anxiety in the refugee group may be due to war-related experiences suffered during childhood or to the environment of highly anxious parents. The differences between the refugee and the Santé Québec groups were not likely to be due to socioeconomic differences, because family income was not correlated to diagnoses in the Santé Québec survey.

The prevalence was quite similar in the Montreal metropolitan area (21.0%) and in the rest of the province (21.7%). Anxiety, suicide attempts, and the omitted diagnosis of simple phobia were more prevalent in the non-metropolitan area and conduct disorders were more prevalent in Montreal. An overrepresentation of Southeast Asians outside of Montreal accounted for a higher rate of anxiety in that region. We cannot therefore conclude if adaptation is easier or not in a big city or in a small town. The team member from Rwanda who had done the higher number of interviews outside of Montreal felt that social integration was easier there and racism weaker, while the in-group pressure to maintain the image of the culture was stronger.

The sociocultural regions, that is, Central American, South America, Eastern Europe, and Southeast Asia, obtained similar rates, between 23 and 27%, with the exception of the Middle East with 16.7%. This latter group included a large number of Iranian families fleeing their country to avoid the military conscription of a son and had been less directly exposed to the horrors of war and persecution.

The quality of parent–child relationships among refugees is closely associated with adolescent mental health (Parker, 1983). In the present research, the level of family abuse and of other forms of maltreatment was similar to that found in a female London community sample with a high rate of depression, using the same instrument (Bifulco et al., 1994). One out of five adolescents reported at least one instance of severe physical violence serious enough to leave a bodily mark for a day. A high level of control manifested either through very strict supervision or strong discipline was also high in 17% compared to 5% in a Quebec French population of the same age. Favoritism or the report that siblings were receiving a more favorable treatment was present in 17% of the sample. Role reversal defined by a parental-like responsibility of the child toward a parent was particularly high concerning the mother, with a rate of 13%. Nearly one third of the families obtained a high score of family discord. All the variables (physical violence, high control, and role reversal), taken independently, were associated with a double rate of psychopathology and favoritism with a triple rate. Severe physical abuse was not associated with psychopathology, however, among respondents who had described the parental behavior as reasonable and legitimate. In a multifactorial logistic regression analysis predicting psychopathology, the only significant factor was favoritism. In conclusion, it appears that it is not so much the level of abuse or other types of negative experiences taken separately that make children vulnerable but a combination of this adversity with the sense that the parental treatment was unjust due to the arbitrary application of the rules. Favoritism in this sample was especially salient among girls who often envied the way their brothers were being handled and given freedom.

The results indicated that the conditions in refugee camps produced long-term effects on the children. For instance, adolescents from families who had suffered from hunger or bad treatment in the camps had 50% more diagnoses than those from families who had not. A long-term separation of more than a year from parents was also associated with difficult adaptation for the children, who had a double rate of psychopathology. The parental separations were not always forced by political situations and could reflect in some cases preexisting tensions between father and mother. Temporary separation certainly caused serious stress on the couples since they were more likely to divorce after the settlement in Canada.

The problems of the refugees are not automatically solved after their arrival in a safe haven. Since most of the refugees are from Third World countries, their socioeconomic integration into the host country during a period of recession has produced difficult challenges. Contrary to the initial hypothesis, downward professional mobility of the father was not associated with psychopathology in the children, probably because it was such a widespread experience in this sample. Only seven fathers had enjoyed upward mobility, but it was not a guaranteed protection either, since three of the children had a diagnosis. The crucial factor was the father's employment status. One in two adolescents had a diagnosis when his or her father had experienced a period of unemployment exceeding 6 months after arriving to Canada. Mothers, who generally started from a lower job status in the country of origin, experienced on average a small upward social mobility. But the main finding was that the majority (57.4%) of the mothers were not in the work market at the time of the interview as opposed to only half that percentage prior to exile. The number of children to care for at home was a likely contributing factor to the decision to not seek work.

Another unexpected finding was that the adolescents who came to Canada after their sixth birthday were slightly less likely to have a diagnosis than those who arrived before that age. This finding ruled out the assumption that adaptation is easier if the child changes culture before being socialized in the school system of his birth country. Moreover, entering a French school after experiencing another system meant in most cases the obligation to attend special classes, often resulting in a delay of 1 academic year. On the other hand, the more recently arrived children may have been in a better position to compare schools and to be more conscious of the advantages of a less authoritarian environment. One important consideration was that Southeast Asian adolescents were overrepresented among the older refugees and Middle East adolescents among the recently arrived.

Most refugee families (85%) used almost exclusively the home country language in parent–child communications. The Canadian policy offers language courses to only one member of the family identified as the main source of family income. According to the adolescent's perception, barely 21% of the mothers could manage an adequate conversation in French on the phone and 15% in English. Another 28% of the mothers could have a functional face-to-face conversation in French. Consequently, this lack of language skills made integration in work and social life more difficult. Though most mothers made up for the lack by having social encounters outside the home, in church, or in other organizations, more than half were quite isolated at home and did not have visitors more than once a week or less. The fact of having few visitors at home as well as an index of mother isolation, however, did not predict adolescent psychopathology. Perhaps these mothers needed only a minimal amount of social life to protect them, they had a good marital relationship to make up for lack of social contacts, or they had more time to devote to their children.

Children of families without any kin contact, either directly through visiting or more indirectly through telephone calls, reported a high rate of psychopathology of 35%, but their number was too low ($n = 17$) to generalize the results. Also, the fact of having family in the same province rather than only family living far away did not have any influence on the child's mental health.

In conclusion, this research showed the high vulnerability of adolescents from refugee families and the high rate of family problems. The results indicated the importance of preexile factors many years after coming to Canada. Southeast Asians and those having experienced difficult camp conditions had the highest rates of psychopathology. But preexile and postexile conditions are not completely independent, because separation between the parents before exile was correlated with later divorce and quality of family life was quite consistent throughout childhood and adolescence. The postexile stress was mainly related to the long-term unemployment of the father.

ADOLESCENCE AND ACCULTURATION

Adolescence is a period of personal and cultural identity formation and this stage of life is thought to be more problematic for those coming from immigrant families. Prediction of successful adaptation is related to a combination of factors, including the attitude toward integration nurtured in the family and the host society reaction to the group. A recent study compared four groups of adolescents raised in Montreal (Greeks, Haitians, Italians, and Vietnamese) and analyzed the interactions between ethnic identity, acculturation attitudes, and scores from the Rosenberg Scale of self-esteem (Sabatier & Berry, 1994). While Greeks and Italians enjoyed a rather positive image among the Quebec population because of their European descent, the Vietnamese attracted the kind of sympathy associated with their war victim status; the Haitians encountered some overt and aversive racism.

The Vietnamese had a slightly higher attachment to Canada than to their home country, while the other three groups showed more attachment to their home country. The federal policy of multiculturalism and a politically correct attitude at the provincial level certainly did play some role to support this pattern of cultural attachment. With regard to ethnic identity, the Greeks scored high on both ethnic and Canadian identity, the Vietnamese obtained middle scores on both dimensions, while the Haitians and the Italians tended to have mainly a strong ethnic identity. This profile helped explain how self-esteem was correlated with modes of acculturation. The Greeks who scored higher on self-esteem were those with a separation attitude, that is, a deeper investment in their cultural group than in the host country. The Vietnamese, on the contrary, fared better when they were more favorably disposed to assimilation. Regarding the association between self-esteem and the attachment to the country of origin and to Canadian culture, three groups, the Haitians being the exception, had a better self-esteem when they were investing in both. Having two strong attachments thus proved to be a source of enrichment rather than neurosis. At the other end of the distribution, Haitians had a lower self-esteem when they were more attached to Canada and the Vietnamese when they were more attached to their own culture. In summary, self-esteem was more related to attitudes congruent with the cultural group than conforming to an abstract universal model.

A similar conclusion came from a series of qualitative studies on ethnic relations and the construction of identity among high school students in Montreal. The least-adapted students were those caught between a traditionalist family and rejection from the dominant culture (Laperrière et al., 1992). In the Haitian group, for instance, the most vulnerable adolescents were those who were unable to negotiate conflicts with their parents when the family concurrently was stressed by tensions from the host society. The often rigid reaction of the parents in that community has been reported elsewhere (Tourigny & Bouchard, 1990). When such frictions occur, the gang then becomes a point of entry to the subculture of deviance. In contrast, the Haitian adolescents who were better prepared by their family to face discrimination were able to associate with the French and other cultural groups, promoting cultural convergence. The young Italians who maintained conservative values were likely to succeed because of the strong economic institutions within their ethnic ghetto. Again, as in Sabatier and Berry's (1994) study, it seems that a separatist attitude is likely to lead to adaptation, given strong support from the group of origin. We may ask if this situation is specific to Montreal or could it be generalized to other bicultural contexts.

THE CHILDREN OF WAR

Refugee children have been the focus of two studies. The first was interested in the aftermath of losing a parent in a civil war among a population of Central American children between 4 and 6 years of age (Rafman, Canfield, Barbas, & Kaczorowski, 1996). On average, the loss of the parent had occurred 2 years before the study. Compared with children having suffered war experiences without any parental loss, those who had lost a parent were still showing significant differences after immigration. In a play situation, they reenacted the orginal scenes of violence with a displacement of the aggressed victim or by altering the context. The theme of imminent danger as well as a certain compulsion toward arranging toys were dominant characteristics of their play. The grief process seemed to develop normally in community children. In general, the surviving mothers had discussed the topic with the child and had entered into a relationship with a new partner. When the community children with a loss were compared with a clinical group having experienced either violence against or death of a family member, several observations differentiated them. The clinical group's productions included more aggressive content, a fragmentation and incoherence in the scenario as well as a sense of destructive moral order, with difficulty in selecting the characters in the drawings who could be trusted. The ability to communicate about the past was also a distinctive trait in the parental behavior. The absence of a silence taboo in the community group contrasted with the secrecy of the clinical group. In conclusion, the authors raised the question as to whether immigration improved the functioning of the traumatized children, and they suggested that a comparison be made with a sample from the country of origin.

Schools that have to integrate child victims of war do not always have the competence to identify their emotional needs and to adequately respond to them. A study of Montreal schools analyzed the relationship between academic achievement and emotional problems among Central American and Southeast Asian children, aged 8 to 12 years and born outside of Canada (Rousseau, Drapeau, & Corin, 1996). Learning difficulties were more often identified by the staff in the Central American group despite the fact that the overall academic performance was similar to the Southeast Asian group. Learning difficulties were associated with hyperactivity, social isolation, and somatization in the Central American group and with aggression, depression, and somatization in the Southeast Asian group. The fact that the Central American students were more often labeled as problematic could be attributed to their more extraverted behavior than to real differences in the emotional adaptation of the two groups.

ADULT STUDIES

This section includes a series of epidemiological community studies among immigrant adults. It indicates that immigration is not a vulnerability factor with regard to mental health and that the isolationist attitude has more payoffs than disadvantages in some groups as we have seen for the adolescents.

The Quebec Health survey did not find any significant difference between the foreign-born and the Canadian-born groups on the Ilfeld symptom scale, excluding those who could neither communicate in French or English (Cousineau, 1991). Women in the Canadian-born population had more symptoms than men, but this sex difference was much smaller in the immigrant group. This lack of difference between the foreign- and the Canadian-born groups may be explained by the fact that, until very recently, most immigrant groups have enjoyed a better economic status than the French group.

A nostalgic desire to return to the home country may delay the grief reaction and be detrimental to mental health. Roskies, Iida-Miranda, and Strobel (1975) found that the Portuguese of Montreal, a majority of them from the Azores, often considered retirement to their island. Contrary to the hypothesis of a progressive adaptation during the immigration period, they reported more symptoms 10 years after than shortly after their arrival, probably due to a protracted mourning reaction. After a few years, they were visiting their birthplace and then confronted the unrealistic nature of their dream and the need to reappraise their future.

The mental health of a middle-class Sephardic North African group took a more positive turn as they gradually confirmed that they had made the best choice by coming to Canada (Lasry & Sigal, 1975). A similar finding was reported in the Montreal Lebanese community (Sayegh & Lasry, 1993). In the latter study, those who had been in the country for less than 5 years had worse

à Montréal [Acculturation, stress and mental health among Lebanese immigrants in Montreal]. *Santé Mentale au Québec, 18,* 23–52.

Task Force on the Mental Health of Immigrants and Refugees (1989). *After the door has opened.* Ottawa: Secretary of State, Multi-culturalism and Health and Social Welfare Canada.

Tourigny, M., & Bouchard, C. (1990). Étude comparative des mauvais traitements envers les enfants de familles francophones de souche québécoise et de familles d'origine haïtienne: nature et circonstances [Comparative analysis of maltreatments toward children in French families from Quebec origin and in Haitian families]. *Prismes, 1,* 57–68.

Tousignant, M., Bastien, M. F., & Hamel, S. (1993). Suicidal attempts and ideations among adolescents and young adults: The role of father and mother care and parents separation. *Social Psychiatry and Psychiatric Epidemiology, 28,* 256–261.

Tousignant, M., Habimana, E., Brault, M., Bendris, M., & Sidoli-Leblanc, E. (1993). Les rapports entre générations dans les familles de réfugiés au Québec [Intergenerational relations among refugee families in Quebec]. *Revue Internationale des Études Canadiennes, Special Issue,* 171–181.

5

Social Stress and Psychological Distress among Latinos in the United States

PETER J. GUARNACCIA

INTRODUCTION

There is little debate in the literature that migration from one country to another and from rural to urban areas of a country is stressful (Desjarlais, Eisenberg, Good, & Kleinman, 1995; Harwood, 1994; Hull, 1979; Kasl & Berkman, 1983; Kuo, 1976; Portes & Rumbaut, 1990; Sanua, 1970). However, there is considerable discussion concerning why migration is stressful, in what ways, and for whom. Not all individuals or groups migrate under the same conditions nor do those migrating under similar circumstances experience the same level of stress. The circumstances surrounding the decision to migrate, the resources of the migrant family, and the response of the host community to migrants all influence the degree to which migration affects health and well being (Cervantes & Castro, 1985; Padilla, 1980, 1994; Rogler, 1994; Rogler, Malgady, & Rodriguez, 1989; Rogler, Cortes, & Malgady, 1991; Portes & Rumbaut, 1990; Portes, Kyle, & Eaton, 1992; Szapocznik & Kurtines, 1980).

No single factor is sufficient for understanding the nature of the stresses created by migration and their consequences for the mental health of migrants and their families. Rather, it is the dynamic interaction of the circumstances

PETER J. GUARNACCIA • Department of Human Ecology, Institute for Health, Health Care Policy, and Aging Research, Rutgers University, New Brunswick, New Jersey 08903.

Ethnicity, Immigration, and Psychopathology, edited by Ihsan Al-Issa and Michel Tousignant. Plenum Press, New York, 1997.

surrounding the migration, the characteristics of the migrant family, and the characteristics of the host community and its service system that produces or prevents the development of the psychological distress commonly associated with migration. In considering this transition, the following points should be underscored:

1. The international context of migration must be analyzed to understand the factors influencing the movement of large numbers of people from one country to another. The historical and political context of the migration will have important ramifications for the resources of migrating groups and the social and institutional response of the receiving society.
2. The stresses of migration do not only lie within the particular family or individual who is migrating, but result from the interaction of families and individuals with both the broader society of origin and US society.
3. The characteristics of migrants—their economic resources, social skills, knowledge of the receiving culture, social supports, etc.—are key factors in determining the stressfulness of migration.
4. The characteristics of the receiving community—its economy, social and class structure, the presence of members of the same ethnic group, the attitudes of individuals and groups toward the migrants—are equally important in determining the adaptation process of new migrants.
5. A key aspect of the receiving society is the institutional support network that migrants encounter on arrival. The responses of economic, social, health, and cultural institutions to new migrant groups greatly influence whether the migrants will adapt successfully or experience psychological distress.

In this chapter, I will review the experiences of various Latino groups along these dimensions and discuss what we know about the consequences of their migrations for mental health.

SOCIAL AND CULTURAL BACKGROUNDS OF LATINOS IN THE UNITED STATES

Latinos are a diverse cultural group; the use of a general label is both conceptually and practically inappropriate. Latino groups differ in national origin and history; in the particular social formations within each country that shape age, gender, and class relationships; in the pressures within each country that have led to migration and the differing waves of migration; and the differing relationships with the United States through time that have affected how those migrants were received (Aguirre-Molina & Molina, 1994; Bean & Tienda, 1987; Melville, 1994; Portes & Bach, 1985; Grenier & Stepick, 1992).

These features have not only created marked differences among the Latino groups but considerable intracultural variation within groups as well. At the same time, changes within United States society and cultures have affected where migrants have gone, how they have been received, the opportunities they have had to develop themselves as individuals and groups, and the cultures of the United States with which the migrants have interacted (Pedraza-Bailey, 1985; Portes & Bach, 1985; Portes & Rumbaut, 1990; Portes & Stepick, 1993; Rogler, 1994).

People of Mexican origin make up the largest portion of Latinos in the United States. Current population estimates are that there are 22.8 million Latinos in the United States and that 64% of them are Mexican (Montgomery, 1994). Mexican diversity results from differences in the generation that migrated, length of residence, legal status, social status, ethnic background, and reasons for migration. A significant portion of the Mexican origin population cannot be considered immigrants. This group, who often refer to themselves as *Hispanos*, established themselves in the southwestern states during the period of Spanish colonialism and were incorporated into the United States through colonial expansion of the United States. At the same time, Mexicans overwhelmingly make up the largest group of new immigrants to the United States (in 1990, 4.3 million foreign-born Mexicans lived in the United States, accounting for 22% of all foreign-born residents).

Wide variations exist in educational level, occupational status, and income within the Mexican-American community. Mexican Americans differ in their knowledge of and preference for use of Spanish and English. While some Mexican Americans actively work in agricultural occupations and make up the largest ethnic group among migrant farm laborers (Chavez, 1992), the overwhelming majority of Mexican Americans now work in the services and industrial sectors of large southwestern cities such as San Antonio and Los Angeles. At the same time, Mexican Americans, because of their proximity to Mexico, their large communities throughout the Southwest, and their continued high rates of immigration, have a strong cultural base from which to reinforce their cultural identity.

Puerto Ricans account for 11% of the mainland Latino population (Montgomery, 1994). While New York City remains the largest mainland Puerto Rican city with approximately 900,000 residents (1990 census), this metropolitan area now accounts for only 33% of the mainland Puerto Rican population. Additionally, Chicago, Philadelphia, Newark (NJ), Hartford (CT), and a number of smaller industrial cities throughout New Jersey, Connecticut, Massachusetts, and eastern Pennsylvania all have sizable Puerto Rican communities. Puerto Ricans experience the lowest socioeconomic status of the major Latino groups. Puerto Ricans are United States citizens, ensuring free movement from the Island of Puerto Rico to the mainland. The United States government plays an active role in controlling the economy and the social life of the island, including a major effort to industrialize the island, starting in 1947, and several attempts to make English the language of instruction in schools and of daily life. In cities like New York, at least a generation of Puerto Ricans have lived all of their lives on the mainland, many of whom use English as their primary language. While Puerto Ricans have easier access to social ties on the island, their ties to an autonomous culture are more tenuous than other Latino groups, because Puerto Rican culture has been more dramatically transformed by almost a century of American dominance.

Cuban Americans, who are concentrated in Miami, Florida, with secondary centers in other parts of Florida and the New York metropolitan area, make up 5% of the mainland Latino population (Montgomery, 1994). While some Cubans migrated to the United States prior to the Cuban Revolution in 1960, the establishment of a large Cuban community postdates the revolution. Much of the intragroup diversity among Cubans mirrors the different waves of emigration from Cuba. The first migrants, who were more educated and professional, received considerable aid from the US government to secure loans to start businesses and to transfer their professional credentials as doctors, lawyers, and so on (Pedraza-Bailey, 1985; Portes & Bach, 1985; Grenier & Stepick, 1992). As a group, Cubans have the highest levels of socioeconomic status of all Latino groups. They also have the highest rate of retention of Spanish as their primary language. Cubans have developed a vibrant ethnic enclave in Miami, where Cubans have become a dominant force in the political and cultural life of the city (Portes & Stepick, 1993).

Migrants from the Dominican Republic comprise another important Latino group from the Caribbean (Garrison & Weiss, 1987; Grasmuck & Pessar, 1991). They have concentrated heavily in the New York metropolitan area, particularly in the neighborhood of Washington Heights. Dominicans come primarily from urban centers of the Dominican Republic, though there is also a significant rural population, many of whom step-migrated through the capital city of Santo Domingo. The Dominican migration began after the assassination of the dictator Trujillo in 1961 and the US occupation in 1965. The US government facilitated the emigration of political dissidents as a political safety valve to reduce the level of protest against the US occupation and the imposition of a pro-US government (Grasmuck & Pessar, 1991). Dominican emigrants are often middle-class individuals who have been frustrated by the lack of jobs and economic underdevelopment in the Dominican Republic. The earlier waves of migrants created a base of legal residents who could bring relatives in a chain migration from the island. While Dominicans often experience downward mobility in terms of job status, the wage differentials between New York and the Dominican Republic are so great that even less prestigious jobs provide the income for acquiring a middle-class lifestyle that would be unattainable at home.

More recently, refugees from several Central American countries have come, fleeing violence, civil war, and social turmoil in their home countries. The largest group comes from El Salvador, and there are also significant communities of Guatemalans and Nicaraguans. Although these immigrants come from areas of extreme violence and many have suffered considerably both at home and on their journeys to the United States, few of them have received official recognition as refugees or asylees. The political relationships of the US government with the governments in each country have been determinant in the treatment of these Central American groups; Nicaraguans have been more likely to be recognized as refugees if they were fleeing the Sandinista government than were Salvadorans or Guatemalans fleeing governments supported by the United States. Other Central Americans come for economic reasons similar to other Latino groups. However, the greater distances and costs of migration make the trip more difficult.

There has also been significant recent immigration from South America, particularly Colombians, Ecuadorans, and Peruvians. These groups come fleeing economic crises and political violence in their home countries. Because of the costs and difficulties of migration, South Americans tend to have more social and financial resources than some of the other recent groups. They also experience more downward mobility in their migration, since they are hampered in finding middle-class jobs by their legal status, lack of programs to facilitate transfer of their credentials, and lack of facility in English (Mahler, 1995). These Central and South Americans make up about 13% of the US Latino population (Montgomery, 1994). However, relatively little is known from a research perspective about these migrants, their experience in the United States, and their mental health status.

EPIDEMIOLOGICAL STUDIES OF PSYCHOLOGICAL DISTRESS AND MENTAL ILLNESS

Several major studies have examined the mental health of Latinos in the United States. These include the Hispanic Health and Nutrition Examination Survey (National Center for Health Statistics, 1985; Moscicki, Rae, Regier, & Locke, 1987), the Los Angeles site of the National Institute of Mental Health (NIMH) Epidemiologic Catchment Area Program (ECA) (Regier et al., 1984; Karno et al., 1987), and the studies in Puerto Rico of mental health and mental health service utilization (Canino et al., 1987; Canino, Bravo, Rubio-Stipec, & Woodbury, 1990; Vera et al., 1991). The major instruments in these studies were the NIMH Center of Epidemiological Studies Depression Scale (CES-D) and the NIMH Diagnostic Interview Schedule (DIS).

Hispanic Health and Nutrition Examination Survey

The Hispanic Health and Nutrition Examination Survey (HANES), a major national study developed to assess health conditions and health needs of the Latino population in the United States, incorporated the CES-D and the depression section of the DIS (see National Center for Health Statistics, 1985, for the details of the development of the survey, the translation of the instruments, and the conduct of the physical examination). The Hispanic HANES, which was conducted between 1982 and 1984, consisted of a medical history, a physical examination, and two measures of depression designed to identify significant pathology in Latino groups. Using self-identified ethnicity, the researchers sampled 7462 Mexican Americans in the five southwestern states, 2834 Puerto Ricans in the New York metropolitan area, and 1357 Cubans in Miami, Florida. The age range of those included in the study was 6 months to 74 years of age. These data are, to date, the best available on the physical and mental health of large representative samples of Latinos in the United States.

Compared to Cuban and Mexican Americans, Puerto Ricans had much higher rates of both symptoms of depression and depression "cases" using the CES-D and a greater prevalence of major depressive episode using the DIS. The weighted prevalence estimates for each group (Moscicki et al., 1987) are presented in Table 1. The higher rates of CES-D scores need to be interpreted with some caution. Recent analyses by Angel and Guarnaccia of the Hispanic HANES indicate consistent differences in the way Latinos conceptualized depression, as reflected in the conflation of poor physical health with psychological distress (Angel & Guarnaccia, 1989) and differing factor structures of the CES-D from those found in other studies (Guarnaccia, Angel, & Worobey, 1989a).

The analysis of the factor structure of the CES-D revealed similar overall structures of the factors among Mexican Americans, Cuban Americans, and Puerto Ricans (Guarnaccia et al., 1989a). Each group yielded a three-factor solution, with a combined affective and somatic factor accounting for the greatest explained variance. These factor analytic results differed from the studies of Radloff (1977) with Anglo-Americans and of Roberts (1980) with a multiethnic sample including Mexican Americans. In both studies, the researchers identified separate factors for depressed affect and somatic/retarded activity. The combined affective and somatic factor identified by Guarnaccia and colleagues fits more closely with other research that has found that Latinos' expressions of distress focus on somatic idioms.

Angel and Guarnaccia (1989) compared reports of depressed affect and of

Table 1. Rates of Depressive Caseness and Major Depression in the Hispanic Health and Nutrition Examination Survey[a]

Diagnosis	Mexicans	Cubans	Puerto Ricans
CES-D caseness	13.2	9.5	27.9
Major depressive episode (lifetime)	4.2	3.9	8.9

[a]From Moscicki et al. (1987).

physical health problems in the Hispanic HANES. For all Latino groups, those who reported the lowest levels of self-assessed physical health had the highest average CES-D scores. Puerto Ricans had consistently higher CES-D scores at all levels of self-reported health. Those Puerto Ricans who rated their health as poor had an average CES-D score well above 16, which is often taken to be a cutoff for depression. Both low levels of education and income were associated with poorer self-assessments of health status. The comparison among Latino groups emphasizes the role of social stressors in declining mental health, as Puerto Ricans exhibited higher rates of unemployment, poverty, and marital disruption than either Mexicans or Cubans.

The Los Angeles ECA Study

The Los Angeles site of the ECA oversampled Mexican Americans to allow for a comparison of their mental health with the Anglo-American sample there and in the other four sites of the national study. The researchers carefully translated the DIS into Spanish for this study (Karno et al., 1987). They collected information on migration history to compare the mental health of recent arrivals from Mexico to longer-term residents and those born and raised in the United States. The overall rates of psychiatric disorder for Mexican Americans were strikingly similar to those of non-Hispanic whites in Los Angeles and to respondents in the other ECA sites. The researchers have argued that these results contradict earlier studies showing higher rates of distress for Mexican Americans using symptom scales rather than diagnostic interviews. At the same time, two findings of the LA-ECA suggest that cultural factors and migration issues played important roles in response to the DIS.

In comparing native-born Mexican Americans to immigrants from Mexico, native-born populations had higher rates of disorder (Burnham, Hough, Karno, Escobar, & Telles, 1987). The immigrants might have been expected to experience greater stress due to migration and lower economic and educational levels. The authors argued that these results support a social selection hypothesis for levels of pathology among Mexican immigrants. They argued that recent immigrants are often the hardiest members of their communities and experience a significant improvement in living conditions compared with their home communities in Mexico. Over time, longer-term residents and US-born Mexican Americans respond with a sense of deprivation after they compare their status to the standards of living in the United States, fitting with a social stress approach. In comparing rates of disorder with non-Hispanic whites, both a social selection hypothesis for recent immigrants and a social stress hypothesis related to frustrated aspirations for natives received some support. Furthermore, they found that acculturation to US society increased the risks of developing both alcohol and drug abuse/dependence disorders, problems that were more prevalent in the non-Hispanic white population.

These findings raise important questions about past studies comparing Latinos in their home countries and in the United States without carefully analyzing migration status and acculturation interactions and poses significant challenges for future studies of Latino mental health. The study shows the varied impacts of immigration and acculturation processes across different psychiatric disorders, arguing for more complex and heterogeneous models of ethnicity and of the relation of migration to mental health.

Escobar, Burnham, Karno, Forsythe, and Goulding (1987) explored a second finding of the LA-ECA. In looking at the somatization items of the DIS, Escobar and colleagues found that Mexican-American women over 40 reported a much larger number of somatization symptoms and that this difference was particularly marked for Mexican-American women meeting criteria for one of the affective disorders. Escobar and colleagues performed a factor analysis of the somatization items. The first factor that accounted for much of the variance included the following symptoms: palpitations, chest pains, shortness of breath, dizziness, and fainting. These symptoms are the most common symptoms associated with *nervios*, an idiom of psychological distress prominent among Latinos (Jenkins, 1988a,b). Escobar and colleagues then created an abridged somatization measure using a cutoff of six or more symptoms (as opposed to 16 symptoms) in the somatization section of the DIS. They found that older (40 years and older) Mexican-American women with low levels of acculturation and a DIS diagnosis of depression/dysthymia reported significantly more somatization symptoms and met criteria for somatization (abridged) twice as often as other Mexican Americans and non-Hispanic whites. They then suggested a cultural explanation for these findings:

> The observation that Mexican-American women over the age of 40 years somatized more than other groups regardless of diagnostic status argues for cultural determinants of somatization. Mexican-American women older than 40 years and who had lower acculturation levels (indicating a strong affinity for the Mexican culture) tended to somatize more than those with higher levels (those who had largely assimilated the values of the host culture). This finding supports previous cross-cultural observations. (Escobar et al., 1987, p. 717)

However, Escobar and colleagues offered no specific cultural explanation. From the perspective of medical anthropology, I would argue that the higher report of the specific somatic symptoms identified in the factor analysis reflect the cultural category of *nervios* (Guarnaccia, Angel, & Worobey, 1989a; Guarnaccia & Farias, 1988; Jenkins, 1988b; Low, 1981). This group of older, less acculturated Mexican-American women respond to the stresses of life in LA through the expression of *nervios*. When they are asked to report their experience using the DIS, one of the few entry points to express their feelings are the somatization items, which reflect the experiences of *nervios*. Thus, the DIS structure led this group of women to disaggregate their experience of *nervios* into a set of symptoms available in the interview.

Other Studies of the Mental Health of Mexican Immigrants

Several other studies of the mental health of Mexican origin populations in the United States have compared Mexican Americans across immigration and acculturation statuses and with other US ethnic populations. Many of these studies have used the CES-D as the primary mental health measure (Burnham, Timbers, & Hough, 1984; Frerichs, Aneshensel, & Clark, 1981; Roberts, 1980, 1981; Roberts & Vernon, 1983; Vega, Warheit, Buhl-Auth, & Meinhardt, 1984; Vega, Kolody, Valle, & Hough, 1986; Vega, Kolody, & Valle, 1987; Vernon & Roberts, 1982; see also Angel & Thoits, 1987, for a review). These studies repeat the finding discussed above that older women who are less acculturated and more recently arrived and those who are separated or divorced have higher depression symptoms scores. Some of these studies have also identified migrant farm worker populations, among whom Mexicans are by far the largest ethnic group, as a high-risk group for psychological distress (Vega, Scutchfield, Karno, & Meinhardt, 1985; Vega, Warheit, & Palacio, 1985). However, when socio-demographic factors are controlled for in these studies, the differences among subgroups are often attenuated or disappear, arguing that the disadvantaged social status of Mexican Americans compared to other ethnic populations underlie the higher rates of depressive symptoms.

Studies in Puerto Rico

Canino and colleagues (1987) designed and implemented the Puerto Rico Island Study at the same time as the ECA studies and used a parallel methodology. This study developed a stratified random sample for all of Puerto Rico. The researchers developed a translation of the DIS specifically for Puerto Rico (Bravo, Canino, & Bird, 1987). The Puerto Rico Island Study, similar to the LA-ECA study, found that there were no major differences between the rates of mental disorder on the island compared to the five ECA studies carried out on the mainland United States (Regier et al., 1984). Puerto Ricans in Puerto Rico were found to suffer from no greater mental disorder than people from a variety of ethnic and social class backgrounds on the mainland United States.

Canino et al. (1990) studied the psychosocial consequences of a natural disaster in Puerto Rico using parallel methodology to their earlier work. The sample built on their earlier study so that they could ascertain the impacts of the disaster on the production of new psychiatric symptoms and disorder by comparing reports of the same individuals both before and after the disaster. They found that a major natural disaster increased symptoms of depressive, somatic, and posttraumatic stress disorder symptoms. Those exposed to the disaster evaluated their physical health more negatively and were more likely to use general medical services more for both physical and psychological distress. This study demonstrated that major stressful life events such as a disaster or the multiple impacts of migration produced an increase in psychiatric symptoms and that this was true particularly in groups that also experienced social disadvantage in terms of low income and education.

The differences, reported earlier between Puerto Ricans and other Latinos in the Hispanic HANES using the DIS depression schedule and the CES-D, indicate more frequent disorder for Puerto Ricans living in the New York metropolitan area than those living in Puerto Rico. These findings suggest a combined social causation and social selection explanation. The significant social disadvantage experienced by Puerto Ricans in New York (compared to other ethnic groups in New York, to Puerto Ricans on the island, and to other Latino groups) indicate that social factors play a prominent role in the production of psychological distress. At the same time, many of those who migrate from Puerto Rico to Manhattan lack the human and social capital to succeed on the island. Because of their lack of human and social capital, they encounter problems in New York as well. Social selection arguments focus on their lack of capital as a key factor in their psychological problems. A more macrosocial analysis argues that Puerto Ricans suffer both on the mainland and the island from the same economic forces that marginalize low-skill workers and leave migration as one of the few economic options available. At this level, the same social stressors are causative of psychological distress in this group regardless of where they reside.

Research by Alegria and colleagues (Vera et al., 1991) on the use of mental health services by poor Puerto Ricans on the island provides an additional comparison. These researchers used the CES-D and DIS depression schedule in their study, allowing for comparisons with the Hispanic HANES. By standardizing the comparison to poor populations both in Puerto Rico and New York, they found similar rates of depressive symptoms and diagnoses. These findings further strengthen the argument that poverty has a direct impact on psychological distress.

A Study of Cuban Refugees

An epidemiological study comparing Mariel Cuban and Haitian refugees from the early 1980s provides further insights into the effects of different characteristics of immigrants, their migration experience, and the nature of the sending and receiving contexts on their mental health and service utilization (Eaton & Garrison, 1992; Portes et al., 1992). These researchers argue that the comparison between the two groups of refugees who arrived in large numbers in Miami during the same period provide a valuable contrast in the contexts of the sending and receiving societies as well as characteristics of the refugees themselves. They propose that the relationship between immigration and its mental health consequences will be context specific across a number of the dimensions outlined at the beginning of this chapter. They note that the relationship between immigration and mental health may vary not only for different ethnic groups in differing social contexts but also for distinct disorders.

The Mariel Cubans left as a result of Cuban government policy that allowed those politically disaffected with the government to be picked up by relatives in the United States. Thus, those who left had official government sanction and were brought to the United States by relatives already residing there. Among this group were a smaller subgroup of residents of psychiatric hospitals and prisons. The Haitian refugees came as a result of social and economic turmoil in Haiti. Private boat owners from Haiti brought many of these refugees; some of the boat owners exploited the opportunity to bring people to the United States at high fees. While neither group was initially recognized as refugees by the US Immigration Naturalization Service (INS), Cubans had a number of advantages compared to Haitians in gaining admission to the United States. The Cuban community was larger, better organized, politically more powerful, and wealthier; most of the Mariel refugees had relatives in Miami, whereas many of the Haitians did not; the Cubans were at considerably lower risk for deportation during the time that their status was being determined; and the Haitian refugees were overwhelmingly black, while a much smaller proportion of the Cubans were black.

The researchers used a design similar to the ECA studies to examine the mental health consequences of migration and they used a modified version of the DIS to measure major depressive disorder, anxiety disorders, alcohol disorder, and a psychosis screen. Their sample included 452 Mariel Cubans and 500 Haitians who entered the United States during the same period. A condensation of data presented by Portes and colleagues (1992) provides instructive comparisons between the two groups and other Latino groups reported on previously in this chapter (Canino et al., 1987; Karno et al., 1987) (see Table 2). The Mariel Cubans experienced more disorders than the Haitians or other

Table 2. Rates of Psychiatric Disorders across Major Studies of Latino Mental Health[a]

Disorder	Mariel Cubans (n = 452)	Haitians (n = 500)	LA-ECA Mexican Americans (n = 1243)	Island study Puerto Ricans (n = 1513)
Major depression	8.3%	4.2%	3.0%	3.0%
Panic disorder	4.3	0.2	1.0	1.1
Generalized anxiety	5.0	5.0	—	—
Phobia	15.6	10.0	7.3	6.3
Alcohol disorders	6.0	1.0	5.3	2.7
Psychosis screen	3.8	0.6	—	—

[a]From Canino et al. (1987), Karno et al. (1987), and Portes et al. (1992).

Latino groups. As a further point of comparison, 3.9% of Cubans met DIS and *Diagnostic and Statistical Manual of Mental Disorders,* 3rd edition (DSM-III) (American Psychiatric Association, 1980) criteria for major depressive disorder in the Hispanic HANES. Mariel Cubans had the highest rates of disorder of any of the comparison groups. The authors argue that a major determinant of these differences are selection factors. Much of the difference in psychotic disorders and some of the difference in other disorders can be attributed to the presence of former psychiatric patients among the Mariel Cubans. At the same time, the investigators argue that the relative health of the Haitian refugees is related to the selection against those prone to psychological distress, given both the high cost and social and organizational challenges of making the journey from Haiti.

Subanalyses indicated the impact of perceived discrimination on mental health for both groups. Eaton and Garrison (1992) report that the Cuban enclave protected the Mariel Cubans in terms of discrimination and racism, although the Mariel Cubans were stigmatized both by the larger society and by the Cuban community to some extent. In contrast, Haitians experienced much more discrimination from the larger society and more alienation from within the Haitian community, in part because the large influx of Haitians in a short time strained the already limited social and economic resources of the Haitian community. Those Haitians who experienced discrimination from whites had higher rates of anxiety disorders due to the perceived threats from the larger society; those who felt stigmatized by the Haitian community felt more depression as a result of social isolation and challenges to self-esteem. The subanalyses indicate that contextual variables have different effects for different disorders. Eaton and Garrison (1992, p. 1412) conclude:

> Enduring cultural differences, enduring individual differences which are connected to social processes initiating the immigration, and the persisting structure of the social environment during and after arrival produce strong effects which are different for each migrant event. They tend to wipe out the more temporary effects of the process of moving, even for immigrations which are outwardly very stressful, such as the two considered here. For the social practitioner or the clinician treating immigrants, the important observation is that the effects are likely to be unique to each distinct immigrant group.

Studies of Central American Refugees

There is relatively little systematic mental health research on other Latino groups from the Dominican Republic and Central and South America. The major body of work focuses on psychological distress among Central American refugees through both community studies (Cervantes, Salgado de Snyder, & Padilla, 1989; Suárez-Orozco, 1990; Suárez-Orozco & Suárez-Orozco, 1994) and clinical ethnographies (Farias, 1991; Guarnaccia & Farias, 1988; Jenkins, 1991, 1994). The research on Central Americans addresses the impacts of the traumas experienced in the home countries as a result of violence and civil conflict and the reinforcement of those experiences through extremely difficult migration experiences and oppressive living conditions in the United States.

The study by Cervantes and colleagues (1989) compared the experiences of Central American and Mexican immigrants to Los Angeles to attempt to sort out the effects of migration alone from the additional effects of being refugees from areas of civil war and high levels of violence. The researchers added the further comparison of Mexican Americans born in the United States who had not experienced migration and Anglo-Americans. They questioned respondents on their reasons for migration, separating the Central Americans into those who explicitly migrated to escape war and those leaving for economic or educational reasons. Mexicans immigrants gave primarily economic or educational reasons. Respondents filled out a number of scales of psychological distress including the CES-D, scales measuring depression, anxiety, and somatization, and a scale created to assess posttraumatic stress disorder (PTSD) based on DSM-III criteria.

Cervantes and colleagues (1989) found that Central American refugees who migrated to escape the war had the highest PTSD scores, closely followed by Central Americans who migrated for other reasons. The context of violence in Central America and the explicit reasons for leaving did not significantly distinguish among the Central American immigrants either in terms of their scale scores or their actual experience of seeing people disappear or killed. The Mexican immigrants had intermediate scores between the Central Americans and the nonimmigrant groups, scoring as high as Central Americas on the CES-D and on some of the symptoms from the PTSD scale such as loneliness and isolation, concentration difficulties, lowered interest levels, and feelings of hopelessness about the future. These symptoms result from trauma and reflect a more generalized demoralization as a result of the migration process. These results confirmed the key role of the effects of war on all Central American immigrants, regardless of their stated reasons for leaving.

Clinical ethnographies of the experience of Central American refugees (Farias, 1991; Guarnaccia & Farias, 1988; Jenkins, 1991, 1994) identify the centrality of trauma in producing their psychological distress and also highlight the cultural category of *nervios* as a key idiom of distress used to express the impacts of those experiences. The traumas of *la situación* (Jenkins, 1991) experienced by Central Americans, particularly Salvadorans, included arrest and torture, threatened conscription into the government and guerilla armies, seeing dead bodies, witnessing the death of neighbors and family members, and rape. They also experienced traumatic journeys in fleeing their home countries over land through Mexico. Refugees relied on *coyotes* who make a living getting immigrants across borders. Many of these *coyotes* can be both financially and physically exploitative. While sometimes protected by family and community ties and support organizations, refugees frequently encounter uncertainty over undocumented legal status and possible deportation, an immigration system hostile to refugee applications from Salvadorans and other Central Americans, fears for the safety of family left behind, demanding work conditions and substandard living conditions, difficult family reunifications after long periods of separation, and fears that members of death squads and government informers will be encountered in the expatriate community. Men reported symptoms such as weakness, fear of falling, nightmares, fear of losing control, and alcohol abuse. Women reported feelings of anger, a loss of tranquility, headaches and other pains, and bouts of crying. Both men and women encapsulated their discussions in the language of *nervios*, a broad idiom of distress, which among refugees is associated with both depression and PTSD (Farias, 1991; Jenkins, 1991).

A MODEL OF THE RELATIONSHIP BETWEEN IMMIGRATION AND MENTAL HEALTH AND ITS APPLICATION TO LATINO POPULATIONS

Researchers have proposed several models of the relationship between migration experience and psychological distress (Cervantes & Castro, 1985; Fabrega, 1969; Portes et al., 1992; Rogler, 1994). Figure 1 presents an integration and elaboration of these models, particularly building on the model developed by Portes and colleagues (1992). I will review the model for each of the major

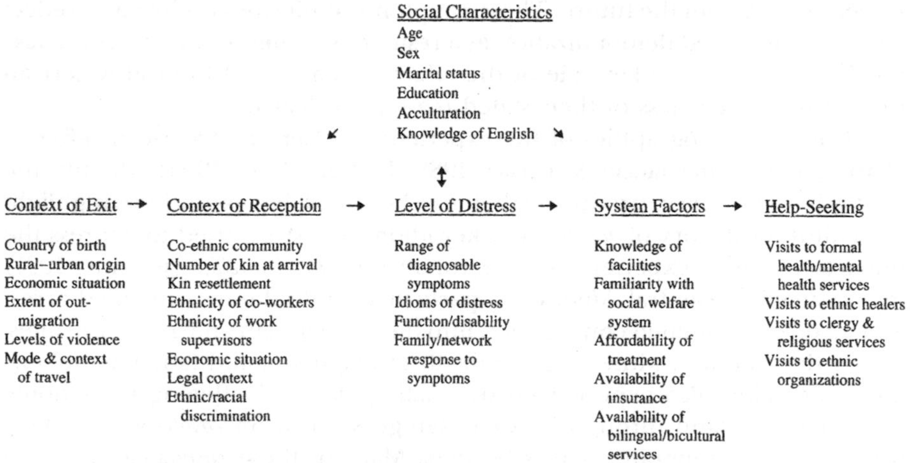

Figure 1. Model of variables affecting psychological distress and help-seeking among immigrants/refugees. (Adapted from Portes et al., 1992.)

Latino groups, highlighting the sources of psychological distress in the migration process and identifying the issues that affect coping with that distress. The model points to key aspects of the migration process and some of the variables that affect the psychological outcomes of those processes. The context of exit from the home country involves a range of factors leading to the decision to migrate. The context of exit also includes the nature of the migration journey. Current researchers argue that the impact of the journey itself on mental health is transitory, even when the trip is arduous and traumatic. However, they do acknowledge that acute consequences from arduous journeys can be quite severe. The contexts of exit and reception have more impact on the long-term adjustment and mental health of Latino immigrants. Important measures of the mental health of immigrants include the range of psychiatric symptoms and diagnoses, the idioms of distress expressed by immigrants, levels of disability from those experiences, and the response of the social network. The social characteristics of the migrant play an important role in shaping the migration experience and determining risk for psychological distress. Knowledge of services and accessibility factors, such as affordability and presence of bilingual/bicultural staff, determine use of mental health services by immigrants. Social network factors also influence access to services; immigrant's networks may be linked to formal health services, to ethnic healers, to church and ethnic organizations, or to any combination of these.

Mexican migrants largely leave economically depressed rural areas, although a significant portion of migrants first go to cities within Mexico. Government policies since World War II that have favored the urban working class over rural populations, economic restructuring programs imposed on Mexico by international lending agencies, and development of an industrial zone in northern Mexico further facilitated by the North American Free Trade Agreement (NAFTA) all have created an economic situation that disadvantages the rural sector. The severe poverty in rural areas has led to the exodus of those most able to organize and finance a trip to the United States and the migration includes a preponderance of young men. The migration process has transformed local social structures at the same time as it has injected more cash and brought more consumer goods into the local economy. The magnitude of the Mexican migration means that many migrants can get information and contacts for making the trip, and even with increased border patrols the number of possible crossings make the trip relatively certain (Massey, Alarion, Durand, & Gonzalez, 1987). The major stressors of the trip are its cost, dealing with unscrupulous *coyotes* and sometimes exploitative Mexican border police (Conover, 1987), and the fears and reality of apprehension by the US border patrol.

Mexican immigrants have found large communities in the United States where they have large numbers of coethnics, frequent kin, and people from their home communities to whom they can turn for aid, and, until relatively recently, a vibrant southwest economy with many jobs in the service sector, manufacturing, and agriculture. Given the poor state of the Mexican economy, Mexican immigrants find a considerable earnings differential, making frequent trips or prolonged stays very attractive. At the same time, the long hours of work, difficult working conditions, and isolation due to work schedules take their toll on immigrants' mental health. In particular, Mexican-American farm workers are at particular risk of psychological problems from the combination of stressful work and living conditions, toxic exposures to pesticides with neurological effects, and substance abuse. Another high-risk group is older Mexican women from lower social class backgrounds, particularly those who have experienced marital disruption and have lost the economic and social support marriage continues to afford.

Second- and later-generation Mexican Americans are at higher risk for developing psychological disorder than new immigrants. By the second generation, issues such as ethnic discrimination, lack of job mobility, economic decline in the Southwest, and frustrated social and material aspirations lead to a rise in psychological distress and disorder. Also, acculturation to the larger society increases the risk of developing substance abuse disorders, as both drugs and drug abuse are more prominent in the United States. These social stressors create higher rates of disorder in second-generation Mexican Americans.

There has been considerable debate about the underutilization of mental health services by Mexican Americans. While the growth of large Mexican communities in major cities throughout the Southwest has led to the development of bilingual/bicultural mental health services, access issues are still significant. Lack of health benefits in the jobs and industries where Mexican immigrants are concentrated, the high cost of services and relatively low wages, pressures of work, and legal status issues all act as barriers to service utilization. Within the community, the stigma of mental illness may also act as a barrier to help seeking in the mental health sector. The extended family system, Catholic and Protestant churches active in the community, and folk sector resources such as *curanderos* and *espiritualistas* provide alternative sources of support for those in distress (Casas & Keefe, 1978; Chavez & Torres, 1994). However, most recent research indicates that use of alternative resources does not deter formal mental health services use, but rather the structural barriers mentioned above are more prominent (Treviño & Rendón, 1994). Ethnographic work suggests that those who use multiple sectors may be the most active help seekers (Chavez & Torres, 1994).

Puerto Rican experiences present a different set of issues. Puerto Ricans are migrants rather than immigrants and Puerto Ricans are citizens. United States government policy and industrial expansion directly affects and even controls Puerto Rican socioeconomic conditions. The major push to emigrate is the lack of employment on the island due to long-term economic policies that destroyed small-scale agriculture and encouraged high-technology industrial development, which created few entry-level jobs for lower-skill workers. For many years, the majority of those who left were poorer Puerto Ricans, many of whom migrated through the San Juan metropolitan area. The exodus of professionals seeking better job opportunities and salary structures in the United States increased in the 1970s and 1980s, particularly to the urban Northeast, but also to Florida and Texas. Poverty is the major stressor on the island, and those with higher rates of distress are in the poorer segments of the population (Vera et al., 1991).

Puerto Ricans have concentrated in the urban Northeast in New York City and surrounding smaller urban centers. A declining employment base with the broad deindustrialization of the Northeast and a rise in poorly paid and limited benefit jobs in the service sector are the major stressors Puerto Ricans face on the mainland. While there are significant Puerto Rican communities in several northeastern cities, Puerto Ricans still experience high levels of discrimination. Urban renewal processes have continued to disrupt Puerto Rican communities so that social networks and community organizations have had to be rebuilt. These social transformations have pushed Puerto Ricans to the least desirable neighborhoods of New York City and to other urban centers in decline such as Bridgeport, CT, and Reading, PA. At the same time, a recent study by Rivera-Batiz and Santiago (1994) indicates that Puerto Ricans born on the mainland are improving their economic status, although a significant proportion (30%) of mainland Puerto Ricans remains in poverty. It is not surprising that the group with the highest rate of psychological distress and disorder is the poorest segment of the population regardless of where they reside (Vera et al., 1991), since Puerto Ricans are exposed to the same politicoeconomic system on the mainland and on the island. Better-educated Puerto Ricans have done well on both the island and mainland and their mental health profile resembles that of the general US population (Canino et al., 1987).

Loss of cultural identity is a prominent issue related to Puerto Rican mental health (Flores, 1993). Decades of efforts to Americanize Puerto Rico have taken their toll on the sense of cultural autonomy Puerto Ricans experience relative to other Latino groups, who draw renewal from relatively intact home cultures. The development of a Nuyorican culture, while a vibrant force on the mainland, has led to discrimination when migrants return to Puerto Rico to live (Flores, 1993). The high rates of circular migration have created a subpopulation who are "neither here nor there." While the implications of these issues are difficult to document in terms of specific mental health outcomes, they provide an important context for understanding the Puerto Rican migrant experience in comparison to that of other Latino immigrants.

Puerto Ricans are relatively high utilizers of health services, particularly the general medical sector. Access to a widespread public health system (until very recently) in Puerto Rico and eligibility for health benefits and federal health programs on the mainland make financial access issues less of a barrier than for other Latinos. Given the high use of the medical sector both in Puerto Rico and the mainland (Treviño & Rendón, 1994; Vera et al., 1991), recognition of mental health problems by primary care providers is a significant issue. Recognition of the idioms of *nervios* and *ataque de nervios* as important signs of psychological distress among many Puerto Ricans, especially those from working-class and poor backgrounds, can contribute to recognition of psychosocial problems in primary care. At the same time, there are not simple translations of these idioms of distress into psychiatric diagnoses; rather, they cut across a range of distress and disorder, requiring careful assessment of both the symptoms and contexts of experience (American Psychiatric Association, 1994; Guarnaccia, Canino, Rubio-Stipec, & Bravo, 1993). Both *espiritismo* and *santeria* continue to flourish in Latino neighborhoods of New York City; their presence is more variable in smaller cities in the Northeast where Puerto Ricans have spread. In epidemiological studies, the use of the folk sector appears limited for mental health problems; however, the long history of rich ethnographic reports of the use of these resources argue for the continued importance of this sector in mental health help seeking (Garrison, 1977; Harwood, 1977; Koss-Chioino, 1992). Less studied, but potentially as important, is the role of both the Catholic and newer Protestant churches, their clergy, and lay organizations in support of people in psychological distress.

The US government has treated Cubans as the classic political refugee group (Pedraza-Bailey, 1985; Portes & Bach, 1985), in spite of the fact that economic issues have always been prominent and in recent waves of Cuban immigrants the most prominent reason for leaving. Both fears of political reprisals and chronic economic distress have provided a powerful push for Cubans to leave. The pulls have been freedom from fear of political persecution, greater range of economic opportunities, and the desire to reunify with family members who had left in earlier waves of immigration. Both the loss of material wealth in Cuba as a result of leaving and the separation of families are potent sources of distress from the leaving process.

Strong family ties, which serve as the basis for bringing new family members to the United States, and a strong ethnic enclave in Miami have made the migration for many Cubans much less stressful. United States government aid for the resettlement of Cubans has also been decisive in their successful adaptation (Grenier & Stepick, 1992). The relatively lower rates of distress and disorder in studies of Cuban mental health result in part from this aid, as well as from the higher premigration social status of Cuban immigrants. The somewhat higher rates of disorder within the Mariel Cuban group are due to the migration of a small subpopulation with preexisting psychiatric disorder as well as the different social characteristics of this group. Those poorer and less connected among the Marielitos experienced more distress and more discrimination than earlier waves of Cubans. While one would expect that the longer stays in detention of this group would adversely affect the mental health of the

Marielitos, the study by Eaton and Garrison (1992) did not support this expectation. One of the most potent sources of emotional distress for Cuban immigrants is the separation of families between Miami and Cuba and the great difficulties of returning to Cuba for important family transitions. However, the epidemiological data do not provide evidence of the impact of this source of psychological distress in symptoms or disorder.

For Cubans, the development of a public and private medical and mental health care system staffed by and, in the case of the private sector, owned and operated by Cubans greatly facilitated access to services. At the time of the arrival of the Marielitos, a Cuban psychiatrist directed the public mental health center in Little Havana, and it had a number of Cuban mental health staff (Portes et al., 1992). Thus, language barriers have been alleviated significantly. In the early phases of migration, financial access was guaranteed by the US government's support package for Cuban refugees. The general high socioeconomic status of settled Cubans makes financial access unproblematic as well. Both *santeria* and *esperitismo* are active in the Latino communities of Miami, though their ongoing role in mental health care is less well documented than for Puerto Ricans.

The Dominican experience is to some extent a mix of the previous experiences. Extreme poverty in the Dominican Republic, even worse than in Mexico in the aggregate, pushes many Dominicans to migrate. Like Cubans, some Dominicans fled political persecution, although from a right- rather than left-wing government. However, unlike Cubans, Dominican political refugees were not officially recognized and did not receive the same aid. Like many working- and middle-class Puerto Ricans, Dominicans leave because of high unemployment on their island, although the situation is more extreme in the Dominican Republic. Many Dominicans come as a result of family reunification efforts as well. Those Dominicans who are undocumented suffer similar stresses to Mexican undocumented immigrants living in urban areas of the Southwest. The Dominican enclave in Washington Heights is quite large but cannot match Miami in its social and economic development. Sources of psychological distress prominently appear in both Dominicans' home communities and in the neighborhoods of New York City where they have settled. However, there is a need for systematic community studies of the mental health of the Dominican community in the United States. The presence of the Columbia Presbyterian medical complex and the New York State Psychiatric Institute (NYSPI) somewhat facilitates access to mental health services. The NYSPI, a state-funded psychiatric treatment, research, and training center, provides specialized in- and outpatient mental health programs for Hispanics, which largely serve the surrounding Dominican community.

Central Americans have suffered the most severe stressors both in their home countries and in the United States. Violence and terror, especially in El Salvador, have produced serious trauma, resulting in PTSD syndromes among this group. The journey itself, well captured in the widely viewed film, "El Norte," is difficult in its length, potential for capture and return across several borders, reliance on *coyotes* at several points, and fears of the consequences of capture and deportation (Farias, 1991; Jenkins, 1991). The migration process screens for those already psychiatrically disabled who would find it difficult to negotiate the long and complex journey.

Once in the United States, Central Americans must compete with other immigrant and to some extent native ethnic groups for jobs in the service, manufacturing, agricultural, and informal sectors. As one of the newest groups to arrive, they have less extensive networks and social resources than other more established groups. Tensions brought to the United States between people on different sides of the civil conflicts in their home countries are a further source of distress. Finally, because most work for low wages and many have significant obligations to send money home to support family members still there, the stresses of working long hours and multiple jobs are often severe (Guarnaccia & Farias, 1988; Mahler, 1995). Community and clinical (Cervantes et al., 1989; Farias, 1991) data indicate high rates of distress and disorder, particularly depression and PTSD, among Central Americans compared to other Latino groups.

Central Americans experience many barriers to help seeking. Their low levels of income, high levels of adult illiteracy, and heavy work schedules impede access to services. Further barriers include high rates of undocumented status and lack of government recognition of refugee status. Those clinical programs that have been developed specifically to serve Central American refugees often lack sufficient financial support. The primary community organizations, especially those developed by the Catholic church and other religious groups, have focused more on broad social services and have had neither the resources nor the expertise to develop specialized mental health programs.

SUMMARY

The Latino populations of the United States are diverse and this is reflected in their mental health status as well. The sources of psychological distress are rooted in both the social dynamics of their home countries and in the particular political and economic relationship of the United States to those countries during the periods of active migration. I have emphasized the important differences and some similarities among Latino groups in the mix of factors that lead to both successful adjustment in the United States and development of psychological distress and psychiatric disorder. Different patterns of stressors also lead to different disorders; the prominent mental health problems within the groups reflect different premigration experiences, different paths to the United States, and different contexts of reception. Similarly, the sources of assistance, both within the community and within the health service system, are shaped by broader political and social forces. While one could always wish for more data, the dimensions of differential risk and differential problems are becoming clearer. Similarly, models exist for reaching out to the different Latino communities. A key issue becomes mobilizing the political will and economic resources to address the mental health needs of those Latinos who suffer from psychological distress and psychiatric disorder.

ACKNOWLEDGMENTS. Dr. Guarnaccia was a Visiting Scholar at the Russell Sage Foundation during the writing of this chapter. He would like to acknowledge the Foundation for its generous support and research assistance in developing the bibliography for this chapter. He would also like to thank fellow Visiting Scholars Alex Stepick and Sara Mahler for their very helpful comments on earlier drafts of this chapter.

REFERENCES

Aguirre-Molina, M., & Molina, C. (1994). Latino populations: Who are they? In C. W. Molina & M. Aguirre-Molina (Eds.), *Latino health in the US: A growing challenge* (pp. 3–22). Washington, DC: American Public Health Association.

American Psychiatric Association. (1980). *Diagnostic and statistical manual of mental disorders* (3rd ed.). Washington, DC: Author.

American Psychiatric Association. (1994). *Diagnostic and statistical manual of mental disorders* (4th ed.). Washington, DC: Author.

Angel, R., & Guarnaccia, P. J. (1989). Mind, body and culture: Somatization among Hispanics. *Social Science and Medicine, 28*, 1229–1238.

Angel, R., & Thoits, P. (1987). The impact of culture on the cognitive structure of illness. *Culture, Medicine and Psychiatry, 11*, 465–494.

Bean, F. D., & Tienda, M. (1987). *The Hispanic population of the United States.* New York: Russell Sage Foundation.

Bravo, M., Canino, G. J., & Bird, H. (1987). El DIS en Español: Su traducción y adaptación en Puerto Rico. *Acta Psiquiatrica Psicológica de America Latina, 33*, 27–42.

Burnham, M. A., Hough, R. L., Karno, M., Escobar, J. J., & Telles, C. A. (1987). Acculturation and lifetime prevalence of psychiatric disorders among Mexican Americans in Los Angeles. *Journal of Health and Social Behavior, 28*, 89–102.

Burnham, M. A., Timbers, D. M., & Hough, R. L. (1984). Two measures of psychological distress among Mexican Americans, Mexicans and Anglos. *Journal of Health and Social Behavior, 25*, 24–33.

Canino, G. J., Bird, H. R., Shrout, P. E., Rubio-Stipec, M., Bravo, M., Martinez, R., Sesman, M., & Guevara, L. J. (1987). The prevalence of specific psychiatric disorders in Puerto Rico. *Archives of General Psychiatry, 44*, 727–735.

Canino, G. J., Bravo, M., Rubio-Stipec, M., & Woodbury, M. (1990). The impact of disaster on mental health: Prospective and retrospective analyses. *International Journal of Mental Health, 19*, 51–69.

Casas, J. M., & Keefe, S. E. (1978). *Family and mental health in the Mexican American community.* Monograph No. 7. Los Angeles: Spanish Speaking Mental Health Research Center.

Cervantes, R. C., & Castro, F. G. (1985). Stress, coping and Mexican American mental health: A systematic review. *Hispanic Journal of Behavioral Sciences, 7,* 1–73.

Cervantes, R. C., Salgado de Snyder, V. N., & Padilla, A. M. (1989). Posttraumatic stress in immigrants from Central America and Mexico. *Hospital and Community Psychiatry, 40,* 615–619.

Chavez, L. R. (1992). *Shadowed lives: Undocumented immigrants in American society.* Fort Worth, TX: Holt, Rhinehart and Winston.

Chavez, L. R., & Torres, V. M. (1994). The political economy of Latino health. In T. Weaver (Ed.), *Handbook of Hispanic cultures in the United States: Anthropology* (pp. 226–243). Houston, TX: Arte Público Press.

Conover, T. (1987). *Coyotes: A journey through the secret world of America's illegal aliens.* New York: Vintage Books.

DeLaCancela, V., Guarnaccia, P. J., & Carrillo, E. (1986). Psychosocial distress among Latinos: A critical analysis of ataques de nervios. *Humanity and Society, 10,* 431–447.

Desjarlais, R., Eisenberg, L., Good, B., & Kleinman, A. (1995). *World mental health: Problems and priorities in low-income countries.* New York: Oxford University Press.

Eaton, W. W., & Garrison, R. (1992). Mental health in Mariel Cubans and Haitian boat people. *International Migration Review, 26,* 1395–1415.

Escobar, J. I., Burnham, M. A., Karno, M., Forsythe, A., & Goulding, J. M. (1987). Somatization in the community. *Archives of General Psychiatry, 44,* 713–718.

Fabrega, H. (1969). Social psychiatric aspects of acculturation and migration: A general statement. *Comprehensive Psychiatry, 140,* 1103–1105.

Farias, P. J. (1991). Emotional distress and its socio-political correlates in Salvadoran refugees: Analysis of a clinical sample. *Culture, Medicine and Psychiatry, 15,* 167–192.

Flores, J. (1993). *Divided borders: Essays on Puerto Rican identity.* Houston, TX: Arte Publico Press.

Frerichs, R., Aneshensel, C., & Clark, V. (1981). Prevalence of depression in Los Angeles County. *American Journal of Epidemiology, 113,* 691–699.

Garrison, V. (1977). Doctor, espiritista or psychiatrist? Health-seeking behavior in a Puerto Rican neighborhood of New York City. *Medical Anthropology, 1,* 65–180.

Garrison, V., & Weiss, C. I. (1987). Dominican family networks and United States immigration policy: A case study. In C. R. Sutton & E. M. Chaney (Eds.), *Caribbean life in New York City: Sociocultural dimensions* (pp. 236–254). New York: Center for Migration Studies of New York.

Grasmuck, S., & Pessar, D. P. (1991). *Between two islands: Dominican international migration.* Berkeley: University of California Press.

Grenier, G. J., & Stepick, A. (1992). *Miami now! Immigration, ethnicity and social change.* Gainesville: University Press of Florida.

Guarnaccia, P. J., Angel, R., & Worobey, J. L. (1989a). The factor structure of the CES-D in the Hispanic Health and Nutrition Examination Survey: The influences of ethnicity, gender, and language. *Social Science and Medicine, 29,* 85–94.

Guarnaccia, P. J., Canino, G., Rubio-Stipec, M., & Bravo, M. (1993). The prevalence of *ataque de nervios* in Puerto Rico: The role of culture in psychiatric epidemiology. *Journal of Nervous and Mental Disease, 181,* 157–165.

Guarnaccia, P. J., DeLaCancela, V., & Carrillo, E. (1989b). The multiple meanings of *ataques de nervios* in the Latino community. *Medical Anthropology, 11,* 47–62.

Guarnaccia, P. J., & Farias, P. (1988). The social meanings of *nervios*: A case study of a Central American woman. *Social Science and Medicine, 26,* 1223–1231.

Harwood, A. (1977). *Rx: Spiritist as needed.* New York: John Wiley & Sons.

Harwood, A. (1981). *Ethnicity and medical care.* Cambridge: Harvard University Press.

Harwood, A. (1994). Acculturation in the post-modern world: Implications for mental health research. In R. G. Malgady & O. Rodriguez (Eds.), *Theoretical and conceptual issues in Hispanic mental health* (pp. 3–17). Malabar, FL: Krieger.

Hull, D. (1979). Migration, adaptation and illness: A review. *Social Science and Medicine, 13A*, 25–36.

Jenkins, J. H. (1988a). Conceptions of schizophrenia as a problem of nerves: A cross-cultural comparison of Mexican-Americans and Anglo-Americans. *Social Science and Medicine, 26*, 1233–1244.

Jenkins, J. H. (1988b). Ethnopsychiatric interpretations of schizophrenic illness: The problem of *nervios* within Mexican-American families. *Culture, Medicine and Psychiatry, 12*, 303–331.

Jenkins, J. H. (1991). The state construction of affect: Political ethos and mental health among Salvadoran refugees. *Culture, Medicine and Psychiatry, 15*, 139–165.

Jenkins, J. H. (1994). Bodily transactions of the passions: *El calor* among Salvadoran women refugees. In T. Csordas (Ed.), *Embodiment and experience: The existential ground of the self* (pp. 163–182). Cambridge, England: Cambridge University Press.

Karno, M., Hough, R. L., Burnham, M. A., Escobar, J. I., Timbers, D. M., Santana, F., & Boyd, J. H. (1987). Lifetime prevalence of specific psychiatric disorders among Mexican Americans and non-Hispanic whites in Los Angeles. *Archives of General Psychiatry, 44*, 695–701.

Kasl, S. V., & Berkman, L. (1983). Health consequences of the experience of migration. *Annual Review of Public Health, 4*, 69–90.

Koss-Chioino, J. (1992). *Women as healers, women as clients.* Boulder, CO: Westview Press.

Kuo, W. (1976). Theories of migration and mental health: An empirical testing on Chinese Americans. *Social Science and Medicine, 10*, 297–306.

Low, S. (1981). The meaning of *nervios*: A sociocultural analysis of symptom presentation in San Jose, Costa Rica. *Culture, Medicine and Psychiatry, 5*, 25–47.

Mahler, S. (1995). *American dreaming: Immigrant life on the margins.* Princeton, NJ: Princeton University Press.

Massey, D., Alarion, R., Durand, J., & Gonzalez, H. (1987). *Return to Aztlan.* Berkeley: University of California Press.

Melville, M. (1994). "Hispanic" ethnicity, race and class. In T. Weaver (Ed.), *Handbook of Hispanic cultures in the United States: Anthropology* (pp. 85–106). Houston, TX: Arte Público Press.

Montgomery, P. A. (1994). *The Hispanic population in the United States: March 1993* (US Bureau of the Census, Current Population Reports, Series P20-475). Washington, DC: US Government Printing Office.

Moscicki, E. K., Rae, D., Regier, D. A., & Locke, B. Z. (1987). The Hispanic Health and Nutrition Examination Survey: Depression among Mexican-Americans, Cuban-Americans, Puerto Ricans. In M. Gaviria & J. D. Arana (Eds.), *Health and behavior: Research agenda for Hispanics.* Chicago: University of Chicago at Illinois.

National Center for Health Statistics. (1985). *Plan and operation of the Hispanic Health and Nutrition Examination Survey 1982–1984.* Washington, DC: US Government Printing Office.

Padilla, A.M. (1980). *Acculturation: Theory, models and some new findings.* Boulder, CO: Westview Press.

Padilla, A. M. (1994). Bicultural development: A theoretical and empirical examination. In R. G. Malgady & O. Rodriguez (Eds.), *Theoretical and conceptual issues in Hispanic mental health* (pp. 19–51). Malabar, FL: Krieger.

Pedraza-Bailey, S. (1985). *Political and economic migrants in American: Cubans and Mexicans.* Austin: University of Texas Press.

Portes, A., & Bach, R. L. (1985). *Latin journey: Cuban and Mexican immigrants in the United States.* Berkeley: University of California Press.

Portes, A., Kyle, D., & Eaton, W. W. (1992). Mental illness and help-seeking behavior among Mariel Cuban and Haitian refugees in South Florida. *Journal of Health and Social Behavior, 33*, 283–298.

Portes, A., & Rumbaut, R. G. (1990). *Immigrant America.* Los Angeles: University of California Press.

Portes, A., & Stepick, A. (1993). *City on the edge: The transformation of Miami.* Berkeley: University of California.

Radloff, L. S. (1977). The CES-D Scale: A self-report depression scale for research in the general population. *Applied Psychological Measurement, 1*, 385–401.

Regier, D. A., Myers, J. K., Kramer, M., Robins, L. N., Blazer, D. G., Hough, R. L., Eaton, W. W., &

Locke, B. Z. (1984). The NIMH Epidemiologic Catchment Area Program. *Archives of General Psychiatry, 41,* 934–941.

Rivera-Batiz, F. L., & Santiago, C. (1994). *Puerto Ricans in the United States: A changing reality.* Washington, DC: The National Puerto Rican Coalition.

Roberts, R. E. (1980). Reliability of the CES-D in different contexts. *Psychiatric Research, 2,* 125–133.

Roberts, R. E. (1981). Prevalence of depressive symptoms among Mexican Americans. *Journal of Nervous and Mental Disease, 169,* 213–219.

Roberts, R. E., & Vernon, S. W. (1983). The Center for Epidemiological Studies Depression Scale: Its use in a community sample. *American Journal of Psychiatry, 140,* 41–46.

Rogler, L. H. (1994). International migrations: A framework for directing research. *American Psychologist, 49,* 701–708.

Rogler, L. H., Cortes, D. E., & Malgady, R. G. (1991). Acculturation and mental health status among Hispanics: Convergence and new directions for research. *American Psychologist, 46,* 585–597.

Rogler, L. H., Malgady, R. G., & Rodriguez, O. (1989). *Hispanics and mental health: A framework for research.* Malabar, FL: Krieger.

Sanua, V. (1970). Immigration, migration and mental illness: A review of the literature with special emphasis on schizophrenia. In E. B. Brody (Ed.), *Behavior in new environments* (pp. 291–352). Beverly Hills, CA: Sage.

Suárez-Orozco, M. (1990). Speaking of the unspeakable: Toward a psychosocial understanding of responses to terror. *Ethos, 18,* 353–383.

Suárez-Orozco, C., & Suárez-Orozco, M. (1994). The cultural psychology of Hispanic immigrants. In T. Weaver (Ed.), *Handbook of Hispanic cultures in the United States: Anthropology* (pp. 129–146). Houston, TX: Arte Público.

Szapocznik, J., & Kurtines, W. (1980). Acculturation, biculturalism, and adjustment among Cuban Americans. In A. M. Padilla (Ed.), *Acculturation: Theory, models and some new findings* (pp. 139–159). Boulder, CO: Westview Press.

Treviño, F., & Rendón, M. (1994). Mental illness/mental health issues. In C. W. Molina & M. Aguirre-Molina (Eds.), *Latino health in the US: A growing challenge* (pp. 447–475). Washington, DC: American Public Health Association.

Vega, W. A., Kolody, B., Valle, R., & Hough, R. (1986). Depressive symptoms and their correlates among immigrant Mexican women in the United States. *Social Science and Medicine, 22,* 645–652.

Vega, W. A., Kolody, B., & Valle, J. R. (1987). Migration and mental health: An empirical test of depression risk factors among immigrant Mexican women. *International Migration Review, 21,* 512–529.

Vega, W. A., Scutchfield, F. D., Karno, M., & Meinhardt, K. (1985). The mental health needs of Mexican-American agricultural workers. *American Journal of Preventive Medicine, 1,* 47–55.

Vega, W., Warheit, G., Buhl-Auth, J., & Meinhardt, K. (1984). The prevalence of depressive symptoms among Mexican Americans and Anglos. *American Journal of Epidemiology, 120,* 592–607.

Vega, W., Warheit, G., & Palacio, R. (1985). Psychiatric symptomatology among Mexican American farmworkers. *Social Science and Medicine, 20,* 39–45.

Vera, M., Alegria, M., Freeman, D., Robles, R., Rios, R., & Rios, C. (1991). Depressive symptoms among Puerto Ricans: Island poor compared with residents of the New York City area. *American Journal of Epidemiology, 134,* 502–510.

Vernon, S., & Roberts, R. (1982). Prevalence of treated and untreated psychiatric disorders in three ethnic groups. *Social Science and Medicine, 16,* 1575–1582.

6

Mental Illness among African Americans

VICTOR R. ADEBIMPE

HISTORICAL BACKGROUND

The evolution of race relations in the United States is uniquely instructive about various aspects of immigration, adaptation, and acculturalation that are of interest to scholars of ethnic coexistence. African Americans involuntarily migrated to the Western Hemisphere during the slave trade. Their social standing remained the same long after slavery was abolished. Racial discrimination persisted into the latter half of the 20th century until legal and social protests achieved official changes in public policy. Before then, African Americans were excluded from the main areas of public life. In many states they were not allowed to vote. For many years they were not represented in Congress by persons of their ethnic group. There were no African-American federal judges. The Army was segregated, with no African-American generals. Their exclusion from financial, professional, legal, and academic leadership circles prevented many generations from playing more than a nominal role in public life. That this period has been described as one of "pervasive tyranny" (Eisenstadt, 1994) is an indication of even more stressful ones that came before it. Important progress has been made in the past 30 years, but the most recent trends in public opinion seem likely to reverse changes that had been designed to make up for past inequalities.

Medical and psychiatric care reflected the socioeconomic climate. Dur-

---

VICTOR R. ADEBIMPE • 320 Fort Duquesne Boulevard, Pittsburgh, Pennsylvania 15222-1616.

Ethnicity, Immigration, and Psychopathology, edited by Ihsan Al-Issa and Michel Tousignant. Plenum Press, New York, 1997.

ing the slave trade and afterward, few provisions were made for the care of mentally ill African Americans. The slaves were usually confined to a separate cottage in the slave quarters of each plantation. Such segregation persisted when state hospitals became available, and mental health professionals seemed to have shown the same attitudes toward their black patients as the larger society showed toward all blacks (Schwab, 1978).

Some of these attitudes are reflected in various debates regarding race, ethnicity, immigration, personality, justice, and equality (Thomas & Sillen, 1972). It is clear from the literature on which various positions were based that the various phases in the evolution of race relations have influenced the choice of research topics, the evaluation of data, the interpretation of findings, and the recommendations made from various inferences and conclusions. Most topics were rarely debated along customary scientific standards of evidence. Therefore, even the most technically sound studies ran the risk of being "scientific proof" of their authors' ethnocentric beliefs.

CHRONIC STRESS AND MENTAL ILLNESS: METHODOLOGICAL ISSUES

One of the most fundamental assumptions about the experience of immigration is that it is almost always stressful, with long-term outcomes being dependent on variables such as the social and cultural background of the group, special risk factors relevant to the circumstances of migration, and the skills of group members in coping with stress. It is also assumed that the interplay of these factors may produce distinct patterns of epidemiology of mental illness and unique needs for treatment.

In the case of African Americans, psychosocial stresses to which other groups are not exposed center around the negative value placed on their skin color and mental ability (Herrstein & Murray, 1994), both of which are still directly related to employability, earning ability (Darity, Guilkey, & Winfrey, 1995), and thus to quality of life, many years after the institutional dependency created by the system of slavery was officially abolished. Black children learn early to cope with the hostilities resulting from this attitude. Then, as adolescents, they struggle with the problems of identity formation, while having few positive adult role models. Black women may be overloaded, but struggle not to be overwhelmed, by multiple role functions as mothers, wives, and breadwinners, quite often as the sole head of the household. Black men may become so desperate in their struggle for survival that they resort to pseudosociopathic lifestyles, including criminality (Shoemaker, James, King, Hardin, & Ordig, 1993). Even the most successful African Americans suffer extra burdens such as the inability to fit in, pervasive lack of respect, being expected to give inferior performance, and ultimately being denied the usual rewards of success (Cose, 1993).

With such a burden, which other ethnic groups do not experience, it would not have been surprising to find distinctive epidemiologic patterns of mental disorder. In the late 1960s, demands for equality in various aspects of American life brought some of these issues to the forefront. It was asserted that

> racist practices undoubtedly are key factors—perhaps the most important ones—in producing mental disorders in blacks and other underprivileged groups, in determining the place where members of these groups receive diagnosis and treatment of these disorders, and in determining the quality of clinical services—accounting wholly or at least in part in the epidemiological differences reported. (Kramer, Rosen, & Willis, 1974)

Given the limited quality of the data then available, this statement, plausible though it was, could not be investigated, confirmed, or refuted at that time. It was not easy to see what needed to be done to rectify the implied deficiencies in social policy. Table 1 shows methodological issues and how failure to address them places constraints on inferences and conclusions that can be drawn from various kinds of studies.

Many of these issues are pertinent to unresolved questions about the universality of mental illness (Patel & Winston, 1994) and to the problems inherent in assuming that categories of mental disorder in one ethnic group are necessarily valid for other groups (Fernando, 1995). They are also relevant to some long-standing debates about the diagnosis and analysis of statistics of mental disorder in the United Kingdom for black immigrants, especially those from the Caribbean.

Even though they are worlds apart, the experiences of black immigrants with blatant hostilities, racial discrimination, unemployment, and lower earn-

Table 1. Constraints on the Validity of Different Study Designs for Research Issues on Ethnicity and Psychopathology

Study design	Deficiencies
Single case studies and single location case studies	Not easily generalized. Often not valid for inferences about the ethnic group as a whole.
Prospective studies	May be contaminated by investigators' preconceived notions or subconscious attitudes.
Studies not controlling for critical variables	Without controlling for age, sex, and socioeconomic status, false racial differences may be found.
Ethnicity categorizations	Subgroups of "black" and "white" may have unique characteristics.
Appropriate epidemiologic indices	Using hospital and clinic data instead of community data risks the contamination of data by a wide variety of variables.
Failure to separate differences from unintended inequalities	Differences may be benign, or harmful to some; unintended inequalities violate public policy, but demonstration usually requires a focused analysis of raw data.

ing capacities elsewhere in Europe (Bainbridge, Burkitt, & Macey, 1995) seem to predict patterns of psychopathology that may be confusing to clinicians who were trained with patients born in the host countries and may involve issues similar to those encountered in the United States (Holtzman & Bornemann, 1990), and the United Kingdom (Leff, 1989). My investigations were originally prompted by the discovery that there was little or no information in standard psychiatric textbooks about populations of African origin (Adebimpe, in press). It seemed to me that African Americans ran a higher risk of being misdiagnosed as suffering from schizophrenia because of cultural distance between diagnostician and patient, stereotypes of psychopathology (Adebimpe, 1981), symptoms that have a different meaning among blacks (Adebimpe, 1982), and psychological tests that were less valid for blacks than whites (Adebimpe, Gigandet, & Harris, 1979). On the other hand, affective disorders could easily be overlooked by the unwary clinician if he or she is overly impressed by somatic symptoms and "depressive equivalents," such as alcohol and drug abuse and sociopathic behavior (Adebimpe, 1982).

In some of the earliest uses of computerized data to compare specific psychiatric symptoms among blacks and whites matched for age, sex, and socioeconomic status, no symptom-based reasons could be detected for the epidemiological differences that had been reported in the literature (Adebimpe, Hedlund, Cho, & Woods, 1982b; Adebimpe, Klein, & Fried, 1981; Adebimpe, Chu, Klein, & Lange, 1982a), and it seemed reasonable to infer that they might have been artifacts of demographic disparities. Such an inference was, of course, contrary to what customary views of these two illnesses and their association with stress would have predicted. It was widely believed that environmental factors precipitated schizophrenic episodes and that such stressors tended to cluster in the 3 or 4 weeks before an episode. In a multifactorial model, life change crises and other forms of stress were thought to bring about episodes of schizophrenia (Blum, 1985). Some studies also demonstrated that stressful life events increased the risk of depression five- to sixfold during the months following such events (Paykel, 1978).

In 1973, the only epidemiological data available were hospital and clinic data (Kramer et al., 1974), and these showed patterns of mental disorder that seemed to reflect popular stereotypes, i.e., severe mental disorders being more frequent among African Americans, while affective disorders were more frequent among whites. The accuracy of such data had been debated without resolution for more than a decade (Pasamanick, 1963; Fischer, 1969).

At that time, the scientific basis for psychiatric diagnosis was rudimentary. There were no epidemiological studies of the frequency of psychiatric disorders in the community, and therefore no comparison with hospital and clinic data was possible. African-American psychiatrists and psychologists doubted the ability of their white counterparts to accurately diagnose mental illness in black patients and they distrusted epidemiological data that seemed convenient in supporting ethnocentric stereotypes.

Table 2. Percentage Distribution of Admissions to Selected Inpatient Psychiatric Services by Race, Hispanic Origin, and Selected Primary Diagnosis: United States, 1980[a]

Race, Hispanic origin, and primary diagnosis	State and county mental hospitals	Nonfederal general hospitals	VA medical centers	Private psychiatric hospitals
White (*N*)	265,442	552,679	125,966	141,209
Alcohol-related disorders	23.8%[b]	7.8%	36.7%	9.4%
Drug-related disorders	5.3	2.8	3.5	2.8
Affective disorders	15.6	33.9	16.4	44.5
Schizophrenia	31.5	22.7	26.4	19.2
Black (*N*)	96,299	102,212	31,245	16,633
Alcohol-related disorders	15.5%	6.4%	25.1%	8.8%
Drug-related disorders	3.1	3.3	11.2	3.7
Affective disorders	7.7	16.8	6.4	30.8
Schizophrenia	56.3	38.0	44.5	35.7
All other races (*N*)	7,308	1,409	1,720	1,525
Alcohol-related disorders	27.2%	8.0%	45.2%	
Drug-related disorders	7.3			
Affective disorders	10.1	23.9	15.1	39.1
Schizophrenia	32.4	31.3	21.0	27.2
Hispanic origin[c]	21,231	33,017	6,410	4,998
Alcohol-related disorders	18.4%	6.0%	21.7%	4.3%
Drug-related disorders	7.5		10.2	
Affective disorders	15.2	27.4	20.8	40.4
Schizophrenia	43.9	36.7	26.6	27.2

[a]Data from Rosenstein, Milazzo-Sayre, MacAskill, & Manderscheid (1987).
[b]Percentages are less than 100% because only selected diagnoses were reported.
[c]Persons of Hispanic origin may belong to any racial group.

For almost a decade, the kinds of direct data regarding the frequency of psychiatric illness in the community, necessary to make definite statements about any racial differences, did not exist. Meanwhile, aggregates of national data continued to reflect previously questioned patterns. For example, Table 2, taken from a government publication showing data collected after a major advance in diagnostic technique, shows higher rates of schizophrenia and lower rates of affective disorders among blacks in four different types of clinical settings (Rosenstein, Milazzo-Sayre, MacAskill, & Mandersheid, 1987).

CHRONIC STRESS AND MENTAL DISORDERS: COMMUNITY-BASED DATA

The types of data needed to make reliable comparisons finally appeared in the literature in the early 1990s. Using the most advanced techniques of psychiatric diagnosis and sophisticated approaches to data analysis, both the

Epidemiologic Catchment Area Study (Robins & Regier, 1991) and the National Comorbidity Survey (Kessler et al., 1994) failed to show a higher rate of schizophrenia among African Americans. Both surveys showed a somewhat lower rate of affective disorder among blacks, but not as pronounced as suggested by the clinic and hospital based reports.

The Epidemiologic Catchment Area Study showed a higher rate of anxiety-related disorders in African Americans but this was not confirmed by the National Comorbidity Survey. Contrary to another popular stereotype, the rates of antisocial personality disorder were equal in both blacks and whites, failing to support the notion of a biological basis for observed differences in crude rates of imprisonment. Taken together, these two studies produced no strong evidence of major ethnic or racial differences in the epidemiology of mental disorders and certainly nothing of the magnitude that had been reported for schizophrenia in the United Kingdom (Adebimpe, 1994a).

In view of widely studied associations between stress and mental disorders, it is paradoxical that affective disorders are found less frequently among blacks. This strongly supports the view that social support systems, including spirituality and religion, and perhaps hitherto unexplored mental mechanisms may have been protecting blacks from developing psychiatric illness from their undeniably more frequent, more persistent, and more traumatic life stresses (Adebimpe, 1984, 1995; Ferraro & Coch, 1994). Now that the epidemiological facts have been established, these possibly ethnicity-specific buffering mechanisms merit intensive study for their potential use in preventive counseling (Appleby, 1991; Cochrane, 1991).

LESSONS FOR CLINICIANS, RESEARCHERS, AND ADMINISTRATORS IN THE BLACK DIASPORA

Despite major advances in diagnostic technique, there is good evidence that problems in the recognition of specific psychiatric illnesses persist. For example, Strakowski, Shelton, and Kolbrener (1993) recently published the results of a retrospective chart review of 173 patients discharged with a final diagnosis of psychotic disorders from a large state hospital. Black patients were significantly more likely to be diagnosed with schizophrenia, and the investigators thought that this might reflect underdiagnosis of affective disorder in blacks. Black patients received higher doses of antipsychotic medications. The same group of researchers found that, at their university hospital, half of the black patients receiving a diagnosis of schizophrenia better met the criteria of mania compared with one third of their white patients. In the United Kingdom, failure to define and control for critical demographic variables may account for some part of the wide differences reported in rates of schizophrenia between blacks and whites. Together with lack of data on the rates of psychiatric disorder in the community, many inferences are at best tentative hypotheses, fueling controversy from different viewpoints (King, Coker, Leavey, Hoare, & Johnson-Sabine, 1994; King, Coker, & Leavey, 1995; Barlett & Fiander, 1995; Bhatnagar, 1995; Bhugra, Leff, & Mallett, 1995; Eagles, 1995; Fernando, 1995; McKenzie, 1995; Perkins, 1995).

In both countries, there are important consequences to not intensively researching, clarifying, and settling these issues (Rendon, 1994; Bell, 1994; Adebimpe, 1994b). For example, inadvertent misdiagnoses have at least three serious consequences. First, the patient who is treated for schizophrenia when he is suffering from mania in bipolar disorder is unlikely to obtain the best benefits from treatment. Second, when sufficient numbers of such misdiagnoses accumulate, erroneous national statistics are generated. Third, such statistics may encourage misleading scientific hypothesis about the etiology of mental disorders (Adebimpe, 1993). Furthermore, failure to identify, rectify, and monitor such patterns may be interpreted as being, in effect if not in intent, discriminatory. It is therefore appropriate that clinicians become familiar with the differential diagnoses of certain psychiatric symptoms in black patients.

Symptoms that may mislead clinicians into diagnosing schizophrenia in black patients include paranoia, abnormal speech, atypical auditory and visual hallucinations, and belief in witchcraft. Paranoid thoughts and behavior may derive from real experiences in the community or in the clinical setting. They may color any cluster of symptoms to simulate paranoid schizophrenia or paranoid personality disorder, in addition to or instead of another disorder. Incoherent speech, frequently found in a patient who is "speaking in tongues," may be abnormal if so interpreted by family or friends, but by itself is not necessarily diagnostic of mania or schizophrenia. A provisional diagnosis of "atypical psychosis" or "psychosis, not otherwise specified" or brief reactive psychosis should be considered. Psychosis secondary to sleep deprivation and prolonged fasting is not uncommon in members of certain churches in the black community. Atypical auditory hallucinations and delusions are well documented in black patients suffering from schizophrenia (Adebimpe, 1982), but clinicians should also be aware that these symptoms are also common in drug intoxications, alcoholic syndromes, dementia (Cohen & Carlin, 1993), psychomotor seizures, as well as bipolar affective disorders. Awareness of comorbidity with some of these disorders is important (Good, 1993). Belief in witchcraft is common everywhere in the black diaspora and may be superimposed on any disease, without being diagnostic of schizophrenia.

In regular medical settings, black patients, like others of lower socioeconomic groups, often present with physical complaints when they are suffering from anxiety or depression, and sometimes they receive treatment for a nonexisting physical illness while the emotional problem persists. Some clusters of physical symptoms are indicative of somatization disorder, which *is* a psychiatric condition and may call for a psychiatric referral (Kirmayer & Robbins, 1991). The differential diagnosis of such symptoms in blacks, especially recent arrivals from Third World countries, includes parasitic or infectious diseases, poor nutrition, and recurrent multisystem conditions.

The basic facts of misdiagnosis among blacks as redemonstrated by Strakowski and co-workers (1993) have been known for more than 20 years. One can only speculate how many patients have been affected, if the percentages documented in research studies (Simon, Fleiss, Gurland, & Sharpe, 1973; Raskin, Crook, & Herman, 1975; Mukhergee, Shukla, Woodie, Rosen, Olatre, 1983) are any indication of what happens elsewhere. Clinical diagnoses are well known to be less accurate in the public and community settings, where most blacks receive treatment, than in academic settings. Time constraints may make use of long diagnostic checklists impractical.

Epidemiologists need to be fully aware of how unsuspected variables can influence the quality of their data and of new standards of data collection, reporting, and analysis. Among the factors that may affect rates in clinical samples are racial differences in help-seeking behavior, legal status of civil commitments (compulsory detention), access to treatment, differences in psychopathology, accuracy of psychological tests, and treatments. Many of these can be addressed by greater attention to clinical policies and procedures, regardless of clinicians' attitudes toward black patients. If there are few or no ethnic differences in the distribution of mental disorders in the community but hospital and clinic statistics show large differences, research into the pathways that lead to this pattern should yield clues about the different experiences of blacks and whites as they seek mental health care. If, on the other hand, there are substantial differences in the community, these may be indications that previously undetected etiological factors are operating differently in the two ethnic groups. It should therefore be self-evident that inferences better suited to community data should not be drawn, without qualification, from clinical samples (Adebimpe, 1994a). For research questions in which adjustment for socioeconomic status is necessary, household income and level of education should be part of routinely collected data. Discussions of epidemiological data in ethnic groups should routinely include information about which of the above factors may have affected accuracy.

Administrators need to be aware that seemingly benign differences may mask unintended inequalities, and that such inequalities may in turn cover up substandard levels of care for black patients, many of whom are in the poor social classes. Concerns in these areas continue to generate heated debates, often with participants basing their positions on data rendered inadequate by the types of deficiencies listed in Table 1. National professional organizations need to be aware that worldwide migration patterns are producing large-scale demographic shifts, and that policies and procedures that were once a matter of voluntary attitude and sensitivity are becoming a matter of knowledge, competence, and accountability.

REFERENCES

Adebimpe, V. R. (1981). Overview: White norms and psychiatric diagnosis of black patients. *American Journal of Psychiatry, 138,* 279–285.

Adebimpe, V. R. (1982). Psychiatric symptoms in black patients, in S. M. Turner & R. T. Jones (Eds.), *Behavior modification in black populations* (pp. 74–82). New York: Plenum Press.

Adebimpe, V. R. (1984). American blacks in psychiatry. *Transcutural Psychiatric Review, 21,* 181–211.

Adebimpe, V. R. (1993). Race and crack cocaine (letter to the editor). *Journal of American Medical Association, 270,* 45.

Adebimpe, V. R. (1994a). Race, racism, and epidemiological surveys. *Hospital and Community Psychiatry, 45,* 27–31.

Adebimpe, V. R. (1994b). Race or ethnicity? (Letter to the editor). *Hospital and Community Psychiatry, 45,* 499.

Adebimpe, V. R. (in press). Participant observer: The experiences of a black transcultural psychiatrist. In J. Spurlock (Ed.), *Black psychiatrists and American psychiatry.* Washington, DC: American Psychiatric Association Press.

Adebimpe, V. R. (1995). *Spirituality and mental health of African Americans.* Seminar presentation, Mercy Psychiatric Institute, Pittsburgh, Pennsylvania.

Adebimpe, V. R., Chu, C. C., Klein, H. E., & Lange, M. H. (1982a). Racial and geographical differences in the psychopathology of schizophrenia. *American Journal of Psychiatry, 139,* 888–890.

Adebimpe, V. R., Gigandet, J., & Harris, E. (1979). MMPI diagnosis of black psychiatric patients. *American Journal of Psychiatry, 136,* 85–87.

Adebimpe, V. R., Hedlund, J., Cho, W., & Woods, J. B. (1982b). Symptomalogy of depression in black and white patients. *Journal of the National Medical Association, 74,* 185–190.

Adebimpe, V. R., Klein, H. E., & Fried, J. (1981). Hallucinations and delusions in black psychiatric patients. *Journal of the National Medical Association, 73,* 517–520.

Appleby, L. (1991). The United Kingdom: Breaking with tradition. In L. Appleby & R. Araya (Eds.), *Mental health services in the global village* (pp. 80–87). London: Royal College of Psychiatrists.

Bainbridge, M., Burkitt, B., & Macey, M. (1995). The Maastrict Treaty: Exacerbating racism in Europe? *Ethnic and Racial Studies, 17,* 420–426.

Bartlett, A., & Fiander, M. (1995). Census categories of ethnic groups are limited. *British Medical Journal, 310,* 332.

Bell, C. C. (1994). Race or ethnicity? *Hospital and Community Psychiatry, 45,* 498.

Bhatnagar, K. (1995). Larger studies are needed. *British Medical Journal, 310,* 333.

Bhugra, D., Leff, J., & Mallett, R. (1995). Numbers are small. *British Medical Journal, 310,* 331.

Blum, B. L. (1985). *Stressful life event theory and research. Implications for primary prevention.* US Department for Health and Human Services ADAMHA DDHS Publication (ADM) 85-1385. Washington, DC: Government Printing Office.

Cochrane, R. (1991). *The social creation of mental illness.* New York: Longmans.

Cohen, C. I., & Carlin, L. (1993). Racial differences in clinical and social variables among patients evaluated in ad dementia assessment center. *Journal of the National Medical Association, 85,* 379–385.

Cose, E. (1993, November 15). The rage of a privileged class. *Newsweek,* pp. 15–19.

Darity, W., Guilkey, D., & Winfrey, W. (1995). Ethnicity, race, and earnings. *Economic Letters, 47,* 401–408.

Eagles, J. (1995). Biological is not synonymous with genetic. *British Medical Journal, 310,* 332.

Eisenstadt, P. (1994, September 19). Jim Crow was a pervasive tyranny. *Wall Street Journal,* p. 39.

Fernando, S. (1995). Study did not deal with "category fallacy." *British Medical Journal, 310,* 331–332.

Ferraro, K. F., & Coch, J. R. (1994). Religion and health among black and white adults: Examining social support and consolation. *Journal for the Scientific Study of Religion, 33,* 362–375.

Fischer, J. (1969). Negroes and whites and rates of mental illness: Reconsideration of a myth. *Psychiatry, 32,* 428–446.

Good, B. (1993). Culture, diagnosis, and comorbidity. *Culture, Medicine, and Psychiatry, 16,* 427–446.

Herrstein, R. J., & Murray, C. (1994). *The bell curve.* New York: Free Press.

Holtzman, W. H., & Bornemann, T. H. (1990). *Mental health of immigrants and refugees.* Houston: Hogg Foundation for Mental Health, University of Texas Press.

Kessler, R. C., McGonagle, K. A., Zhao, S., Nelson, C. B., Hughes, M., Eshelman, S., Wittchen, H., & Kendler, K. S. (1994). Lifetime and 12 month prevelance of DSM-III-R psychiatric disorders in the United States. *Archives in General Psychiatry, 51,* 8–19.

King, M., Coker, E., Leavey, G., Hoare, A., & Johnson-Sabine, E. (1994). Incidence of psychotic illness in London: A comparison of ethnic groups. *British Medical Journal, 309,* 1115–1119.

King, M., Coker, E., & Leavey, G. (1995). Reply to comments on "Incidence of psychotic illness in London": A comparison of ethnic groups. *British Medical Journal, 310,* 333.

Kirmayer, L. J., & Robbins, J. M. (1991). Three forms of somatization in primary care: Prevalence, co-occurrence, and sociodemographic characteristics. *Journal of Nervous and Mental Disease, 170,* 647–655.

Kramer, M., Rosen, B. M., & Willis, E. M. (1974). Definitions and distributions of mental disorders in a racist society. In C. V. Willie, B. M. Kramer, & B. S. Brown (Eds.), *Racism and mental health.* Pittsburgh: University of Pittsburgh Press.

Leff, J. (1989). The psychiatric epidemiology of ethnic minority groups. In *Report to Council of the Special Committee on Psychiatric Practice and Training in British Multiethnic Society* (pp. 59–72). London: Royal College of Psychiatrists.

McKenzie, K. (1995). Accuracy of variables describing ethnic miniority groups is important. *British Medical Journal, 310,* 333.

Mukhergee, S., Shukla, S., Woodie, J., Rosen, A. M., & Olatre, S. (1983). Misdiagnosis of schizophrenia in bipolar patients. *American Journal of Psychiatry, 140,* 1571–1574.

Pasamanick, B. (1963). Some misconceptions concerning differences in the racial prevelances in mental disorder. *American Journal of Orthopsychiatry, 33,* 72–86.

Patel, V., & Winston, M. (1994). "Universality of mental illness" revisited: Assumptions, artifacts, and new directions. *British Journal of Psychiatry, 165,* 437–440.

Paykel, E. S. (1978). Contribution of life events to categorization of psychiatric illness. *Psychological Medicine, 8,* 245–253.

Perkins, R. (1995). Some ethnic groups may be more vulnerable to extremes of social deprivation. *British Medical Journal, 310,* 332.

Pilay, H. M. (1983). The concepts "race," "racism," and "mental illness." *International Journal of Social Psychiatry, 10,* 29–39.

Rendon, M. (1994). Race or ethnicity? (Letter to the editor). *Hospital and Community Psychiatry, 45,* 498.

Robins, L. N., & Regier, D. A. (Eds.). (1991). *Psychiatric disorders in America: The Epidemiologic Catchment Area Study.* New York: Free Press.

Rosenstein, M. J., Milazzo-Sayre, MacAskill, R. L., & Manderscheid, R. W. (1987). Use of inpatient services by special populations. In R. W. Manderscheid & S. A. Barrett (Eds.), *Mental health, United States, 1987.* Washington, DC: US Government Printing Office.

Schwab, J. J. (1978). Nineteenth century studies of mental illness in Southern blacks. *Interaction, 1,* 21–25.

Selten, J.-P. (1995). Data on Surinamese patients in the Netherlands support study results. *British Medical Journal, 310,* 331.

Shoemaker, W. C., James, C. B., King, L. M., Hardin, E., & Ordig, G. J. (1993). Urban violence in Los Angeles in the aftermath of the riots with implications for social reconstruction. *Journal of American Medical Association, 270,* 2833–2837.

Simon, R. J., Fleiss, J. L., Gurland, B., & Sharpe, L. (1973). Depression and schizophrenia in black and white mental patients. *Archives of General Psychiatry, 28,* 509–512.

Strakowski, S. M., Shelton, R. C., & Kolbrener, M. L. (1993). The effects of race and comorbidity on clinical diagnoses in patients with psychosis. *Journal of Clinical Psychiatry, 54,* 96–102.

Thomas, A., & Sillen, S. (1972). *Racism and psychiatry.* New York: Brunner/Mazel.

7

Hutterite Colonies

Stress and Coping in the Context of Communal Life

PETER H. STEPHENSON

INTRODUCTION

The Hutterian people, like the Amish and Mennonites, were part of the Anabaptist movement that arose in German-speaking lands in the early 16th century. All of these groups practice adult baptism, which was the basis of their shared persecution (as well as their cultural identity) through the ages. All three groups are drawn together in strongly group-oriented communities and practice some degree of mutual support that ranges from communal living (the Hutterites), through mandated mutual assistance (the Amish and Old-Order Mennonites), to tithes and community work (most Mennonites). The Hutterites, Amish, and Old-Order Mennonites are all densely concentrated, regional, rural, endogamous, genetic, and cultural isolates, and hence they have often been employed (along with others, such as the Mormons) as population models in quasi-experimental comparisons. The Hutterites, who are further subdivided into three endogamous groups (*Leute*), have often been employed and described by many authors as "a natural laboratory" for the study of: (1) mental disorders (Eaton & Weil, 1955); (2) personality (Kaplan & Plaut, 1956); (3) model therapeutic communities (Schenker, 1986); (4) genetic, demographic, and microevolutionary studies (see Hostetler's summary, 1985); (5) economic development collectives (Dorner, 1976); (6) a nostalgic model of

PETER H. STEPHENSON • Department of Anthropology, University of Victoria, Victoria, British Columbia, Canada V8W 2Y2.

Ethnicity, Immigration, and Psychopathology, edited by Ihsan Al-Issa and Michel Tousignant. Plenum Press, New York, 1997.

German "folk" culture (Holzach, 1982; Mumelter, 1986); and (7) a precedent for minority legal rights and cultural pluralism (Janzen, 1990). For major descriptions of Hutterian culture, see Stephenson (1991), Peter (1987), Hostetler (1974), and Bennett (1967).

THE HUTTERIANS AND MENTAL DISORDERS

The Hutterian people have long been of special interest to psychologists and anthropologists interested in mental disorders and social stress. Few studies of the Hutterites have been as widely cited as Eaton and Weil's (1955) initial landmark survey of Hutterite mental disorders, which was broadly influential in the fields of culture and personality studies, epidemiology, demography, and population genetics. More recent studies conducted by Brunt and colleagues (Brunt, Reeder, Stephenson, Love, & Chen, 1995a,b; Stephenson, 1985) have concentrated on the risk factors associated with stress-related physical disorders such as heart disease and stroke in the context of communal work. The topic of stress and cardiovascular diseases will be taken up later in the chapter after it has been illuminated by an initial discussion of stress and coping related to mental disorders.

Although Eaton and Weil (1955) made a series of predictions about changes in frequencies of certain disorders that they hoped subsequent researchers would test, these have never been systematically assessed with a second large-scale survey. Predicted changes included increases in the frequency of certain disorders (schizophrenia and senile dementias), which the authors thought would be consistent with aging and the stresses associated with an assimilating population. Recently, the need for follow-up studies of such "special populations" (including the Hutterites) has been persuasively argued by Torrey (1987) in a review of 77 prevalence studies of schizophrenia published since 1948. Only a very few studies of psychosocial behavior and change among the Hutterians have been undertaken during the last 36 years, despite such an important baseline study (see, in particular, Peter & Whitaker, 1984; Stephenson, 1983–84; Schludermann & Schludermann, 1969a, 1971). Indeed, there is only one ethnopsychiatric case study (Stephenson, 1979) that explores the most frequent mental illness category (depression) discovered in Eaton and Weil's initial survey. Eaton and Weil (1955) concentrated on the 2.33% of the Hutterite population that were or had been diagnosed as mentally ill at some time. They noted that this number was especially significant because it meant that more than 97% of Hutterites living had probably never experienced a mental disorder. Kaplan and Plaut (1956) amplified this finding by noting that, indeed, most Hutterites were well adjusted and could moreover actually be described as happy or content.

Eaton and Weil (1955) compared the Hutterites to nine other cultural groups for which sufficient data existed and used a simple actual versus expected frequency model for their comparisons. The Hutterites had higher frequencies of depressive symptoms that could be categorized along a gradient from serious (psychotic) to mild (psychoneurotic) than did the other groups in their comparison set. In terms of schizophrenia, the Hutterites had by far the lowest percentage of diagnosed cases of all groups (and one of the lowest ever recorded). Eaton and Weil (1955, pp. 86–89) invoked social cohesion as the major explanatory factor influencing the inversely correlated frequency of depression and schizophrenia in both their samples and other studies directed at one or another of these forms of mental illness. They simply noted that the highest rates of schizophrenia and lowest rates of depression in their sample (the northern areas of Sweden) occurred in the most dispersed and least cohesive group, whereas the highest rates of depression and lowest rates of schizophrenia (the Hutterites) were found in the least dispersed and most cohesive group. As such, social isolation and social disorganization were associated with a disarticulated self and cognitive and personality disorganization (schizophrenia). In addition, a rather total social incorporation of individuals and orderliness were associated with guilt, low self-esteem, and despair (e.g., depression) (see Stephenson, 1979).

Interestingly, Eaton and Weil (1955) noted that 16 of 39 Hutterite cases of what they termed "manic-depressive reaction cases" (depression) were closely related to at least one other individual suffering from the same disorder. In addition, while none of the schizophrenic persons were related to one another, two of them had a close relative with depression (pp. 90–91). One could argue that the degree of consanguinity in psychoses revealed by the study suggests that an underlying genetic basis for temperament exists, including mental instability. However, the results of the study also suggested to Eaton and Weil that the form such instability might take is directly related to the social form and cultural arena of expression within which an individual who possesses such a psychological makeup lives.

Eaton and Weil (1955) themselves concluded that,

> Hutterite mental patients with a variety of functional disorders reflected Hutterite cultural values in their symptoms of illness. There was little free-floating anxiety among the people who had grown up in this highly structured social system. Dominance of depression and introjection rather than acting out or projection of conflicts was found in both manic–depressive reaction and psycho-neurotic cases. Nearly all patients, even the most disturbed schizophrenics, lived up to the strong taboo against overt physical aggression and physical violence. Paranoid, manic, severely antisocial, or extremely regressive symptoms were uncommon. Equally rare or completely absent were severe crimes, marital separation, and other forms of social disorganization. People had interpersonal problems rather than anti-social manifestations. Hutterites showed evidence of having aggressive impulses in projective tests, but these impulses were not manifested overtly as acts physically harmful to others. (p. 211)

Thus, early and influential studies identified communal life as two-sided: it was a context within which care and healing could take place but was also associated with significant risk of depression. However, the specific sources of both the caring response and the stresses that result in illnesses have received little ethnographic attention to date.

THERAPEUTIC COMMUNITY RESPONSES TO ILLNESS: THE HUTTERITES AS A CASE STUDY

Many Hutterian practices and the belief system that underlies them greatly ameliorate the serious consequences of mental disorders or disability for individual Hutterites, their families, and their communities. Additionally, other forms of disability that make individuals dependent on fairly intensive care (stroke, heart disease, accidents) are accommodated within the communal life of Hutterite colonies. The movement toward therapeutic communities has even used the Hutterites as an example to advance their case (see, most recently, Schenker, 1986). It is to the ethnographic particulars of therapeutic aspects of Hutterite culture that we shall now turn. However, one must keep in mind that the same intensely social context that ensures care may be the source of considerable stress as well. This last aspect of communal life is more difficult to assess, but we shall return to it in the final discussion.

Hutterite Ethnopsychiatry

The Hutterites recognize something like depression in their own vernacular but term it *Anfechtung*, which best translates as "temptation" (implicitly, by the devil). Behaviors generally associated by the Hutterites with *Anfechtung* include withdrawal from social interaction, crying and seeking solitary places, loss of appetite, troubled sleep and dreams, pacing back and forth, and extreme worry. These symptoms correspond closely to our diagnostic category of depression in psychiatry, but the Hutterite category has dynamic features particular to their own culture, which further discussion will serve to clarify.

The Hutterites recognize physical characteristics of people who belong to specific kindreds and connect these to susceptibility to diseases and to mental disorders, including *Anfechtung*. Peter and Whitaker (1984) argue that within the communal context of Hutterite life, where individuals and families cannot easily be differentiated by material differences in wealth or by clothing, the referent used to differentiate between people is their physical appearance. The Hutterian term for this is *Sabot*, which designates a set of closely related individuals with distinguishing traits: height, complexion, morphology, hair growth (pattern baldness, beard), voice, and susceptibility to both mental and physical illness. Personality characteristics are ascribed to various *Sabot*, which are further utilized in identification of others, identity formation, and self-identification. Therefore, when a particular person, who in all likelihood is closely associated with similar individuals (the *Sabot*), falls ill with *Anfechtung*, by definition they are not isolated. Rather, de facto, they are part of a set of persons (*Sabot*) in a series of sets within the larger group in which others have had similar experiences. Therefore, from the outset, the person suffering from *Anfechtung* is included within a common category rather than assigned to a new one.

As soon as the behavior associated with *Anfechtung* begins to be displayed, the local group (colony and family) enfolds the suffering individual within a set of supportive individuals and practices that act to limit the experience. First, there is no categorical reassignment or associated stigma attached to the problem, which is regarded as temporary from the outset, because with sufficient faith in God the problem should be overcome. Who, the Hutterites would ask, has not been "tempted?" There is great empathy for individuals who only represent a nonviolent threat to themselves—the depressed, disabled, or epileptic individual is not blamed for his or her difficulty. Except in the most extreme cases of schizophrenic behavior, a Hutterite with a mental disorder will not be isolated from others by being sent away from the colony or segregated within the colony. Nearly all treatment occurs within the community itself and the individual becomes the center of increased attention within the family and the colony. A person stays with the individual at all times as a "nurse." The affected person is also encouraged to work at something enjoyable, because work brings the individual into contact with others and confers meaning to experience. "Work" in the colonies is not an activity that easily translates into the alienating experience of work in most industrial societies. It is not differentially rewarded with money, so it is not an inherently "unrewarding" activity. It is almost always a group activity, often accompanied by songs or conversation. Moreover, the most enjoyable forms of Hutterite work often involves being outside and/or involved in some physical exertion that leads to relaxation and, no doubt, endorphin release when it is completed. See Stephenson (1986) for a description of differences in Hutterite work and non-Hutterite labor.

A recovered person can expect to achieve any position in the colony and will never be limited by his or her previous experience. On the contrary, recovery is the hallmark of someone who has overcome his or her own weakness with faith in God. It is important to recognize that this form of treatment is in no way comparable to the deinstitutionalization of mental patients. First, the individuals have never been institutionalized and, most importantly, maintaining an individual in community care in an accepting Hutterite colony is a far cry from releasing them into an hostile inner-city slum.

Massage, a form of chiropractic activity, is still used, and if an Hutterite adept is not available (it is a traditional role still occasionally found in some of the colonies), then non-Hutterite chiropractors or massage therapists may be sought. This is said to relieve neurasthenic complaints. Herbal teas, particularly chamomile, nervine, valerian, and other soporifics, are sometimes used to help with sleep. Special visits with distant relatives and friends now living away from the individual in other colonies are arranged and these may involve considerable travel. Prayer and confession are widely employed by ministers who visit the individual confronting *Anfechtung* to pray with them, to hear their confessions, and to recommend scriptural readings. The stories of early Hutterites will be recounted to the individual as well and will involve people in great personal distress who overcame their adversity with the help of God. Inspirational parables are recited, and so the individual is made to confront the clearly articulated and demonstrated fact that they are not alone. Confession, if it results in the admission of a serious or imagined transgression of Hutterite norms, leads to a formal statement before the entire colony at church. As long as repentance is regarded as genuine, complete exculpation results. In these ways guilt and the associated stain of stigmatization are removed. There is genuine celebration at the return of individuals to the colonies when they have been abroad in the "outside world" as well. The metaphor of "the prodigal son" is widely used, and life begins anew.

The treatment of individuals in their colony is regarded by the Hutterian people as far superior to the custodial care of their mentally ill in institutions. In my experience, a few individuals seek assistance from psychiatry and use drugs such as antidepressants, but this is connected to the treatment preferences of local physicians more than the demands of the Hutterites themselves. This can mean that a significant number of individuals from one colony may have prescriptions for antidepressants at one time, but those prescriptions may be restricted to that region (and prescribing physician). It is thought to be a great tragedy if someone has to be removed from care in the colonies, and the individual will be visited as often as possible, often for many years. Very few individuals are known to be isolated entirely; the few exceptions are those severely defective from birth who do not really have social interactions with anyone.

Evil Eye Beliefs (*Pshrien* or *Beschrien*)

Anfechtung is related to the Hutterian belief in "evil eye," which they term *Beschrien* or *Pschrien*, which I have described in detail elsewhere (see Stephenson, 1979). Briefly, individuals are thought to have the power to harm others, particularly young farm animals and babies, should they envy them. The behavior and attendant beliefs are grounded in scriptural description. Envy is a serious antisocial emotion associated with the self-absorbed individual in this antimaterialist communal culture, and so it may occasion strong feelings of guilt in individuals who have been censored for or suspected of casting the evil eye. In the colonies where I worked, women were thought to be more susceptible to casting the evil eye. There are important differences between Hutterite beliefs in the evil eye and those of other groups. These stem mainly from the lack of any real material differences between individuals that could stand as the basis for envy. Instead, it is the emotion itself that is to be feared, particularly when it is focused on another relatively helpless human being or animal. As well, Hutterite episodes of evil eye accusation serve not only as the rationalization and explanation of misfortune, they are actually grounded in observed social interaction. In one such case, the invidious gaze was probably responsible for a panic or anxiety reaction that I observed (Stephenson, 1979). Neither *Anfechtung* nor *Pschrien* are associated with fear of death, which represents a stark contrast with most other cultures (see Stephenson, 1983, 1985). Furthermore, although *Anfechtung* is relatively common, it is not associated with suicide, which is very uncommon among Hutterites. As well, although loss of appetite is a symptom of *Anfechtung*, disturbed body images and eating disorders (anorexia nervosa, etc.) are simply unknown. Since it is fear of an emotion itself (envy) rather than a focus on the material manifestations of envy (acquisitions), there is always an implied scrutiny of ones motives. Thus, while material life may be simple in the Hutterian commune, the web of interpretations made on behavior is complex and scrutiny is more or less constant. Indeed, withdrawal is thought to be one of the first symptoms of *Anfechtung* itself.

CARDIOVASCULAR DISEASES AND CARE

Hutterite society is highly structured and socialization of its members creates a remarkably similar inter- and intragenerational lifestyle (Hostetler, 1974; Morgan, Grace, Kemel, & Robson, 1983). This means that habits and personal behavior patterns that may have an impact on risk of coronary heart disease (CHD) and stroke are strongly influenced by group norms. Smoking is officially forbidden, but limited smoking has been observed, particularly among young Hutterite men (Brunt & Love, 1992). Moderate alcohol consumption is permitted and many colonies are known for their homemade wines and beer. Although alcoholism does not appear to be commonplace, it is certainly found in a number of colonies. All major meals are taken communally, with men, women, and children each eating in separate groups. The usual diet is high in animal fat and regularly includes pork, goose, beef, cheese, fried potatoes, butter, baked goods, and eggs (Hostetler, 1974; Stephenson, 1991). Leisure-time aerobic exercise (e.g., running) for adults is virtually unknown and the highly mechanized farming techniques used by Hutterites also has led to a reduction in aerobic work-related exercise (Brunt & Love, 1992; Brunt et al., 1995b).

In a recent study by Brunt and colleagues (1995a) found that significant differences in measures and in the distributions of measures for many conventionally hypothesized CHD risk factors exist when several of the three subgroups (*Leute*) of Hutterites are compared, and these in turn are more marked for males than females. Since there is little intermarriage between these groups (they are endogamous) yet they are culturally highly similar, differences between them likely reflect genetic differences. As well, because there is a fairly rigid division of labor in Hutterite society, significant differences between men and women may represent differences in men's and women's lives, as well as reflect some fundamental biological differences between men and women. Since the Hutterites are communal, all colony members are served a common diet and engage in similar activities that are made distinct mainly by virtue of sex or age. For example, compared to the *Lehrerleut, Dariusleut* males in the study had higher mean values of body mass index (BMI), total cholesterol (TCHOL), low-density lipids (LDL), diastolic blood pressure (DBP), and systolic blood pressure (SBP). *Dariusleut* females also had significantly higher mean values of BMI, DBP, and SBP than did their *Lehrerleut* equivalents (Brunt et al., 1995a,b).

A similar pattern of mixed, gender-related differences in the distributions of the same measures (prevalence) between *Leute* was also observed. This means not only were the levels significantly higher, but there were more individuals with those higher levels in one group than in the other. *Dariusleut* males had a significantly greater prevalence of elevated BMI, TCHOL, and LDL. In contrast, the only significant inter-*Leut* difference between the female distributions was in relation to elevated TCHOL (*Leherleut* > *Dariusleut*). In order to explain these gender specific inter-*Leut* differences, we explored the influence that lifestyle (diet and exercise in particular) and genetic factors may have on the anthropometric, lipid, and blood pressure measurements of Hutterites. However, we concluded that lifestyle differences in diet and activity were not significant enough to explain inter-*Leut* differences in the anthropometric, lipid, and blood pressure profiles of the two groups. However, gender differences in lipid profiles levels may partly reflect differences in energy output based on a strict division of labor that favors mechanization in men's tasks. Frequent childbearing/lactation in this highly fertile group, along with a longer stage of physical labor in the work lives of women, may also serve to ameliorate their risk until they cease having children. However, after they withdraw from childbearing, childrearing, and colony work, Hutterian women appear to plummet in their overall level of fitness and exhibit a marked increase in BMI. Indeed, Hutterian women die at almost exactly the same age as do Hutterian men. I (Stephenson, 1985) have hypothesized that Hutterite women may die of multiple subclinical cardiovascular diseases within a cultural context where the fear of death is nearly unknown and a social context where long deathbed scenarios reunite older women with their dispersed daughters.

Inter-*Leut* differences in population genetics have been well documented in the past for the *Schmiedeleut* and the *Lehrerleut* (see Hartzog, 1971), but not until now for the *Dariusleut.* All three *Leute* populations have been endogamous subsets of the overall Hutterian population since about 1910. Both the *Dariusleut* and *Schmiedeleut* Hutterians formed as communal entities prior to migrating from Russia to the United States. The *Lehrerleut,* however, formed their first colony after arriving in the Dakota territories (Hostetler, 1974, pp. 119–133). If we may rule out environmental–subcultural factors, then we can conclude that the differences in BMI, blood pressure, and lipid measures probably reflect genetic differences. These genetic differences should be derivative from genetic drift in the form of founder effect, which is maintained by relatively high coefficients for inbreeding reported by many other authors (see Hartzog's summary, 1971). Founder effect, as the name implies, means that a significant difference in the original settlers of a region has persisted due to a number of factors including genetic drift. Genetic drift is differentiation that stems from pure chance rather than elimination of some forms through natural selection. It may increase or even eliminate gene frequencies, yielding very distinctively different populations recently descended from a common ancestral group. This form of divergence occurs most often in the settling of island archipelagoes, extreme population loss, and migration. These are all contexts where separation and sudden chance reduction to small numbers creates a likelihood that recently connected and closely related groups may not resemble one another (in genetic terms). The Hutterian people have experienced two of these (depopulation and migration) and now live in three endogamous units that, rather like islands, experience little intermarriage.

The greater support for inter-*Leut* laboratory and physical measure differences in males, vis-à-vis females, also may be partially explained by the patrilocal nature of Hutterite society. Colony lineages are established through the males of a family. Thus, in any given colony the males are more closely related than are the females (Morgan et al., 1983).

It is important to recognize that although we hypothesized that the *differences* in the physical and laboratory measures that were found reflected genetic differences in these two populations, diet, exercise, and certain stresses inherent in contemporary commercial farming are still important causal agents (stressors) in CHD. For example, many Hutterite men have told me that a simple error in decision making today might cost their colony as much as $100,000. Such decisions are related to the volatile characteristics of food commodity prices and the unpredictability of weather on the northern prairie. Decisions about what kinds of animals to keep, what to plant, and the timing of planting and harvesting are critical to the economic success of the colonies.

Increased mechanization also carries with it some psychological stresses that are not immediately self-evident. For example, when one is harvesting using a massive combine or planting with a high-speed pressure seeder, the work can (and does) go on around the clock using shift labor and artificial lights. During especially intense periods, men in smaller colonies may even work for 18 or 24 hours without sleep. While discussing this, one older Hutterite preacher said to me, "In the old days when the horse got tired, you had to quit! Today you work longer hours and that just isn't good. If you aren't working, you can still be productive: Help take care of others, think, and pray." Exhaustion (both physical and mental) and distraction due to worries over farm management may also play important roles in debilitating or lethal accidents. Farming is an extremely dangerous occupation and those who survive getting a leg caught in an augur, falling into a running combine, or severe electric shock are often disabled for the rest of their lives. Like those who survive stroke, major heart attacks, or those who are mentally disabled, care of accident victims is extended by the colony. The community response may involve finding appropriate, part-time work, or it could even involve continually rotating home care for years. This is often the case for stroke victims or the frail elderly residents of a Hutterite colony as well.

Custodial care of the disabled is collective and maintained by colonies for as long as possible. Those engaged in this kind of work most often are women and young adolescent children (both boys and girls). Regular visits by men, especially relatives and friends, are commonplace as are visits from preachers. The Hutterian responses to stress and stress-related disorders of all kinds rest on the simple premise that people should not be isolated because loneliness is itself thought to be an extremely stressful experience for them. Coping techniques for all forms of illness are strongly connected to the nature of communal work obligation and are influenced by notions of cause that are rather fatalistic but which do not "blame the victim." Thus, stigmatization and fault-finding are minimized in a social context where care is realized and recovery potentiated. Individual motivation to change higher-risk behavior, however, is problematic because of the highly collective nature of work, recreation, and eating.

CONCLUSION

The Hutterites are communal and so they live in what can only be described as a dense human sphere that both creates and resolves problems in a dynamic that also reproduces a common set of notions about human nature. Human beings are thought to be essentially weak and vulnerable to the temptations of acquisitive and selfish behavior that are mitigated by living communally. There are psychological costs in communal living owing to constant scrutiny and worry over motivation based on selfishness rather than meeting an idealized concern for others. Indeed, the first manifestation of these worries (a desire to be alone) is regarded as an early stage of mental distress. Yet, when individuals suffer this, they are also enfolded into a caring community that increases its focus on the individual, but shifts from simple scrutiny to more supportive measures. These measures in turn do not stigmatize individuals but are inclusive, categorizing them with others as a vulnerable human being susceptible to temptation. Recovery and cause are thus intimately linked in communal life and beliefs. The modern agricultural life of Hutterite colonies breeds additional stress related to the basic insecurities of intensive industrial farming, and this too has consequences for the risk of stroke, CHD, and accidents. The specific risks of cardiovascular diseases related to diet and low levels of physical activity are also compounded for some people by genetic factors. Highly collectivized care is extended to all forms of disability and individual responsibility for illness is minimized. This avoids stigmatization but may also undermine individual motivation to change higher-risk behaviors.

Acknowledgments. I am particularly grateful to John Bennett, Howard Brant, Joseph Eaton, and Fiona Jeffries for helpful discussions around these topics. Jennifer Hopkinson and Hartmut Krentz also provided supportive information during fieldwork in the Hutterite Heart Health project.

REFERENCES

Bennett, J. W. (1967). *Hutterian brethren: The agricultural economy and social organization of a communal people.* Stanford, CA: Stanford University Press.

Brunt J. H., & Love, E. (1992). Hypertension and its correlates in the *Dariusleut* Hutterite community in Alberta. *Canadian Journal of Public Health, 83,* 362–364.

Brunt, J. H., Reeder, B., Stephenson, P., Love, E., & Chen, Y. (1995a). A comparison of physical and laboratory measures *Leute* and the rural Saskatchewan population. *Canadian Journal of Public Health, 85*(5), 299–302.

Brunt, J. H., Reeder, B., Stephenson, P., Love, E., & Chen, Y. (1995b). The Hutterite and rural Saskatchewan heart health surveys: A comparison of physical and laboratory measures. In H. H. McDuffie, J. A. Dosman, K. M. Semchuk, S. A. Olenchock, & A. Senthilselvan (Eds.), *Agricultural health and safety: Workplace, environment* (pp. 513C–520). New York: Lewis Publishers.

Dorner, P. (1975). *Cooperative and commune: Group farming in the economic development of agriculture.* Madison: University of Wisconsin Press.

Eaton, J. W., & Weil, R. J. (1955). *Culture and mental disorders: A comparative study of the Hutterites and other populations.* Glencoe, IL: Free Press.

Hartzog, S. H. (1971). Population genetic studies of a human isolate. Doctoral dissertation, University of Massachusetts, Amherst.

Holzach, M. (1982). *Das vergessene Volk: Ein Jahr bei den deutschen Hutterernin Kanada.* Munich: Deutscher Taschenbuch Verlag.

Hostetler, J. A. (1974). *Hutterite society.* Baltimore: Johns Hopkins University Press.

Hostetler, J. A. (1985). History and relevance of the Hutterite population for genetic studies. *American Journal of Medical Genetics, 22*(3), 453–462.

Janzen, W. (1990). *Limits on liberty: The Experience of Mennonite, Hutterite, and Doukhobor communities in Canada.* Toronto: University of Toronto Press.

Kaplan, B., & Plaut, T. F. A. (1956). *Personality in a communal society.* Lawrence: University of Kansas Press.

Morgan, K. H., Grace, T. M., Kemel, M. S., & Robson, D. (1983). Patterns of cancer in geographic and endogamous subdivisions of the Hutterite brethren of Canada. *American Journal of Physical Anthropology, 62,* 3–10.

Mumelter, G. (1986). *Die Hutterer: Tiroler Taufergemeinden in Nordamerika.* Innsbruck: Haymon-Verlag.

Schlenker, E. H., Parry, R. R., & McMillan, M. J. (1989). Influence of age, sex and obesity on blood pressure of Hutterites in South Dakota. *Chest, 25,* 1269–1273.

Peter, K. A. (1987). *The dynamics of Hutterite society: An analytical approach.* Edmonton: University of Alberta Press.

Peter, K. A., & Whitaker, I. (1984). Hutterite perceptions of psychophysiological characteristics. *Journal of Social and Biological Structures, 7,* 1–8.

Schenker, B. (1986). *Intentional communities: Ideology and alienation in communal societies.* London: Routledge & Kegan Paul.

Schludermann, S., & Schludermann, E. (1969a). Developmental study of social role perception among Hutterite adolescents. *Journal of Psychology, 72*(2), 243–246.

Schludermann, S., & Schludermann, E. (1969b). Social role perceptions of children in Hutterite communal society. *Journal of Psychology, 72*(2), 183–188.

Schludermann, S., & Schludermann, E. (1971). Adolescents' perception of themselves and adults in Hutterite communal society. *Journal of Psychology, 78,* 39–48.

Stephenson, P. H. (1979). Hutterite belief in evil eye: Beyond paranoia and towards a general theory of invidia. *Culture, Medicine, and Psychiatry, 3,* 247–265.

Stephenson, P. H. (1983–84). "He died 'too quick' ": The process of dying in a Hutterian colony. *Omega: Journal of Death and Dying, 14*(2), 127–134.

Stephenson, P. H. (1985). Gender, aging, and mortality in Hutterite society: A critique of the doctrine of specific etiology. *Medical Anthropology, 9*(4), 355–365.

Stephenson, P. H. (1986). On ethnographic genre and the experience of communal work with the Hutterian people. *Culture, VI*(2), 93–100.

Stephenson, P. H. (1991). *The Hutterian people: Ritual and rebirth in the evolution of communal life.* Lanham, MD: University Press of America.

Torrey, E. F. (1987). Prevalence studies in schizophrenia. *British Journal of Psychiatry, 150,* 98–108.

III

Ethnic Groups and Migrants in Europe

8

Psychosocial Stress and the Process of Coping among East German Migrants

HARRY SCHRÖDER

TYPES OF PRESSURES TO CONFORM FACING EAST GERMANS

In light of the significant political developments that have occurred in parts of eastern Europe and the rest of the world, the last 50 years of German history have been characterized by a multitude of changes, altering the lives of its citizens, new and old. Recent circumstances have created certain pressures to conform to new standards and have necessitated coping with the corresponding new demands in their lives. These pressures served to induce a massive migratory movement, which, in its dimensions, sometimes has been compared with the European Barbarian migrations in the middle of the last millenium.

When considered from the period between the inception of the two German states in 1949 up until their unification on October 3, 1990, migration tendencies followed a relatively constant route, namely one leading from East to West. During these 40 years, 5.2 million people left what is now the defunct German Democratic Republic (GDR). In the same period, only 471,000 persons chose to migrate to the GDR, a small figure in comparison. Furthermore, this exodus did not proceed at a constant rate. By the time the Berlin Wall was constructed on August 13, 1961, thereby indefinitely closing the inter-German

---

HARRY SCHRÖDER • Department of Clinical and Health Psychology, Institute of Applied Psychology, Leipzig University, 04275 Leipzig, Germany.

Ethnicity, Immigration, and Psychopathology, edited by Ihsan Al-Issa and Michel Tousignant. Plenum Press, New York, 1997.

border, 2.6 million people had fled East Germany. From this point onward the numbers decline considerably. By the end of 1988, only 610,000 persons managed to escape, 6.5% risking their lives in doing so by crossing the heavily guarded state border without permission (Haberland, 1991). In addition, 30,000 prisoners serving time in East German institutions were released to West Germany during this time.

As the domestic political situation in the GDR reached crisis proportions in 1989, migratory activities came to a quantitative as well as qualitative climax. The mounting pressure to leave East Germany became itself a decisive factor for change at this time, serving as a catalyst for the eventual demise of the entire regime. In that year, 343,854 East Germans fled to the Federal Republic of Germany or West Berlin, representing an overall 2.6% of East Germany's workforce (Wendt, 1991). Furthermore, between 1989 and 1992, as many as 1.3 million people moved into the western part of what is now a united Germany, a process that has, by no means, come to an end.

In order to facilitate further analysis of migrant stress characteristics, the types of individuals involved in such processes of transition and coping can hereby be divided into two groups. The first group are those who managed to escape the former GDR, utilizing a variety of methods. Their experiences involved combating state authorities; fleeing illegally across state borders, thus risking their lives; occupying embassies to eventually cross open borders into neighboring countries; and, of course, those who have since legally moved to the West since the fall of the wall. The second group is made up of those who remained in East Germany, yet who, nevertheless, found themselves drawn into a radical transformation process after 1989; a process that not only otherthrew the existing political structures, but which also deeply affected the life of each individual involved, bringing subsequent gains and losses. Perhaps a few general comments would best articulate these situations, and although they may seem somewhat simple, they still aptly characterize these people's endeavors to adapt and adjust to new challenges and thereby determine their futures. The first is, "They have emigrated without leaving their country," and the second, "Nothing new in the West, nothing old in the East."

THE RESETTLERS' NEED TO CONFORM AND THEIR SUCCESS IN COPING WITH CHANGES

For the most part, it was former East Germany's young and healthy who took it upon themselves to carve out a completely new existence in the West and to accept the challenges such a bold move brings. On average, their alcohol consumption before they left was less than that of those who remained at home. They can be described as highly motivated and competent individuals, capable of dealing with the psychophysical burdens they were determined to undertake (Schwarzer & Jersusalem, 1994).

The source of motivation for these East German migrants became, over the course of time and especially after 1989, less and less a factor of internal expulsion as of external western attraction. For many, new products, opportunities, and possibilities available in the western world simply could not be overlooked. In other words, the decision to make a fresh start in the West was the result, more or less, of independent choice and was made with the ultimate intention of assimilating themselves into a largely stable and well-established political system. Theirs, though far from easy, was perhaps the more fortunate situation when compared with that of those who remained in East Germany. These people were suddenly confronted with a new, imported world, which for years to come will remain a provisional one in which the prospects for the future are vague at best. The circumstantial pressure to conform was total and acute, for in their everyday familiar lives, everything became new and unfamiliar.

Fear of losing rank in the East German state hierarchy was hardly a concern for most of the resettlers, because not only did they lack ambition to integrate themselves into this political system more than was necessary, but they also felt that they were being marginalized. Unfortunately, the same did not hold true in the social domain. Those who fled the former GDR did so at great personal cost. They had to abandon family and friends, a network of social relations that remained largely intact for those who stayed behind. Yet, in retrospect, the imminent political upheaval in the GDR combined with the difficult transformation period that followed invariably justifies the initial losses suffered and tips the scale in favor of the decision made by those who left for West Germany. These individuals at least had the opportunity to reestablish social ties again once the wall came down. There exists some empirical evidence that corroborates this general assessment. It was obtained through a panel study (Schwarzer & Jerusalem, 1994) conducted at the Freie Universität of Berlin between the years of 1989 and 1991, and it examined the situation of those who left East Germany to resettle in the west. A corresponding study was conducted, using a sample of 508 individuals in Saxony, who had remained in the former East Germany. This was achieved through a collaboration with psychologists at the University of Leipzig (Schwarzer & Jerusalem, 1994).

The Network of Social Relations

As could be expected, the losses sustained in the social network were high (on average, three family members), with the spread ranging from no loss (in the case of 56 resettlers) to 14 family members (in the case of one individual) in a total number of 1083 people surveyed. However, compared with those who escaped before the fall of the wall, the number of family members resettlers lost is smaller. Aside from family members, resettlers also left behind, on the average, 13.9 friends and distant relatives.

How did these people integrate socially into their new surroundings? They demonstrated a remarkable readiness to make new friends. During the period studied (1989–1991), the openness of male resettlers to new contacts was only slightly greater than that of female resettlers. At the beginning, the latter even preferred more friendly relations with men than women (1.24 : 0.78). Halfway through the study, the differences were still similar (2.14 : 1.7), whereas by 1991, same-sex friendly relations predominated (2.35 : 2.15).

Such empirical studies lend support to the assumption that new friends have a positive effect on emotional well-being. With the addition of friends, depression, loneliness, and anxiety scores declined considerably. It is also noteworthy that women derived more benefit from friendly relations with women than with men. These results suggest that making friends must be looked at as an active coping strategy for resettlers (Auhagen & Schwarzer, 1994).

Perceptions of Stress and Coping with Stress

When various stress-relevant cognitions of resettlers are considered, the overall outcome is favorable: resettlement is more often evaluated in a positive light in terms of gains and challenges than in a negative light in terms of losses and threats. This depends directly on the resources resettlers are able to draw upon, which assume various forms, for example, self-efficacy, having a job, or the presence of a partner. Resettlers who had neither a partner nor were employed represented a risk group for whom stress levels intensified with time.

Similarly, the ability to actively cope with stress is contingent upon the availability of resources. This was studied right after resettlement in 1989 and again in 1990 and 1991. Throughout all three test periods, the entire test group demonstrated more of a go-getter or aggressive attitude, which predominated over or overshadowed their emotional side. It was only on the third occasion, following a period marked by extended external coping activities, that efforts toward emotional integration began to emerge.

Health Hazards

When comparing resettlers with those who continued to live in East Germany in terms of smoking, alcohol consumption, and use of medications, interesting differences emerged. Among the resettlers, a high proportion of both sexes turned out to be addicted, and thus at risk for health-related concerns. Smoking seems to fulfill a coping function that controls emotions without the disadvantages caused by increased alcohol consumption. Following the three testing periods (1989, 1990, 1991), the percentages of male resettlers who smoked were as follows: 69.4%, 72%, and 70.2%, whereas the proportions of the female resettlers were 62.3%, 63.3%, and 61.7% respectively. Ultimately, of those who had remained in eastern Germany, almost 50% of the men and approximately 30% of the women were smokers.

Conversely, the women in the two populations (resettlers and those who stayed in East Germany) drank much less pure alcohol on a daily basis (approx. 40 grams) than their male counterparts. Eastern Germany's men drank the most, with daily intake ranging from 140 and 160 grams, in contrast to the 80 to 100 grams representing the consumption of the resettlers (Mittag & Schröder, 1994).

Interpretations and Conclusions

The study that compared resettlers with "true" eastern Germans yielded quite unexpected results. Although it was assumed that precisely because of resettlement the new demands of daily life combined with the disruption of social relations would define resettlers as a group at risk, what was actually found was quite the opposite. The sample consisting of resettlers proved to be a well-selected group. Those who comprised the group were younger and in better mental and physical condition than those who stayed in eastern Germany. They viewed the new demands life brought them as opportunities and challenges, and were successfully beginning to determine their futures. Over the 2-year period of observation, they reported increasingly fewer symptoms.

In contrast, the conditions of those who remained were less favorable. Compared with the resettlers, they were of a much less determined nature and lacked necessary and healthy psychological characteristics such as "optimism," "anger," and "expectation of self-efficacy." While the quality of adjustment achieved by most of the resettlers can be regarded as very positive, the process by which eastern Germans are coping with stress factors and their effects on their health must be examined more thoroughly.

THE STRESSFUL SITUATION OF EASTERN GERMANS FOLLOWING THE POLITICAL CHANGES

A tentative global assessment of the amount of stress to be managed by those who continue to live in the former GDR is based on the relationship between the new demands in their environment and their psychophysical abilities and resources available to cope with them.

A qualitative characteristic of the strains imposed, at least temporarily, on all sections of eastern Germany's population lies in the pervasiveness of the changes that have occurred. In other words, the political upheaval of 1989 was not restricted to the political system; rather, it also affected individual economic foundations, the administrative abilities, and the jurisdiction and social structures, including specific social relations. People had to redefine their concept of self and reevaluate the meaning of their past, their present, and their future. Not only were world outlooks and value systems challenged, but also necessitated reconstructing. Each individual was forced to accept a completely new environment and to somehow integrate themselves into the new and complicated social system or otherwise face the consequences if they failed to do so.

When confronted with a new situation, even for someone who did not grow up in the former East Germany, it is natural to develop, at least temporarily, acute states of stress. Nevertheless, because of the fundamental structural changes that have occurred, there seem to be special socializing effects that lead one to ask the following questions: How are individuals who grew up under the particular East German conditions equipped to cope with the new demands life is now making on them? Have particular behavioral patterns and attitudes, which were once useful and important, become dysfunctional and have they become the targets of psychological interventions? A wide variety of evidence, some of which was empirically obtained or confirmed, points to favorable coping effects, and, for the most part, the differences found in comparisons of East German and West German samples (Becker, Hänsgen, & Lindinger, 1991; Schwarzer & Jerusalem, 1994) were negligible. However, there are some personality characteristics that for the population as a whole appear only as trend, but greatly lower coping potentials when focusing on specific individuals (cf., among others, Schröder, 1990a,b). Of these let us note the following:

1. The difficulty of individuals in switching from a highly differentiated cognitive analysis of a situation to a more flexible course of action when confronted with a problem situation. Because of this, they fail to utilize and take advantage of available possibilities to remedy the problem and ultimately limit their scope of action.
2. A basic human characteristic that only allows an individual to enjoy a carefree life without anxiety if it can be guaranteed that optimal financial security and a positive outlook for the future exist; if this is not the case, central or governmental assistance will be sought for solutions and guidance. Furthermore, for such individuals, it is nearly impossible to accept instability and insecurity as facts of life, and they find it difficult to assume the responsibilities for managing their own lives.
3. The almost complete lack of ability to cope with stress and a failure to use available resources in a systematic, useful way. Such individuals remain far behind on the path to a healthy psychosocial development and competence.

We should also be aware that a number of personality characteristics (especially when compared with the population in the old states in West Germany) prevailed that are likely to have facilitated the adjustment processes. These include patience with and a great measure of tolerance for situational crises and provisional states of affairs; the talent for improvising in everyday life; the ability to make do with shortages; in general, modest aspiration levels as far as property, luxury, and a person's individuality are concerned; prosocial attitudes, enabling individuals to feel sympathy for others; experience in coping with authorities; the ability to offer various kinds of resistance, including indirect and flexible forms; and prominent formal virtues such as punctuality, dependability, and steadfastness to principles (Becker et al., 1991).

On the individual level, discrepancies between society's demands and the possibilities for coping with them are reflected in emotions. If the balance is unfavorable, this will result in an impaired state of well-being and in an increased outbreak of emotions, which, from a psychological point of view, must be described as critical. These emotions are invariably connected with the biological–organismic level, and they serve to indicate the onset of pathophysiological and pathobiochemical conditions. Statistical meta-analyses (Booth-Kewley & Friedman, 1987; Otto, 1992) emphasize that negative emotions have important pathogenous relevance if they occur frequently, last for a long time, and are of high intensity. The following emotional states were identified as sickness-incurring: dejectedness, anxiety, anger, hostility, and aggression. They are triggered by the following types of stressful situations: "helplessness," "uncertainty about a course of action," "incompetence to act," "hopelessness," "frustration," "ambiguity," and "loss of the ability to make sense of life." A serious pathogenous effect arises from challenges in which the eventual outcome alternates between a sense of hope and one of defeat, the so-called pendulum, or Sisyphean syndrome (model by Henry, 1983; cf. also Schröder, 1992).

In empirical studies of the emotional states of East German samples conducted since 1989 (some of which were compared with West German samples), the presence of emotionally critical states repeatedly turned out to be high (Becker et al., 1991; Kasielke, 1991). This is due in part to problem groups and in particular to life crises, but may still be interpreted here as evidence of a real incongruity between society's demands and the population's corresponding ability to deal with them.

EPIDEMIOLOGICAL TRENDS

Outcome variables of pathogenous processes, morbidity, and death rates can also provide information about the extent to which people successfully adjust to new conditions following critical changes in their lives. This statistical evidence also reveals clues about the supportive, compensatory, and palliative influence of health systems and the efficacy of health policy measures. However, the prevailing diseases do not develop from one causal factor, but rather through a multitude of physical, chemical, ecological, and psychosocial factors, and that manifest only after passing through various multisymptomatic stages, requiring many years before their effects can be interpreted. Also, such interpretations will always depend on the available statistical data, and even the causality of clear quantitative changes may still be difficult to evaluate. Sometimes statistical entries are incomplete, certain categories of diseases are not reportable, and statistical data may not be accessible. In such cases, only general statements about trends can be made.

A general review largely confirms the time trends and regularities that were observed in various countries. The suicide rates in the new states of Germany (former East Germany) and eastern Berlin, based on high rates in eastern Germany, especially in Saxony and Thuringia, reached an all-time high in 1991 (36 per 100,000 inhabitants, compared with 22.3 in the old states in western Germany). This figure then decreased considerably in 1992 and 1993. Statistics corresponding to cardiovascular diseases experienced an abrupt increase in 1991, when 56% more cases of myocardial infarction were reported in Germany's eastern states. Later, the sharp rise was said to be a result of coding errors. The eastern German percentage of cancer mortality rose between 1991 and 1992, increasing from 23.1% to 24%. In most major areas of diagnosis, appreciable differences continue to exist between the old and the new states of reunited Germany. It has been reported (Geyer, 1992) that the number of patients suffering from mental illness has again reached preunification levels. There are new cases of bulimia nervosa and of people suffering from chronic psychosomatic functional disorders due to their recent downward social mobility. In addition, there are many patients above age 40 who are diagnosed as having an abnormal personality condition in its first stages of manifestation, characterized by ego weakness (*Ich-Schwaeche*) and an inability to bear and/or solve conflicts. These individuals used to derive social support from the repressive political regime in former East Germany. Now that they have been forced to endure critical changes to their environments, they tend to decompensate by developing narcissistic depressions, psychosomatic syndromes, or psychotic behavior. But no change has occurred in the incidence of psychotic diseases in the general disease statistic tables.

HEALTH RISK CONSTELLATIONS

Upon examining pathogenic and sanogenic criteria, the eastern German population has begun to split up. Health and disease statistics, which attempt to analyze a population as a whole, and generalizations about pathogenic psychosocial constellations in such a large, anonymous group tend to balance out and reduce what are otherwise significant, sometimes enormous differences and therefore cannot be used as a base for preventive measures or other types of interventions. Moreover, positive and negative developmental effects particular to certain subgroups tend to cancel each other out, thus making it difficult to accurately define risk groups. In contrast, an analysis that takes into consideration specific sociodemographic criteria, the interrelationship between demands, the ability to cope with them, and available resources yields results that point to special risk groups and in turn helps to determine the overall health of the population. The following are key words used to differentiate a population under examination: sex, age, employment situation, economic status, economic prospects for the region, state of health, critical events in life, and fateful accumulation of risks.

In order to identify risk groups, one can use the following criteria: loss of control and motivation, loss of the ability to make sense of life, pathogenic emotions (especially depression, anxiety, anger resulting from helplessness, and hopelessness), social and material losses or threats of such losses, and psychophysical symptoms.

A first and rather large risk group consists of those who identify themselves as being "losers" during the reunification transition in East Germany. These are unfortunate individuals who have experienced losses in every sense of the word and who no longer foresee a chance to better their situations. This group includes senior citizens, single mothers, persons who were forced to take an early retirement, those unemployed for long periods of time (especially young adults), persons undergoing retraining, and those who live in economically less-developed areas with little chance of finding employment. The announcement by the DGB, a German trade union, that in the new eastern states, more than 80% of those above 51 years of age are jobless and that only 4% of those between the ages of 60 and 63 have jobs, drastically shows the uneven distribution of the losses that have occurred.

This first group also includes those who until well into the 1989–1990 period of transition personified the administrative, security, and governmental structure and who afterward failed to adjust to the new developments. Because of their former positions of power, they lost their standing in society, their world vision, their self-esteem, and their friends. As the first political changes became apparent, they became the targets of *Schadenfreude*, disdain, and vindictiveness. Embittered and suffering, they have taken refuge in anonymity. This group of persons must be categorized under their own heading of "politically unemployed," although some of them have already retired and are surviving on minimum pensions.

According to surveys, such as the one conducted in Leipzig in 1992, 20% of the population have some problem that requires specific help. Those individuals whose situation is more problematic had a number of risk factors to contend with. Four percent of those surveyed stated factors such as loneliness and loss of control. A further 9.3% stated loss of control and said that they had no friends. In all groups, the ratio men to women was 1 to 2, putting women at a disadvantage.

Another risk group is represented by "chronically destablized" persons, i.e., persons who have long been awaiting a solution to unemployment or housing problems (e.g., the settlement of a property dispute). A lack of restricted scope for action often exacerbates such lingering fears and uncertainties. In the long term, waiting for a decision or a change in conditions over which those ultimately affected have no control and which they perceive as fateful can be an extremely stressful experience and, again, one in which emotions characteristically range from hopefulness to negative resignation (the pendulum syndrome). All those who have temporary or nonstandard employment (i.e., all intermediate patterns on the employment–unemployment scale), especially those who expect they will lose their jobs, belong to this category. This group also includes people undergoing retraining who stand little chance of permanent employment.

Psychophysiological health risks are also taken by people we perceive as "dynamic." Often these types of individuals take personal risks by becoming involved in projects such as founding or taking over a business. On the surface, they are among those whose prospects are good even though they are not necessarily the winners of the new era. Their behavior and lifestyles meet the phenomenological "type A" syndrome description, whose main characteristics include orientation toward work, striving for success and recognition, a compulsion to do things quickly while working under a tight schedule, and a tendency to compete with others. These behavioral patterns alone are, for the most part, positive and would not themselves warrant the prediction that they are a health risk factor. However, in eastern Germany, as in other industrialized countries, this group seems to include a high percentage of individuals whose exterior competence is merely a cover for internal weakness. They pretend that they are more socially and professionally self-assured than they truly are. Often such persons are described as having inconsistent identities, feelings of self-doubt (sometimes going through crises), repressing past events and emotional control, and lacking methods of overcoming stress. This ultimately results in their exploiting their own psychophysical resources. This risk group can be found at all times of socioeconomic unrest and change, and it is an important target group for preventive measures.

UNEMPLOYMENT AND POVERTY AS NEW STRESS COMPLEXES

Job market developments in the new East German states are characterized by nonstandard types of work and by an unprecedented loss of labor. As early as

1992, it surpassed the dimensions of the Great Depression of the 1930s. Unemployment rates range between 14 and 18%. Through the use of various job market mechanisms unheard of in the Federal Republic of Germany, it has been possible to keep unemployment rates under control. For example, for every 100 persons who were registered as being without work, there were 121 persons involved in creating new jobs, training, and retraining programs. The situation would be much worse if those who left were still living in eastern Germany, if there were not 600,000 who have taken work in the old western states and West Berlin, and if early retirement schemes and a host of measures designed to stimulate the job market did not exist.

Inadequate psychosocial abilities of the eastern Germans in dealing with emotionally stressful situations add to the psychophysical stress caused by unemployment and vulnerability in the job market. There are several ongoing studies about the long-term consequences of unemployment in eastern Germany and how its adverse effects on personal health manifest themselves. In some aspects, these studies have already yielded results. A study by Dauer, Wagner, Hennig, and Morgenstern (1992) on unemployment and health involved 600 jobless persons and found that for 20% of the males and 25% of the females who had not reported symptoms or medical and psychological treatment 66.1% were frequently depressed, and that almost three quarters of those surveyed (73% of the males) were drinking alcohol with a frequency ranging between daily and often to almost daily, with 27.1% of the males admitting drinking more alcohol than they had in the previous year. Of the unemployed persons surveyed, 82.6% could not imagine a future without work. The close relation between unemployment and social distress is further highlighted by regional statistics. In the city of Leipzig, for example, almost 70% of those who were receiving supplementary benefits in 1991 stated that unemployment was the reason for requesting help, according to a statistical report published in 1992. In West German cities, unemployment is also the main reason that subjects had requested social benefits, though to a much smaller extent than in Leipzig.

From this information we may infer that with the extension of West Germany's socioeconomic system to East Germany, impoverished conditions will plague the same sections of the populations that have suffered impoverishment and "marginalization" in West Germany. The 1994 poverty report by the Deutscher Geverkschaftsbund (German trade unions) and the Paritätischer Wohlfahrtsverband (public welfare committee) (Hanesch, Adamy, & Martens, 1994) clearly documented that poverty in its various aspects affects eastern Germany to a greater extent than in western Germany. Nonetheless, as far as overall income and property trends in the new eastern states are concerned, prosperity rather than poverty is expected to increase, a trend that does not necessarily express itself linearly in an increase in satisfaction with life and emotional well-being.

LOOKING AHEAD

In our analysis of the stressful status of eastern Germany's population and how it has since managed to cope since the historical changes almost 6 years ago, we have chosen a health science perspective. In doing so, we have focused mainly on the individual health results, arising from major transitions in life. The reason for this emphasis is to develop preventive, palliative, and therapeutic measures to combat adverse effects of such experiences. A wide variety of such measures are currently being taken, although they are most effective when adapted to specific economic and health policy settings.

Such efforts range from social policy measures from the governmental level to psychological training techniques developed to protect individuals from the deleterious effects of life crises (Schröder & Reschke, 1994). The areas to which such methods of coping can be applied is not restricted to attempts to enhance the individual's current ability for action, but also can be extended to efforts to enable him or her to organize his or her future by projecting his or her zone of subsequent development. This is accomplished by connecting the three time perspectives of a person's life, namely the past (awareness of one's origin, reinterpretation, consistency), the present (identity, individuality, special abilities, control of emotions), and the future (quality of one's concept of the future in terms of the criteria differentiation, realism, and proximity to action, utilizing scopes for action, resource development). This method can be applied to the motivational level and the level at which individuals make sense of life.

Even if the overall coping capacities of those who continue to live in eastern Germany are less developed than those of the resettlers, we must not lose sight of the fact that, as most East Germans themselves emphasize time and again, their gains still have been tremendous. This means that even if the tendency to gloss over the past in a nostalgic manner grows stronger, no one is seriously determined to politically restore the collapsed regime. In this respect, the situation in eastern Germany differs from that in other central and East European countries (as in Russia or Hungary). While in eastern Germany psychosocial stress to conform and stress reactions can be seen as transient phenomena in the evolution of its society and population, these same factors in eastern Europe not only hamper the process of political reform, but also seriously jeopardize it.

REFERENCES

Auhagan, E., & Schwarzer, R. (1994). Das unsichtbare Netz [The invisible network]. In R. Schwarzer & M. Jerusalem (Eds.), *Gesellschaftlicher Umbruch als kritisches Lebensereignis* (pp. 105–121). [Social change as a critical life event]. Weinheim: Juventa.

Becker, P., Hänsgen, K.-D., & Lindinger, E. (1991). Ostdeutsche und Westdeutsche im Spiegel dreier Fragebogentests [East Germans and West Germans as shown by three questionnaires]. *Trierer Psychologische Berichte* [Trier Psychological Reports], *18*, H.3.

Booth-Kewley, S., & Friedman, H. S. (1987). Psychological predictors of heart disease: A quantitative review. *Psychological Bulletin, 3*, 343–362.

Dauer, S., Wagner, G., Hennig, H., & Morgenstern, J. (1992). Arbeitslosigkeit und Gesundheit—Erste Ergebnisse einer empirischen Studie [Unemployment and health—Preliminary results of an empirical study]. In T. Kieselbach & P. Voigt (Eds.), *Systemumbruch, Arbeitslosigkeit und individuelle Bewältigung in der Ex-DDR* (pp. 248–267) [Change in the political system, unemployment and individual coping in the former East Germany]. Weinheim: Deutscher Studienverlag.

Geyer, M. (1992). Neue Länder—Alte Patienten? [New lands—Old patients?] Paper presented at the 13th Psychotherapy Congress, September 4–5, 1992, Leipzig.

Haberland, J. (1991). Eingliederung von Aussiedlern und Zuwanderern: Sammlung von Texten, die für die Eingliederung von Aussiedlern aus den osteuropäischen Staaten von Bedeutung sind (5.überarbeitete und erweiterte Auflage) [Integrating resettlers and immigrants: A collection of texts dealing with the integration of resettlers from East European countries (5th revised and enlarged edition)]. Leverkusen: Heggen-Verlag.

Hanesch, W., Adamy, W., & Martens, R. (1994). *Armut in Deutschland* [Poverty in Germany]. Hamburg: Rowohlt.

Henry, J. P. (1983). Coronary heart disease and arousal of the adrenal cortical axis. In T. M. Dembrowski, T. H. Schmidt, & G. Blümchen (Eds.), *Biobehavioral bases of coronary heaert disease* (pp. 365–381). Basel: Karger.

Kasielke, E. (1991). Vergleichende Untersuchungen neuroserelevanter Persönlichkeitsmerkmale in Bevölkerungsgruppen Ost- und Westdeutschlands. Vortrag auf dem 1.Deutschen Psychologentag vom 19.–22.9.1991 in Dresden [Comparative studies on neurotic personality traits in sections of the East German and West German population. Paper presented at the 1st Congress of German Psychologists in Dresden from Sept. 19–22, 1991].

Mittag, W., Schröder, K. (1994). Gesundheitliches Risikoverhalten [Health risk behavior]. In R. Schwarzer & M. Jerusalem (Eds.), *Gesellschaftlicher Umbruch als kritisches Lebensereignis* (pp. 199–225) [Social change as a critical life event]. Weinheim: Juventa.

Otto, J. (1992). Ärger, negative Emotionalität und koronare Herzkrankheit [Anger, negative emotionality and coronary heart disease]. In U. Mees (Ed.), *Psychologie des Ärgers* (pp. 74–86) [Psychology of anger]. Göttingen: Hogrefe.

Schröder, H. (1990a). Individualität, Identität und Befindlichkeit des DDR-Bürgers im Umbruch (pp. 163–176) [The individuality, identity and emotional status of the East German citizen at a time of change: Research on socialization and the sociology of education]. Weinheim: Juventa.

Schröder, H. (1990b). Staatliche Repression und psychische Folgen—DDR-Bürger in der Wende [State repression and psychological consequences—East Germans at a time of change]. *Gruppendynamik* [Group Dynamics], *21*(4), 341–356.

Schröder, H. (1992). Emotionen—Persönlichkeit—Gesundheitsrisiko [Emotions—personality—health risk]. *Psychomed, 4*, 81–85.

Schröder, H., & Reschke, K. (1994). Psychosoziale Gesundheitsrisiken im Transformationsprozeß [Psycho-social health risks during the process of transformation]. *Reader der KSPW Halle.* Reader published by the Commission to study political and social change in the new lands of Germany (KSPW), Halle.

Schwarzer, R. & Jerusalem, M. (Eds.) (1994). *Gesellschaftlicher Umbruch als kritisches Lebensereignis* [Social change as a critical life event]. Weinheim: Juventa.

Wendt, H. (1991). Die deutsch-deutschen Wanderungen—Bilanz einer 40jährigen Geschichte von Flucht und Ausreise [Inter-German migrations—A record of 40 years of escape and emigration]. *Deutschland Archiv, 24*(4), 386–395.

9

The Mental Health of North Africans in France

IHSAN AL-ISSA and MICHEL TOUSIGNANT

North African countries—Algeria, Morocco, and Tunisia—have a special relationship with France. They are not only across the Mediterranean Sea from France, but they are also its former colonies. There are 3 million Muslims in France; and with the exception of 200,000 Turks concentrated in the eastern part, the remaining Muslims are mainly North Africans. There are, however, more Algerians than other North Africans in France (700,000 Algerians and 1 million with double nationality, excluding a large number of illegal immigrants) (Stein, Kerchouche, Pasquire, & Amine, 1995). Yet there is very little systematic empirical research on Algerians or other North Africans. For example, our search of two special issues on immigration of two major French psychiatric journals, *Psychologie Médicale* (1981, Vol. 13) and *Annales Médicopsychologiques* (1982, Vol. 146), revealed only clinical and case studies with no well-designed research. Therefore, this chapter reflects the available descriptive data that are mainly based on case studies and clinical observations. We deal first with the sociocultural background and traditional concepts of mental illness of North Africans. This will be followed by a review of clinical data on mental illness and its manifestation in North Africans. Finally, we discuss a major ethnopsychiatric approach to the treatment of North African patients in France.

IHSAN AL-ISSA • Department of Psychology, University of Calgary, Calgary, Alberta, Canada T2N 1N4. **MICHEL TOUSIGNANT** • Laboratory for Research in Human and Social Ecology, University of Quebec at Montreal, Montreal, Quebec, Canada H3C 3P8.

Ethnicity, Immigration, and Psychopathology, edited by Ihsan Al-Issa and Michel Tousignant. Plenum Press, New York, 1997.

SOCIOCULTURAL BACKGROUND OF NORTH AFRICANS

Throughout the major part of its history, North Africa has been exposed to various invasions such as those from the Phoenicians, Romans, Vandals, Arabs, Spaniards, Turks, and French. However, the Arab invasion and French colonialism have left indelible effects on North African countries and their people. The Arabs in the seventh century brought with them Islam, which still remains one of the major forces in the life of North Africans. Arabic, which is the language of the Koran, the Muslim holy book, became the national language of these countries after their independence from the colonial rule of France. French colonialism had drastic effects on the social and cultural life of the native inhabitants. This is particularly true for Algeria, which was considered part of France before its independence and where consistent efforts were made to eradicate its old cultural traditions and integrate it with the mother country. Being dispossessed of cultivated land during the French colonial era, the majority of Algerians became daily workers on the farms of the colonialists. Lack of employment in the countryside forced them to migrate to the large urban centers to live in shantytowns on the outskirts of cities. It is the degrading poverty of these peasants described by Camus (1962) that had driven a large number to join the French army or emigrate to France to work in the coal mines. However, despite the cultural and material poverty of North Africans and particularly Algerians during the colonial period, many cultural and social features of the society resisted change. Algeria as well as other North African countries remain a Muslim society, with religion a strong unifying factor among Arabs and Berbers, who are the native North African population. Islam provided the poor peasants during the colonial era with a spiritual outlet from a miserable existence and a hope for a better afterlife. This society has also remained loyal to the extended family, where the father or the oldest son holds absolute power for decision making.

Thus, the majority of North African immigrants to France and their children are poor and uneducated peasants who lack the experience of urban living and have a strong commitment to Islamic religious practices and the extended family. Most North African immigrants are concentrated in the largest French cities of Paris, Lyon, and Marseilles, and thus have to deal with an urban, secular, and individualistic society. These immigrants are often secluded in ghettolike communities with high unemployment rates among the young and are often exposed to police repression, leading to sporadic outbursts of violence.

Cultural differences may create fewer problems in a multicultural society where the values of ethnic groups could be preserved and respected. However, with the French immigration policy of assimilation, cultural differences between North Africans and the native French population have become a source of constant conflict. For example, in 1989, the French ministry of education supported the dismissal of Muslim girls from school because they were wearing head scarves. Since the head scarf is part of the cultural identity of Muslims, the French legislation against it has deprived a large proportion of citizens of the right to be different. The exclusion of Muslim female students who wear the head scarf from public school has sharpened the division between Muslims and the rest of the population. The rebirth of a strong national right-wing movement in France and the support of some Algerians in France of the Islamic fundamentalists have intensified tension between North Africans and the French population. A recent opinion poll (Tinco, 1994) reveals that the French tend to identify Islam with fanaticism, submissiveness, and rejection of Western values. On the other hand, Muslims in France consider Islam as the religion of democracy, justice, and liberty. In the same opinion poll, the young, the educated, and recent immigrants among Muslims expressed worry about their ethnic identity.

France provides an excellent example of the failure of assimilation when there are wide cultural and ethnic differences between immigrants and the host culture. Typical responses of North Africans during recent interviews are the following:

> Anyway, it is difficult to be completely integrated, people will never consider you as their equal. (Stein et al., 1995, p. 23)

> Integration. I am fed up with talking about integration. I arrived here at the age of 3. I studied child care at the university. I live and work here. My family and my friends are here. Explain to me how I can be integrated any more. It is not integration that one should talk about. It is acceptance. Acceptance by others is when they stop blaming us for our name, our skin and our face, and stop confining us in rotten neighbourhoods far from everybody else. When people become less racist, things will get better. (Backmann & Aichoune, 1994, p. 4)

North Africans in France are not only reacted to as French by the native population, but they are also considered as Arabs, Muslims, Algerians, Beurs (North Africans born in France), and Harkis (children of North African army veterans), as well as pejoratively called *bicots* (little goats) and *ratons* (little rats). As Stein et al. (1995) pointed out, these multiple identities are too much for one person to bear. The stereotype of North Africans as fanatics seems incompatible with the finding that three quarters of Muslims in France do not object to a member of their family having a non-Muslim spouse (Tinco, 1994). Many North Africans in France do not define themselves as Muslims, yet they are perceived as such by French society (Solé, 1994).

Those with North African racial traits have to face strong prejudices as well as frequent police harassment. A study of a sample of 128 young French Muslims, between ages 16 and 25, has shown that their psychological problems as well as their experience of rejection by the native French white society was associated with the color of their skin (Bouneb, 1985). In a survey reported by

Amar and Milza (1990), 55% of a national sample considered the Algerians as the most difficult nationality to integrate into French society.

NORTH AFRICAN CONCEPTS OF MENTAL ILLNESS AND TREATMENT

North Africans use the Arabic word *ginoon* for madness, which is derived from *ginn* (demons). The patients are considered to be possessed (*maskoon*) by supernatural beings that may control their behavior, thoughts, and desires. Thus, the causes of madness are regarded as exterior to the person and often considered as a result of persecution and sorcery. Although the symptoms of mental illness are believed to be caused by possession, precipitating factors are intimately linked with social relationships and the position of the individual in society. Consider, for example, *tankir* (denial), which explains indifference to one's social environment such as social withdrawal or loss of interest in the social environment. This state is induced by a witch and may be used by a woman to regain the lost love of a man, or by a parent to bring back a son who left the extended family to live separately with his wife, or by a wife to reduce the influence of the husband's family on the daily life of the couple. The evil eye, another precipitating factor, is considered a means of sanction against anybody who exceeds the limits put by the community on positive attributes such as wealth, health, beauty, and happiness. It is often motivated by envy, jealousy, or even admiration by an enemy or a friend.

There are three traditional therapists in North Africa: the taleb, the marabout, and the clairvoyant. The taleb functions both as a religious teacher and a healer, and his practices are more related to Muslim religion than that of other healers. In therapy, he may recite phrases from the Koran or give the patient an amulet (*herz*) to carry around or may soak a paper with religious writings in water for the patient to drink. The marabout is more like the sorcerer in black Africa and is regarded as a saint, an exorcist, and a healer. Exorcism consists of conversing with the evil spirit through the patient, using appeal or threat by repeating a religious–magical formula, burning incense, or offering a sacrifice such as a black cock. Beating the patient with a stick may be the last resort to get rid of the evil spirit. The North African countryside is dotted with shrines of marabouts that are visited by patients, honoring him with offerings and food festivities (Zerda or Casaa). During the shrine visit a descendant of the marabout may carry out a therapeutic session (Hadra), which includes exorcism. Finally, the practices of the clairvoyant are more regarded as related to magic than to Muslim religion. He is particularly specialized in dealing with sexual and emotional problems such as impotence, frigidity, sterility, and contraception. In addition to these three traditional therapists, the patient may contact any imam in a neighborhood mosque for help (the imam is the equivalent of a Christian priest).

PSYCHIATRIC DISORDERS

One problem faced by clinicians is whether the French diagnostic system should be applied to North African immigrants (Ey, Bernard, & Brisset, 1973). One difficulty is that in general the clinical picture of North African patients tends to change throughout the course of the illness, with no stable pattern to conform to French nosology (Benadiba, Adjedj, Horber, & Sichel, 1980). "Delusions" and "hallucinations" may simply be an exaggeration of normal cultural tendencies in the general population rather than related to mental illness. For example, it has been observed that the most frequent mechanisms used in health and illness by the general population in North Africa are flight into fantasy and imagination, external attribution, and the experience of morbid jealousy and hostility. The delusion of persecution of North African immigrants in France may thus be a "normal" response precipitated by prejudice and discrimination (Al-Issa, 1990). Similarly, the belief in spirits (*ginn*) among North Africans makes the distinction between hallucinations and culturally sanctioned visions quite difficult (Al-Issa, 1995).

Depression

Somatic symptoms tend to dominate the manifestation of depression among North African patients. For example, the "hypochondriacal" depression described by Chauvot, Pascalis, and Champanier (1981) accounts for one third of the psychiatric diagnoses of North Africans. Various types of pain complaints are characteristic of this syndrome. The episode often follows a work accident and requires a long absence from work. Similar episodes may also occur to the same patient many years later without any apparent maladaption in the patient's occupational or social functioning. However, such a situation could sometimes easily lead to repeated claims for disability pension, making the prospect of returning to work rather grim. The illness behavior involved in this type of depression is usually labeled *sinistrose* by French clinicians.

The provision of a pension and the possibility of retiring back in Algeria can lead to the remission from hypochondriacal depression. For North African immigrants, work accidents are an acceptable way to leave a stressful occupation and yet maintain one's status in the family and the clan in the home country (Chauvot et al., 1981). The predominance of somatic symptoms in depression among North African immigrants is also reported by North African psychiatrists (Boucebci, 1985; Bensmail, Bentorki, & Touari, 1981). In contrast, the mood of sadness is either minor or not verbalized by these patients (Boucebci, 1985; Marie-Cardine, 1981).

Marie-Cardine (1981) reported three groups of depressive patients among North Africans in France. One group is characterized by psychomotor inhibition: "my body is heavy, it cannot move anymore." This type of depression is dominated by physical symptoms that appear after a work accident and are quite similar to the hypochondriacal depression described by Chauvot et al. (1981). The syndrome is pejoratively labeled as the "Mediterranean syndrome" by French psychiatrists. It tends to have a good prognosis.

A second group of depressed patients expresses object loss: "my soul remains with my parents; I am like a dog that had lost its owner; my mind remains there, at home." The syndrome is seen among acculturated North Africans who have been living in France for a long period of time. This depression is usually precipitated by an accident at work or a current illness. The patients find it difficult to resume their work and end up in a psychiatric hospital. They stop eating and become withdrawn and disoriented. These features are quite similar to those seen in autistic withdrawal or melancholic stupors. Whenever the patients are induced to communicate with the psychiatrist, they indicate that part of themselves remains in their home country. This clinical picture often resists medical treatment. Patients are sometimes reacting to real bereavement or to a negative life event in the family or may be simply grieving the loss of their culture.

Finally, the third group expresses affect associated with possession by the spirits, *ginn*, which are controlling their body, or by the devil, driving the spirit out of the body. The illness takes the form of *bouffées délirantes*, with an acute and expressive onset. The clinical picture is related to possession and animistic beliefs that are widespread among disadvantaged lower social class North Africans in France. Contacts with a marabout, the North African native healer, tend to bring a relief of symptoms.

A type of depression among North African immigrants that is similar to *bouffée délirante* and is characterized by paranoid delusions is also reported by Papeta, Junod, Ballereau, and Moutet (1990). This is similar to "delusional depression," a subtype of depression diagnosed in North Africa (Douki, Moussaoui, & Kacha, 1987). Delusional depression is characterized by delusions of persecution, bewitchment, and possession and poisoning, sometimes associated with aggressive behavior. It is often confused with *bouffées délirantes* and schizophrenia, but it tends to respond to antidepressives rather than to neuroleptics (Al-Issa, 1990). The presence of delusions of persecution in depression is found not only among North African depressive patients in France and North Africa but also in other Arab countries (Bazzoui, 1970; El-Islam, Moussa, Malasi, Suleiman, & Mirza, 1988). This suggests that there may be a general tendency to respond to stressors by developing delusions of persecution, which are triggered by racial prejudice and discrimination in France.

Suicide and Attempted Suicide

Similar to traditional North African society (Al-Issa, 1990), suicide is very rare among recent North African immigrants and tends to occur only among those with psychiatric illness such as depression (Chauvot et al., 1981). However, suicidal behavior as a means of communication with the environment is seen among immigrants who have been in the country for a long period and are assimilated into French society. Attempted suicide is most prevalent among second-generation adolescent girls. Entrapment and confinement to the home are suggested as a factor underlying the high rate of attempted suicide among girls. In many cases, young North African girls come to France to live with their fathers, leaving their mothers in the home country. They are expected to do the housework as well as work outside the home. They are also exposed to conflicts between European values and the rigid, conservative values of their fathers. Another stressor associated with suicidal behavior among girls is simply to avoid a marriage arranged by the father. In contrast to girls, boys tend to react to stressors by showing academic failure, drug abuse, and delinquent behavior (Chauvot et al., 1981; Moussaoui & Sayeh, 1982). The patriarchal structure of the North African family where the father or the oldest son holds absolute power in decision making may contribute to the high rate of attempted suicide among acculturated North African adolescents in France as well as among Westernized youth in urban settings in their countries of origin (Al-Issa, 1990).

Psychoses

More is written on major depression than psychosis in North Africans in France (Chauvot et al., 1981). Psychosis tends to manifest itself predominantly in the form of acute *bouffée délirante*, paranoia, or acute schizophrenia. Psychosis tends to be polymorphous and unstable at first, and thus more difficult to label and integrate within Western nosology. The contents of symptoms are related to possession by the *ginn* and the belief that the body is impure or being attacked or dismantled. These symptoms are often accompanied by delusions of persecution with or without hallucinations. Traditional themes of psychosis tend to be more predominant among first-generation immigrants than second- or third-generation immigrants, who manifest the typical symptoms of psychosis. In general, fear of racism is more intensely expressed in the symptoms of North African patients than other ethnic groups (Chauvot et al., 1981).

Bouffée délirante is one of the most frequent psychotic reactions among immigrants from North Africa and black Africa (Johnson-Sabine et al., 1983). It is characterized by a sudden onset with vivid hallucinations, delusions, clouding of consciousness, and rapid mood swings. Among North Africans, the themes of delusions are related to religion (prophetic inspiration, divine revelation, messianic conviction, end of the world, and resurrection), sexuality, jealousy, poisoning, forced marriage, sexual abuse, and incest. One type of *bouffée délirante* specific to North African women is nuptial psychosis, which happens after the wedding night as a result of stresses involved in arranged marriage and usually is experienced by the bride (Pfeiffer, 1982). The Anglo-Saxon classification of mental illness has no category that is equivalent to *bouffée délirante*, but its symptoms are similar to brief psychotic disorder or schizophreniform disorder in the *Diagnostic and Statistical Manual of Mental Disorders*, 4th edition (American Psychiatric Association, 1994).

Other Psychological Disorders

Based on previous surveys, Ahami (1991) suggested that psychophysiological disorders are more prevalent among North African immigrants than French subjects, particularly after the first year at work. Analyzing a series of 30 hospitalized cases, suffering mostly from asthma and peptic ulcer, he attributed the illness to a burnout consequent to long working hours without personal involvement in the job. Using a control group of North African migrants, he found that most of the hospitalized sample (28 of 30) reported a need for affection as compared with the control group (6 of 30). Other large differences from the control group were lack of peer socialization and family care during childhood. The social life of the patients was almost nonexistent: none reported going out for entertainment and only two had regular contact with friends, with the remaining 28 patients complaining of loneliness. Ahami (1991) also pointed out that the patients had no dream life and the absence of fantasy was compensated for by the rigid ritualization of their religious life.

Traumatic neurosis, a diagnosis similar to posttraumatic stress disorder, was reported to have a high incidence in the migrant population. In a study of 95 clinical cases in which 75% were of North African origin, the symptomatology was characterized by reenacting of the trauma, repetitive requests for medical attention, rumination, depressive affect, lack of interest in the social environment, and loss of sexual desire (Biznar, 1991). This disorder was also accompanied by gastrointestinal disturbances, anxiety reaction, and *délire de revendication* (a delusion with a sense of entitlement to claims). Most of these migrant patients were men (85%). Unlike the burnout type of reaction described earlier by Ahami (1991) among patients with psychophysiological disorders, in a majority of cases, traumatic neurosis starts 10 to 15 years after arrival to France. Most of these patients described by Biznar (1991) had suddenly stopped work and were either self-declared sick or given a diagnosis by a physician, even though they had been functioning normally at work. Nearly half (46%) of their episodes were provoked by surgery and another 30% by work accidents. Many of the patients had very recently experienced a loss of a family member (a parent or a child) or had a newly born child. As many as 60% had lost a parent through death before the age of 10. Biznar (1991) attributed the cause of the traumatic state to a delayed culture shock. North African immigrants, because of isolation from the dominant culture, may rely more on the family for social support and the definition of the self, and thus are more vulnerable to the effects of a family loss. For these patients, the birth of a child is also an additional stressor because of the absence of the support of the extended family and the difficulty of transmitting their culture in a foreign environment.

Sexual disorders, especially impotence among males, is a recurrent theme of many clinical reports (Benadiba et al., 1980). Sexuality is considered as an expression of life in this culture since a large number of children in the family is highly valued. According to Ben Jelloun (1977), the Moroccan novelist, the concept of the self (*nafs*) in North Africa refers to life, which is located in the heart and expressed through sexuality.

A large number of North African immigrants are married men who left their families in the home country. The mental status of children in the families left behind was studied by Boucebci (1981) who found that Algerian families of migrant fathers working in France tend to have a high risk of mental illness. This is particularly true of the oldest son who replaces the father in taking responsibility for the family and tends to have the highest risk for psychosis and other psychiatric disorders. A study of Moroccan children reported by Charbit and Bertrand (1985) reveals more enuresis, sleep problems, and aggressive behavior among children whose fathers work in France.

Although anorexia nervosa is very rare in North Africa, a case of a North African girl was reported in France by Chazot, Lang, and Pellet (1989). Nora was hospitalized at age 19 with a history of anorexia nervosa since age 15. She comes from a relatively acculturated family that still keeps some of the Muslim tradition. The illness started during the fasting month of Ramadan in which Muslims abstain from taking food and drink from dawn to sunset. In this case, the disturbance may be considered as an exaggeration of the Muslim rule of fasting in a prosperous environment where food is plentiful.

PSYCHOTHERAPY WITH NORTH AFRICAN PATIENTS

There have been some attempts in France to take into consideration the cultural background of North African patients during therapy. One example is the ethnopsychoanalysis of Tobie Nathan, a consultant in ethnopsychiatry in Paris (Nathan, 1988, 1994). In the treatment of ethnic groups and immigrants he replaces individual analysis with a group of co-therapists from different ethnic backgrounds to participate in the therapy. A co-therapist from the cultural background of the patient uses the patient's mother tongue, which is conducive to better understanding. During therapy, Nathan attempts to re-create the village atmosphere in the traditional society of the patient where all members of the group become involved in the patient's problems. Members of the patient's family also become involved in the patient's treatment. The presence of the co-therapists as well as the participation of the patient's family reduces the tendency of patients to perceive the threat of sexual abuse or bewitchment seen in individual psychotherapy of North African patients. Traditional beliefs in the *jinns*, the evil eye, and sorcery are also used by the co-therapists in their interpretation of the symptoms of patients.

Unfortunately, ethnoanalysis also attempts to impose psychoanalytical interpretations on the cultural beliefs and customs of patients and ignores the influence of socioeconomic status and cultural conflicts of patients in French society. We give as an example the case of Zahra, a 22-year-old daughter of a lower-class Algerian worker, to illustrate the working of ethnoanalysis in contrast to native healing (Pierre, 1993).

Zahra contacted the ethnoanalysis clinic with the complaint that she was seeing flashes of a camera with a man taking her picture as if she were a prostitute. She reported the delusion that the psychiatrist she saw previously knew everything about her and even read her thoughts. She also reported a dream during one therapeutic session: While she was in a garden, she escaped from some unknown danger by hiding herself in a pumpkin. In the traditional North African rural society, a pumpkin is not only used for food but also for churning milk: a small opening is made and the milk is poured through it and churned by a pestle (mothers also tend to rock their babies while churning the milk). The ethnoanalyst interpreted the pumpkin in Zahra's dream as representing the mother's stomach ready to receive the male semen and to bear babies. Such interpretation ignores the family and social conflicts that may be the source of the problems of this young Algerian girl.

One conflict Zahra had with her father was that she could not participate in sports in school. The ethnoanalyst was aware of the belief that exercise and other physical activities are forbidden for North African girls because they may interfere with their virginity. Sports are conceived by the ethnoanalyst as symbolic of masturbatory practices. For Zahra's father, sports do not exist in the rural Algerian environment and they may represent to him strange and unfamiliar practices with no symbolic connotations.

There is no cooperation between therapists and native healers in France. However, on the insistence of her parents, Zahra went to see an imam who dealt directly with the contents of her vision: "If the man in your vision asks you to marry him, you should say no. Surely he intended to ask you to marry him since he was tapping his feet on the ground as if he were taking a marriage photo. You are stronger than him since you can escape from him by lowering your head when he tries to take your photo." The imam also told her that she became sick because she walked in dirty water. Since it is believed by Algerians that dirty water is a preferred location for the *jinn*, the implication is that the man of her vision is a *jinn* and the imam himself can deal with him. In contrast to ethnoanalysis, only a few consultations with the imam were needed for the disappearance of the patient's visions.

SUMMARY AND CONCLUSION

North African immigrants in France are predominantly uneducated peasants who have to deal with and adapt to an urban European life. Added to culture shock is their exposure to the French government policy of assimilation into French society on the one hand and social exclusion and rejection by French society on the other. Young North African children are torn between a patriarchal traditional Muslim home environment and the French secular school system. Clinical research reveals that these stressors take their tolls in delinquency, attempted suicide, and drug abuse among the young and in depression among adults. Symptoms of depression as well as the prevalence of delusions among patients seem to be related to the immigration experience of this minority group. Psychotherapeutic intervention with immigrants in France is influenced by psychoanalytical theory with a tendency for using psychoanalytical interpretations to understand the cultural beliefs of immigrants and ethnic groups. There is little cooperation between psychiatrists and native healers in the treatment of mental illness.

REFERENCES

Ahami, A. T. (1991). Facteurs et situations impliqués dans l'apparition des désordres psychosomatiques chez les malades nord-africains en France [Factors and situations related to the onset of psychosomatic disorders in North Africans in France]. *Annales Médico-Psychologiques, 149*(7), 573–580.

Al-Issa, I. (1990). Culture and mental illness in Algeria. *The International Journal of Social Psychiatry, 36*, 230–240.

Al-Issa, I. (1995). The illusion of reality or the reality of illusion: Hallucinations and culture. *British Journal of Psychiatry, 94*, 368–373.

Amar, M., & Milza, P. (1990). *L'immigration en France au XXe siècle* [Immigration in France in the twentieth century]. Paris: Armand Collin.

American Psychiatric Association. (1994). *Diagnostic and statistical manual of mental disorders* (4th ed.). Washington, DC: Author.

Backmann, R., & Aichoune, F. (1994). Violence urbaine: La cote d'alerte. *Le Nouvel Observateur, No. 1568*, 4–8.

Bazzoui, W. (1970). Affective disorders in Iraq. *British Journal of Psychiatry, 117*, 195–203.

Benadiba, M., Adjedj, J. P., Horber, M., & Sichel, J. P. (1980). Quelques problèmes particuliers posés par la pathologie mentale des transplantés Nord-Africains [On some special problems raised by the mental pathology of transplanted North Africans]. *Annales Médico-Psychologiques, 140*(6), 588–592.

Ben Jelloun, T. (1977). *La plus haute des solitudes* [The greatest of solitudes]. Paris: Editions du Seuil.

Bensmail, B., Bentorki, H., & Touari, M. (1981). La depression en Algérie: Aspects culturels et evolution epidémiologique. *Psychiatrie Francophone, 0-4e trimestre*, 10–19.

Biznar, K. (1991). Les névroses traumatiques des migrants: Une quête compulsive de sens. Résultats d'un recherche systématique sur 95 cas cliniques [Traumatic neuroses of immigrants: A comprehensive survey. Results of systematic research on 95 clinical cases]. *Psychologie Française, 36*(4), 341–350.

Boucebci, M. (1981, June–July). Santé mentale du fils de migrant. *Compte rendu du Congrès de Psychiatrie et de Neurologie de Langue Française, LXXXIX Session.* Colmar, France.

Boucebci, M. (1985, May). Le handicap mental: Aspects épidémiologiques de prise en charge et preventifs en Algérie. *Compte rendu de Congrès Medical Meghrébin,* Monastir, Tunisia.

Bouneb, K. D. (1985). Adaptation et identité culturelle des jeune Français Musulmans. *Cahiers d'Anthropologie et Biométrie Humaine, 3,* 1–21.

Camus, A. (1962). *Actuelles III chroniques Algériennes 1939–1958.* Paris: Gallimard.

Charbit, Y., & Bertrand, C. (1985). *Enfants, familles, migrations dans le bassin méditeranéen* [Children, families, migrations in the Mediterranean region], Institut National d'Études Démographiques. Paris: Presses Universitaires de France.

Chauvot, B., Pascalis, G., & Champanier, J. P. (1981). Psychopathologie du migrant adulte et jeune dans la région de Reims [Psychopathology of adult and young migrants in the Reims region]. *Psychologie Médicale, 13*(11), 1801–1803.

Chazot, L., Lang, F., & Pellet, J. (1989). Réflexions sur un cas d'anorexie mentale: Nohra. *Psychologie Médicale, 21*(2), 193–197.

Douki, A., Moussaoui, D., & Kacha, F. (1987). *Manuel de psychiatrie du praticien Maghrébin.* Paris: Masson.

El-Islam, M. F., Moussa, M. A. A., Malasi, T. H., Suleiman, M. A., & Mirza, I. A. (1988). Assessment of depression in Kuwait by principal component analysis. *Journal of Affective Disorders, 14,* 109–114.

Ey, H., Bernard, P., & Brisset, C. L. (1973). *Manuel de Psychiatrie* (5th ed.). Paris: Masson.

Johnson-Sabine, E. C., Mann, A. H., Jacoby, R. J., Wood, K. H., Peron-Magnan, P., Olie, J. P., & Deniker, P. (1983). Bouffée délirante: An examination of its current status. *Psychological Medicine, 13,* 771–778.

Marie-Cardine, M. (1981). La relation médecin-malade entre psychiatre et maghrébin migrant. *Psychologie Médicale, 13,* 1709–1713.

Moussaoui, D., & Sayeh, A. (1982). Les enfants de migrants ou l'impossible identité [Migrant children or the impossible identity]. *Annales Médico-Psychologiques, 140*(6), 588–592.

Nathan, T. (1988). *Le sperme du diable.* Paris: P.U.F.

Nathan, T. (1994). *L'influence qui guérit.* Paris: O. Jacob.

Papeta, D., Junod, A., Ballereau, J., & Moutet, H. P. (1990). Antidépresseurs. Manifestations psychotiques aiguës et transculture [Antidepressant drugs, acute psychotic manifestations and transculture]. *Psychologie Médicale, 22*(4), 330–332.

Pfeiffer, W. M. (1982). Culture-bound syndromes. In I. Al-Issa (Ed.), *Culture and psychopathology* (pp. 201–218). Baltimore, MD: University Park Press.

Pierre D. (1993). Approche psychothérapeutique de patients migrants de première ou deuxième génération: Apports de l'ethnopsychoanalyse de Tobie Nathan. *Acta Psychiatrica Belgica, 93,* 97–117.

Solé, R. (1994, October 20). La France et l'Islam: Si proche et si loin. *Le Monde: Sélection Hebdomadaire,* p. 1.

Stein, S., Kerchouche, D., Pasquire, S., & Amine, N. (1995). Les leurs venues d'Alger. *L'Express, 2312,* 22–24.

Tinco, A. (1994, October 20). Une religion mal aimée, des fidèles mieux intégrés. *Le Monde. Selection Hebdomadaire,* p. 1.

10

Turkish Immigrants in Belgium

A. GAILLY

This chapter deals with the health and medical needs of Turkish immigrants in Belgium. The Turkish migration to Belgium and their social organization and living conditions in Belgium are first described, with special attention given to first- and second-generation immigrants. The second part of the chapter deals with the health problems and the ethnopsychiatry of Turks in Belgium and with the results of our research on somatoform disorders.

TURKISH IMMIGRATION TO BELGIUM

Turkish immigration in Belgium started in the 1960s. Three types of immigration can be distinguished: immigration as a result of recruitment by the Belgian government, the immigration of "tourists," and the arrival of political refugees. The first type of immigration was organized by an international agreement between Turkey and Belgium and was due to economic factors. Turkish immigrants, mostly from eastern Turkey and the Black Sea region, were welcomed in Belgium as guest workers. They settled in industrialized areas and were allowed later to bring in their families. As unskilled laborers, they hoped to make a fortune in a short time and then return to Turkey. But things moved more slowly than expected, and a chain of immigration developed over the years.

The phenomenon of the "immigrant as a tourist" started in the 1970s when Turks, mostly from the Afyon area in Turkey, came with a tourist visa to

---

A. GAILLY • Centrum voor Welzijnszorg, E. Delvastraat 35, 1020 Brussels, Belgium.

Ethnicity, Immigration, and Psychopathology, edited by Ihsan Al-Issa and Michel Tousignant. Plenum Press, New York, 1997.

Belgium. Upon arrival they looked for work and tried to legalize their status as laborers. The presence of these tourists created a "black market" labor force so that on two occasions the government had to legalize their status. Once they obtained the status of "guest workers," they could bring in their family. In the 1980s, immigration to Belgium for economic reasons was forbidden by law. The only legal way to take up residence in Belgium was by family reunion (which was only applicable to members of the nuclear family of a guest worker) or by marrying someone who was a Belgian citizen, whether a Turk or not.

Generally, villagers in Turkey do not seem to be very happy with the immigration of tourists. They contend that they obtain almost no profits from this emigration and during summer when emigrants return home for holidays, life becomes very expensive. Moreover, since most tourists were young, the land was no longer being worked and older people were left behind in poorer conditions than before the emigration. Manifest conflicts in the family and the village or with the government are more related to the emigration of tourists than guest workers, whose emigration is related to poverty and attempts to provide for the family.

Another possible motive for coming to Belgium is to apply for the status of an asylum-seeker upon arrival. After a judicial inquiry the status of a political refugee can be obtained and the refugee is allowed to stay in the country. When the application is rejected, the asylum seeker is supposed to be sent back to his country. Since this entails legal as well as practical problems, many remain as "illegals" in Belgium. Turkish asylum seekers come from all over Turkey, with some belonging to minority groups in the country (Kurds, Armenians, etc.). Other asylum seekers are Turkish minority groups in Eastern Europe (Bulgaria and Macedonia). Asylum seekers and political refugees are not considered to be immigrants. Therefore, the mental health problems of and the therapy with refugees are dealt with elsewhere (Gailly, in press; Leman & Gailly, 1991; Westermeyer, 1989).

TURKS IN BELGIUM

The 90,000 Turkish immigrants constitute an important group in Belgian society that is socioeconomically much more homogeneous than the host society. Most immigrants come from rural, underdeveloped areas where they had little contact with the Western urbanized Turkish culture. By Belgian standards, most of them belong to the lower socioeconomic class.

Most of the Turkish immigrants are settled in the Flemish region, while only 25% in the Walloon region and in the Brussels-Capital region (Table 1). They are concentrated mostly in the poor quarters of the cities. The proportion of the Turks in the cities seldom exceeds 3% of the total city population (except for Limburg, with its defunct mining industry where the proportion for some

Table 1. Belgian and Turkish Population in Belgium and in the Three Regions, January 1994[a]

	Belgium		Flemish region		Walloon region		Brussels–Capital region	
	N	%	*N*	%	*N*	%	*N*	%
Belgians	9,538,249	90.9	5,565,885	95.2	2,946,353	89.2	667,825	70.4
Non-Belgians	920,568	9.1	281,137	4.8	358,186	10.8	281,245	29.6
Turks	88,302	0.9	44,602	0.8	21,872	0.7	21,828	2.3
Total	10,458,817	100.0	5,847,022	100.0	3,304,539	100.0	949,070	100.0

[a]From the National Institute for Statistics, January 1, 1994.

cities is about 7%). Turks from the same region in Turkey also tend to congregate not only in the same city but also in the same quarters. In this situation, Turks organize their social life according to the traditional notions of *memleket* (native land) and *hemşeri* (fellow countrymen), separated by urban boundaries such as a square, an avenue, a railroad, or a river. This implies that Turks from the same region in Turkey frequent only the shops in their neighborhood and have little or no contact with Turks from another *memleket.* This segregation enhances the reciprocal mistaken ideas between the *hemşeri* of different *memleket* and hinders the development of a sense of political and social community.

The Turks are a highly visible group in Belgian cities. They determine the character of their neighborhood by the way they dress and organize or use public space, by their shops, and by the way they decorate their homes. The schools are populated with Turkish children who spend most of daily life in the streets. One could say that Turkish traditional village life goes on, but it has been transplanted into a totally different context (Gailly, 1991a; Manço & Manço, 1992).

Most of the Turks in Belgium are Muslims and have had only a few years of formal education, generally primary school, in Turkey. If employed in Belgium, they work as unskilled laborers in the agricultural and industrial sectors and in construction. Due to the economic recession, however, many are trying to improve their social position by becoming self-employed.

Turkish women, on the other hand, usually stay home as housewives. This means that their participation in Belgian society is indirect and restricted to the family at home. Men and children participate in Belgian society through their job or school attendance. At present, however, women are beginning to look more for jobs (cleaning, for example) because of the unemployment of their husbands.

About 1500 Turks are shopkeepers (most being grocers), barbers, or café owners. Others run import–export shops (gifts, carpets, textiles, or electronic equipment), *döner kebab* snackbars, or insurance or travel agencies. Some Turks are doctors in general practice and others are lawyers. There are also about 25 Turkish enterprises that employ 20 or more Turkish workers. Most of the Turkish shopkeepers were born in Turkey (first-generation immigrants) and arrived in Belgium in the 1970s. They have had more years of formal education than the average immigrant (about 50% of them had graduated from high school). Generally, Turkish shops are very cheap in order to attract Belgian customers, which makes competition very keen. Because profits are low and the shopkeepers usually lack the skills needed to run a shop, many go bankrupt and the shops change owners very often.

Due to the economic recession, participation in Belgian society is decreasing and the Turkish society is becoming more and more self-contained. Within the Turkish community, there is a religious revival (Koran schools and religious organizations centered around mosques), and many Turkish independent organizations (sociocultural clubs, sport clubs, etc.) are being founded. Although these organizations focus on the Turkish community, some also develop intercultural activities. Lack of participation in Belgian society enhances the ethnic feelings of belongingness. Turkish immigrants try to preserve their own culture, and social control is very strong. The cultural tradition and religion they claim and use as an ethnic marker, however, differ a great deal from what can be found in their home villages.

Nevertheless, the Turkish immigrants want to acquire a maximum of Western products and material culture. Indeed, the material and technical culture was the major reason for immigration: social security, health care, machinery, luxury goods, and participation in the high-tech society. Turkey, however, remains the most important frame of reference for Turkish immigrants and for their children (second generation) and grandchildren (third generation). They build their dream houses in the almost-deserted villages of their fathers to which they return each year for holidays, and they continue to have their sons circumcised and to marry their children to someone who had been brought up in Turkey. The immigrants continue, subjectively and psychologically, the life and the traditions of their parents. They do not refer to Turkey as it is today but to the country they left behind and as they perceive it from the perspective of an immigrant in Belgium.

Unlike Turks in Turkey, immigrants are not involved in the dynamics of the larger Turkish society, nor do they fully participate in the Belgian society. Immigration generates a new culture. Describing life in this new reality as "living between two cultures," as is often done for children and adolescent immigrants, is misleading because it suggests the existence of a cultural vacuum that could be seen as a transitional stage in a linear evolution from a traditional to a modern culture.

Participation in Belgian society depends largely on the educational opportunities one has. The kind of school one can enter is very important and being successful in school means more than just graduating. It opens the way to a number of social domains in the Turkish and Belgian society, and it can lead to changes in sex role patterns and one's social level. Most Turkish children go to "immigrant" or "black" schools, which are usually of low quality and where most of the pupils are Turkish and Moroccans. Research (Gailly, 1991b; Timmerman, 1992; Phallet, 1993) shows that most of the children in these schools are not really interested in school work. Nevertheless, most Turkish children, especially the girls, like to go to school where they are free of parental authority. Parents are not very interested in higher education, because it would cut their children off from Turkish culture and tradition. This is one reason why most Turkish children enroll in technical and professional schools. In 1993, only 443 Turks were enrolled at the universities and other institutions for higher education (this is only 0.16% of the Belgian and non-Belgian student population at these institutes). Education, then, does not affect the traditional role pattern that parents choose for their children. Girls are expected to become good housewives after their marriage, which will be arranged by their parents. Young girls hope that their future husband will earn enough money so that they can stay at home where they belong.

Low academic and professional aspirations, however, are typical for lower socioeconomic class children in general, regardless of their cultural background. Therefore, it might be that the comparison between Belgian and Turkish migrants idealizes the Western part and omits the discrepancy between an ideal Western culture and the subjective culture of many Western youngsters.

This does not mean that some parents do not encourage their children to study. In the field of sociocultural public life (which has to do with self-fulfillment, motivation to study, and professional aspirations) these children display attitudes and ambitions that are attuned to Western values. In the realm of the family (family structure and intrafamily dynamics), leisure activities, and the private community, the traditional lifestyle and values prevail.

These ambiguities can create serious problems when children marry, for they usually marry a "pure" Turk, someone who has grown up in Turkey. When the partner is educated, he or she comes to Belgium to live with the parents-in-law. He or she does not speak the language, has no job, is controlled by the parents-in-law, and must show gratitude for being able to come to Belgium. When the partner is not educated, problems arise when he or she marries a Belgian Turk who has education. In any event, whatever marriage is arranged, the tradition is maintained.

THE HEALTH AND MEDICAL NEEDS OF TURKISH IMMIGRANTS

In Belgium, there are no nationwide or regional epidemiological studies available on immigrants. Studies about health and medical needs, as well as the immigrants' knowledge and attitude toward health, illness, and care, are limited to private medical practices. Differences in research topics and methodology make it difficult to draw any general conclusions. Most studies deal with Turkish and Moroccan immigrants, and almost no studies are available on other minority groups, political refugees, and asylum seekers.

Studies cover various topics ranging from methodological novelties, health status, preventive behavior, risky habits, primary health care visits, intake of medications, medical views, and conceptions of how the Belgian health system functions. Over the last 10 years, the researchers' attention has moved beyond case reporting and the descriptive work that set out to give a cultural explanation for the way ethnic minorities deal with health problems. The main achievements are methodological development, prenatal care work, subjective and objective health status work, an analysis of the medical needs practice, psychosomatic problems, and assessment of the quality of care.

A survey of the available scientific literature on the health and the medical needs of and the services to immigrants in Flanders and Brussels (Van de Mieroop, Peeters, & De Muynck, 1989; De Muynck & Peeters, 1994) reveals some general hypothetical trends that need further research. Turks and also autochthons define perfect health as "not being ill." Moreover, autochthons as well as Turks regard climate and natural causes such as age as the primary causes of ill health. The burden of ill health, a yardstick for several ailments and lingering complaints, does not appear to differ much between Flemings and Turks but rather between men and women. By and large, Turkish women feel the most unhealthy, while Turkish men feel the most healthy.

On the whole, Turks usually wait longer to see a doctor than autochthons, but with increasing acculturation, allochthons are more apt to go sooner to their doctor. Autochthons are more inclined to have a regular general practioner, whereas Turks are more likely to put their trust in "medical shopping." A possible explanation for medical shopping is communication problems. Turks do not feel that they have understood everything after a consultation with their doctor and think that he or she could prescribe better drugs. This does not reduce the client's concern and undermines trust in the doctor. As a result, the client then wants to consult other doctors. When compared with Turks, autochthons generally use more medication on prescription, demonstrate less patient compliance, use more sleeping pills and sedatives, and practice less self-medication. Furthermore, autochthons make more use of specialist services than do Turks. Referral by the general practitioner to specialists is more likely to occur as a function of the patient's age and sex than ethnic origin.

The perinatal mortality rate among immigrants of Turkish origin (17.7%) is considerably higher than that of the indigenous population (10.7%). This is not attributable to a low birth weight or to a higher incidence of premature births. It is striking, in this respect, that Turkish women exhibit suboptimal prenatal consultation behavior. Abortion is also prevalent among Turkish women, usually as a means of birth control.

With children, problems are found especially with rachitis (rickets) and other diet-related (malnutrition and overfeeding) complaints, caries, and problems surrounding vaccinations and avoidable accidents (especially burns at home). Problems of a more psychosocial and psychological nature are, in particular, anxiety disorders, enuresis, problems at school, and behavioral problems. The latter are often accompanied by relational problems between the parents. With adolescents, too, there are problems as a result of avoidable accidents (especially road accidents) and the prevalence of fugues (periods of memory loss). There are some indications of an increasing prevalence of schizophrenia and other psychotic disorders among Turkish adolescents. This is explained by the fact that the Turkish community becomes more self-contained, which would entail more oppressive socialization practices. There is still too little systematic data available about lifestyle and habits of life and about awareness and behavior with regard to sexuality, particularly among young people. The same exists for the problem of risky behavior, such as attitudes toward and the use of drugs for adult males, alcohol (leading to dipsomania), compulsive gambling, and the peddling of drugs. Attention should also be drawn to the fact that second-generation junkies (i.e., youngsters on heroin) belong to the underclass (i.e., the underprivileged); they have problems in several areas but chiefly in finding work and accommodation and in running afoul of the law. Discriminatory social and environmental factors make immigrants more of a high-risk group for drug abuse. In the case of adult males, alcoholism and compulsive gambling often lead to relational and other problems.

As a rule, the overall complaint pattern and diagnostic profile of adult autochthons, Turks, and Moroccans does not vary, apart from a few exceptions. Turks are slightly more inclined to seek medical advice for infections and problems with the digestive system, tuberculosis, diabetes, and diet-related disorders (obesity, hypertension) but less inclined for mental disorders. Turkish women suffer from chronic health complaints (somatoform disorders).

For elderly Turks, the profile of health and ill health behavior still has to be determined. The population of elderly Turks in Belgium is very small. In 1991, the proportion of Turks within the age group 45–64 of Belgians and non-Belgians was only 0.4% and in the age group 65+ only 0.02%. Therefore, little is known about the specific problems that aging Turkish immigrants might present in the future. Some trends, however, are already clear. Migration is not only a process of mobility in space but also in time. Elderly persons live in a culture other than the one they were born into. In this sense, elderly Turks experience double migration, and their problems are those faced by elderly people of whatever ethnic culture combined with the problems of being a foreigner.

This perspective enables us to understand conflicts between young people and parents/grandparents as conflicts between generations. The participants then attribute these conflicts to external factors. Parents in Turkey ascribe the refusal of arranged marriages to the American shows their children watch on television. Parents say that their children are affected by Belgian society.

Most Turks, whenever they came to Belgium, still nurture the dream of "going back to Turkey." Children and grandchildren who do not want to return may be the cause of one-parent families. Retired men realize their dream by spending most of the time in their home village. Women, however, cannot leave their children behind, although they also would like to return to the home country. Leaving their children seems much more difficult than leaving their parental home some 35 years previously.

In the literature frequent mention is made of more psychological disturbances (i.e., mental disorders) among Turks compared with the indigenous population. This cannot be inferred, however, from the level of medical consumption, since immigrants are admitted in even fewer numbers than autochthons to psychiatric hospitals. The Centers for Mental Health also have very few allochthons among their clientele. Nonetheless, the primary care sector complains that they are not able to refer immigrants with psychological problems. In addition, alleged language problems and cultural differences encountered by the care provider but also by the patient can affect the transference and feedback to such an extent that a therapeutic process becomes very difficult if not impossible. So allochthonous clients are looked upon, a priori, as clients that cannot be helped (Leman & Gailly, 1991). In spite of communication and other problems, both public services and individual providers of care, apart from a few exceptions, appear to be little concerned about improving the communication with the allochthonous patients in order to improve the quality of the care provided to them or about involving allochthons in the discussion of the provision of medical care (Peeters, Gailly, & De Muynck, 1994).

THE ETHNOPSYCHIATRY OF TURKISH IMMIGRANTS

When confronted with suffering Turks in Turkey and in Belgium, people rely on scientific, medical, as well as traditional healing systems in order to give meaning to and to get help for diseases. The Turkish ethnopsychiatric causes and healing processes for diseases are presented in Table 2 (Gailly, 1982, 1986).

The classification used in Table 2 is too static, as if there were clearly demarcated and mutually independent systems and subsystems. People do not differentiate between systems and the distinction only facilitates an analytical approach. In the center of Table 2 is the *falcı kadın,* a woman seer who can be consulted, makes a diagnosis, and prescribes a suitable therapy. Such seers do not do therapy and can only be consulted by women who can consult also on behalf of their close male relatives.

Table 2. The Ethnopsychiatric Explanations and Therapies for Illnesses

- Interpretation of illnesses
  - Personalistic explanations
    1. Human beings
       - The evil eye
       - Sorcery
    2. *Cin*
    3. The devil and God
  - Naturalistic explanation
    - Humoral interpretation

Falcı kadın

- Therapies
  - Personalistic system
    1. Prayers and religious texts
    2. *Nazar boncuğu*
    3. Pilgrimage to the tomb of a saint
    4. The *hoca* as mediator
  - Naturalistic system
    - Metaphoric principles

The Naturalistic System

In the Turkish humoral belief, illness is attributed to an influencing of the fine balance between hot–cold and wet–dry that creates a humoral imbalance. A therapy is then devised in which one seeks, by means of a diet, a series of baths, and the like, to restore the humoral balance. Natural and climatic factors, choice of diet, and other objects that are associated metaphorically with the qualities of wet, dry, hot, or cold are not only regarded as causes of diseases but used as healing factors. They are also used as preventive measures on condition that they are monitored and used in the culturally prescribed manner. For this reason Turks go to Turkey in order to restore their body or nourish it with "good water" or "good air."

Turks have great difficulty in recognizing the psychological causes of their illness. They do associate experiences, emotions, "bad" behavior, grief, and the like with illness, but these are only considered as factors that bring about the ultimate cause of the illness, a change in the humoral equilibrium. Thus, psychological factors can only indirectly contribute to the actual cause of the illness (which is localized in the body).

Consequently, expression of emotions and other psychological experiences in somatic forms, the scant use of psychological jargon, and the process of somatization in the above-mentioned sense are not the result of a psychological defense mechanism or a pathological disregard or repression of intrapsychic factors. Somatization is functional because it makes it possible, in case of illness, to set the healing process in motion using physical tools such as baths, diets, and drugs, and the process explains the intensive and extensive use of medical examinations (to "see" the cause of the disease).

But somatization is functional not only because it makes a disease naturalistic but also because it has another social function when compared with magic, bewitchment, or a psychological explanation of the disease. The latter brand other persons as the root cause of the illness and localize the cause of the illness in interpersonal or intrapsychic conflicts. Somatization, on the other hand, pinpoints the cause of the illness as being in nature, away from other people, so that potential interpersonal conflicts are avoided.

Somatization is not only a way of thinking but also a complex, symbolic process in which metonyms, the symbols for etiology, are metaphors for the humoral imbalance, the ultimate cause of the illness. The causes of illness often cited by Turks such as grief, nerves, suspended menstruation, hardening of the arteries, cold, microbes, and so on are metonymic for and therefore syntagmatically related to the causes of illness. The association, however, between these causes of illness and the ultimate cause of the illness—the humoral imbalance—is paradigmatic and metaphorical. In other words, there is a continual transformation and contratransformation of metaphors and metonyms.

The Personalistic System

In a personalistic explanation of a disease one relies on spirits, human beings, and superterrestrial creatures. People can cause misfortune and illness directly, by means of the evil eye, as well as indirectly by means of intermediary objects of magic. Somatoform disorders (hysterical disorders) and mood and anxiety disorders are usually explained in terms of the evil eye or magic.

In order to bring about indirectly someone else's misfortune, one consults a *hoca,* an expert on the Koran, or an elderly woman. Tools to cast the spell are plants, stones, earth, soap, wax, and the like. These can be treated with needles, hair, olive oil, lard (from unclean swine), honey, sugar, or salt. The intermediary objects, the carriers of the magic, are usually bewitched with religious incantations or charmed to ensure that they work and to heighten the effect. Amulets of poisonous seeds or a piece of paper on which a curse is written and which is hidden in a house or hung in a tree can also be used. A spell can also be put on somebody by means of a charmed drink or food.

The evil eye, or *nazar,* is a natural power with which individuals (particularly those with blue or green eyes) can directly injure other people and damage objects by simply staring at them, whether intentionally or not, or by thinking or saying something about them. The main reason given for objects or people being struck by the evil eye is envy.

The *cin* (plural: *cinler*) is a spirit that can make people ill. Born invisible, they are created by Allah, recognized by the Koran, and can take on a vegetable, animal, or human form. They are very mobile and usually aggressive beings that haunt ruins, woods, crags, caves, deserted houses, fireplaces, chimneys, and damp places such as bathhouses and sewers. There are both male and female *cin* and they constitute a reflection of human society; they have their own social order, live in houses, have families, get married, and have children. They can also seduce people and enter into a sexual relationship with them. In their whims or out of revenge they can make things very difficult for people. The existence of *cin* is also an important socialization measure. Children are not allowed to go out alone in the dark and are often made fearful of the punishments and aggression of the *cin*. People can be possessed by a *cin* without reason, but mostly it is a punishment for violating taboos or for the nonobservance of rules surrounding *cin*. Not treating bread with respect, not washing oneself after sexual intercourse, or cursing Allah, a father, or a mother will incur the wrath of a *cin*. Other acts such as urinating, sitting down, or pouring water are preceded by incantations so as not to offend any *cin* and to protect oneself from their vengeance. Anxious people, in particular, and those in an unclean state or in transitional situations (following childbirth or marriage, for example) are vulnerable to *cin* and not infrequently are beaten. Acute mental disorders such as psychotic disorders are often interpreted in terms of *cin*.

A superterrestrial pathogen is the devil (*Şeytan*). Offending the devil can cause major calamities and illness and he can even possess someone. Allah and the other saints can also cause illness. It is then usually a punishment for infringing on religious rules in which it is not necessarily the offender himself but perhaps one of his closest acquaintances who suffers.

For diseases with a personalistic cause, numerous therapies exist that are used in combination or otherwise. First, there is individual prayer, which may be accompanied by sacrifices or pilgrimages to graves of saints or to other places that are credited with supernatural healing power. A prayer is said at the place of pilgrimage. Afterward, the sick person or his companion ties a ribbon of cloth or seamless linen to the place of pilgrimage while expressing his wish. At the same time, a sacrifice has to be made or pledged. Usually a sheep, a goat, or a cock is slaughtered, after which the meat is served.

A sick person can be exorcised, perhaps on the advice of his entourage, by a *hoca* or have a *muska* written for him in which the spoken word as an incantation and the written word can be therapeutic. *Muska* are amulets of extracts from the Koran written on a piece of paper by a *hoca* combined with ritual symbols that are used therapeutically or as a preventive measure against disease, spells, and evil. What kind of *muska* are written and what the sick person should do with them depends on the diagnosis that the *hoca* makes on the basis of the letters from the mother's first name and the patient's first name. *Muska* are usually packed in a metal box and worn on a necklace or under the arm. In order to absorb the curative power of the writing, some muska have to be placed in water so that the ink flows out, after which the sick person drinks for several days from the water or uses it each time he or she washes. Other *muska*, sometimes with herbs, are burnt while the sick person inhales the vapors.

Before a sick person has himself exorcised, he has to undergo the ritual washing. The exorcism itself is done in Arabic and in between the *hoca* blows over the sick person. Sometimes *hocas* also do a laying-on of hands while they knock on the wall. In this connection, the *hoca* acts as a medium through whom the pain flows out into the wall. Another much-used technique is the pouring of molten lead into a bowl of water positioned above the sick person's head. The shape of the solidified lead allows one to determine the identity of the avenged *cin* or to tell someone's fortune. In the case of diseases caused by *cin* or demons, *hocas* can contact the pathogen so as to exorcise the latter from the sick person's body. Certain *hocas* consult the devil in order to discover the cause or the perpetrator of certain negative incidents.

Men, women, and children also protect themselves with all kinds of talismans from the evil eye. The most widely used is a blue bead on which an eye is painted and which is pinned to the cot or the clothes of children. Objects that might arouse envy are usually painted with a hand whose fingers are outstretched and where the palm of the hand, which may have an eye painted on it, is turned to the front (the hand of Fatma).

Diseases caused by magic can be cured by magical counterpractices. Here, too, one can invoke all kinds of religious incantations in order to increase the power of the carriers.

SOMATOFORM DISORDERS

Physical complaints for which there is no diagnosed medical condition are very common among Turkish immigrants in Belgium. Since many care providers interpret these complaints as vague and incomprehensible, we present some of our research findings in this field (Gailly, 1988, 1991b).

We studied the frequency and the significance of the complaints by means of a closed, standardized questionnaire administered orally to a random sample of 244 adult Turks in Antwerp. The study involved a list of 52 complaints (including modes of behavior that are difficult to accept, and so were presented in the form of complaints) encountered in our practice. The questionnaire was presented in Turkish, and the subjects were instructed to respond "yes" or "no" to the question "Do you suffer from ..."

The statistical model chosen for processing the responses had to permit a dynamic interpretation of the results. To this end, we used a structural problem grid (De Boeck, 1986; De Boeck & Rosenberg, 1988), which allowed us to establish a configuration of complaints within which complaints are structured by graded groups. Figure 1 gives the results of the statistical analysis.

Figure 1 indicates that seven groups of complaints were thus divided into three levels, containing distinct groups. The base level consists of three groups. Group 1 contains only one complaint (sore mouth) and can be ignored, since its incidence rate is relatively low. Group 2 contains hitting, dissension, fits, excitation, and the like, and can thus be defined as aggression. Group 3 contains apathy, sore feet, weakness, chest pain, bone pain, muscle aches, heart palpitations, and painful and numb limbs. Thus, it is a matter of somatic complaints that approach a framework of hysteric complaints of the conversion type. The essential characteristic of these complaints consists of a clinical picture in which the predominant disturbance is a loss or an alteration of a physical function. This disturbance, although it suggests a somatic problem, seems to be the expression of a conflict or a psychological need.

The average level also has three groups. Group 4 consists of depressive signs, group 5 consists of backache, and group 6 consists of oppression in the chest (*bunaltı*). The highest level (group 7) consists particularly of backache and the *sıkıntı*, which can be translated as general anxiety.

Some Reflections on the Interpretation of the Results

Depression Is Grafted on Aggression. This fact could indicate that, in the Turkish culture, aggression is expressed by depression and that this form of expression is determined by the culture. Fernando (1969) and Kendell (1970) reported that depression is more frequent in cultures that strongly inhibit aggressive impulses. In the Turkish culture, the inhibition of aggression is exercised essentially toward women. Thus, it would be interesting to study the potential difference between the sexes on this level.

It is also important to note that the aggressiveness is expressed at the moment of an anger fit. A fit of uncontrollable anger permits emotional expression, since the person in crisis cannot be held responsible for his or her acts at the moments. Indeed, among the Turks, only men have the right to show aggressiveness, but women are allowed to be aggressive when they are sick. In other words, the sickness is used to express behavior more relevant to relational problems than the depression itself. Since this syndrome is seen only among Turkish immigrants, we can call it a culture-bound syndrome. Some of the depressive complaints are expressed in somatic symptoms. This is not surprising, since in many cultures, Occidental and otherwise, depression is often somatized (Kleinman & Good, 1985).

The question arises of knowing how many of the subjects examined among the 244 subjects express other complaints that could also be taken into account,

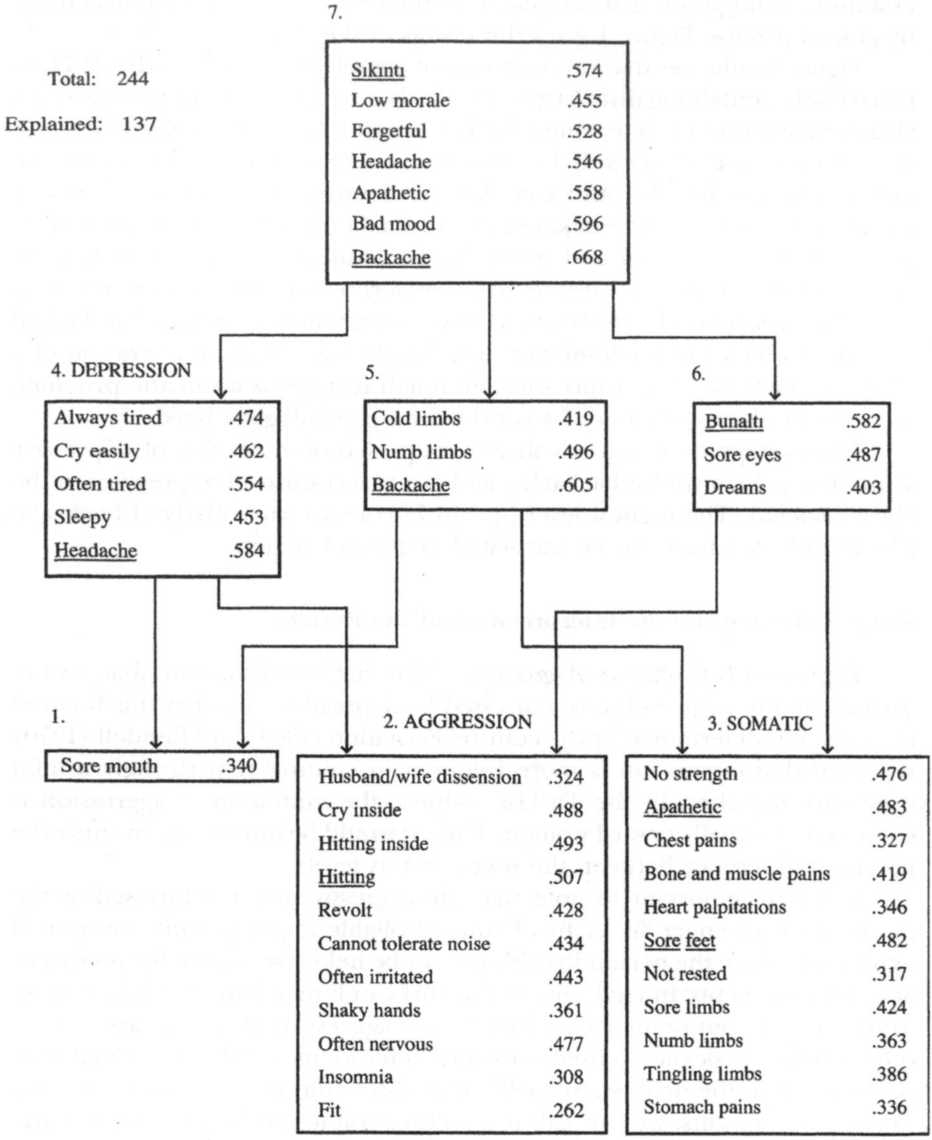

Figure 1. Configuration of somatic complaints. The numbers indicate the relative importance of the complaint within its group. The hierarchical relations between the groups are indicated by arrows.

such as the simple fact of having a cold. Even if the 244 subjects express such complaints, it must be noted that 137 of them situate themselves in this syndrome. It thus accounts for more than 50% of the responses obtained from a nonselected sample.

Extension of the Questionnaire. The first study was limited to research of a configuration of complaints (or of behaviors experienced as such). Another study (Gailly, 1988) was conducted by associating this configuration of complaints with situations related to their complaints, such as the relationship with family members and in-laws, immigration status, living conditions, and so forth. From this study, it must be noted that no complaints were associated with the fact of immigration.

However, somatic complaints of women are usually linked to relational problems with their children and in-laws and especially with their spouse. As a result of the unemployment situation, Turkish men can no longer identify with their work. While they used to be "miners" they are now "Muslims." This means that they no longer can claim an identity in terms of participation in Western society. The result is that they are thrown back on their own society and end up in a vacuum, where the fall is often cushioned by a "fun and games" economy (frequenting public houses, gambling, prostitution, drinking, dating East European women, and so on). Women look upon this kind of husband as a child, as an adolescent with a fool's blood, and as totally incapable. Children also acquire a very negative father image. In the Turkish culture, the public world is seen as the man's space, while in the home the mother represents the positively valued father to the children. However, this situation creates a symbolic absent father figure, and gives rise to an absence of fixed rules and laws. Women have to take on simultaneously the male as well as the female role, which results in a chronic high level of stress.

It can be concluded that immigration cannot be considered as a direct cause of somatoform disorders. It may be considered as an indirect cause since it alters the intrafamily relationships in such a way that they become too stressful and result in somatic complaints.

Extension of the Research to Other Populations. The study in Antwerp concerned a homogeneous Turkish population with a low socioeconomic level. The questionnaire was later administered to a homogeneous Belgian population of the same socioeconomic level. It emerged that socioeconomic differences between the care givers and the care receivers seem to dominate over cultural differences of ethnic origin.

Dobbels (1991), in his comparative study, has shown that no difference exists between Turkish first-generation immigrants and Flemings from the same socioeconomic class with regard to the complaints and the situations associated with them. However, Dobbels did not examine the relationship of the complaints and situations or determine whether the class structure is the same in both populations.

Such a study would be very useful because it would be possible, in combination with a semantic anthropological analysis, to examine cultural differences in meaning of somatic complaints between Turks and Belgians. The semantic approach (Devisch & Gailly, 1985b) considers the processes by which a culture patterns and is patterned by body acts, and thereby shapes the subject in relation to his social and natural world. It studies each human phenomenon as a process that produces meaning in and through action inserted into the social and natural domains (my world as it appears in my world vision).

By focusing on the body, Devisch (1985) is mainly concerned with the phenomenal body, that is, with what a person evokes or expresses in his or her overall, culturally shaped pattern of body acts and physical appearance. The body is regarded as the space within which an individual experiences his or her limitations and from which an individual extends to the outer world by his or her capacity to open to social relationships. The body limits the subject spatially within the bodily surface and temporally between birth and death. It also constitutes the medium of individuation by which the subject inserts him- or herself in the outer world. This twofold function of the body forms the underlying dynamic of a person's universe construction. The body provides the most immediate and tangible frame of reference within which the person constitutes and interprets him- or herself in relation to the social and the natural order. The twofold function of the body shapes both the individual's uniqueness (difference) and likeness (mediation). Hereby the body is experienced as a duality: as limitation and as openness, as a closed space and as a space of exchange. The body actualizes its creative capacities and intertwines the various bodily and sociocultural levels through symbolic relationships of mediating and differentiating within and between the bodily, social, and natural levels. These multidimensional relationships in and through the physical and social bodies are symbolic when they integrate the bodily, social, and natural spheres by linking and separating, by mediation and differentiation. When they are disintegrative, dualistic, or fusional, however, they may be pathological and may give rise to symptoms. Our hypothesis is that a disturbance of mediation on one level, such as penetrating or oppositional relations between spouses or with children, can be expressed somatically via a disturbed bodily mediation function.

We investigated (Gailly, 1985; Devisch & Gailly, 1985a; Gailly & Devisch, 1984) how the symbolic dimension of bodily reaction represents irreducibly the space and the history within which the individual gives meaning to his or her socialized individuation, social belonging, physical or existential well-being, and illness. Thus, a disturbance in the bodily space corresponds to a disturbance in the outer space such as pathological relationships or dualistic and fusional patterns operating between the bodily manifestation and the family-related sociocultural context of the patient. This is not a causal relationship but a semantic one. Attention is given to the way in which the cultural system shapes a relationship between the body in its psychosomatic dimension and the body in its psychosocial dimension. It is within this relationship that the body as a bounded space of organic and sensory functions receives a meaning dimension.

Since a semantic approach does not take into account the intrapsychic dynamics of pathology, we combined the semantic interpretation of the symbolic cultural processes with a psychological interpretation (Gailly, 1988; Gailly, Devisch, & Corveleyn, 1985). From these studies it can be concluded that the psychological and semantic analyses of somatoform disorders corroborate each other.

CONCLUSION

Migration, whether in space or in time, involves a discontinuity, a rupture with the culture of the homeland, or a restructuring of filiation. This is accompanied by a deterioration of operational models so that immigrants have to be creative. The religious and family domains seem very suitable for establishing continuity. This makes the migrants' culture not only different from the culture in their homeland but also makes immigrant groups more self-contained, with little or no participation in the host society. Rigidity of culture hampers the possible interaction between culture and psyche and the ability to think by way of association. Therefore, it should not be surprising that psychotherapy with immigrants is not very efficacious, because Western therapies are based on intrapsychic associative processes. Psychotherapy with immigrants can only start after reactivating their culture of origin or by a process of rerooting.

REFERENCES

De Boeck, P. (1986). Methoden en technieken van onderzoek in de context van therapie [Methods and techniques for research and data analysis in the context of therapy]. In J. W. G. Orlemans, P. Eelen, & W. Harisman (Eds.), *Handboek voor Gedragstherapie* (pp. A-16-1–A-16-38). Deventer: Van Loghum Slaterus.

De Boeck, P., & Rosenberg, S. (1988). Hierarchical classes: Model and data analysis. *Psychometrika, 53*, 361–381.

De Muynck, A., & Peeters, R. F. (1994). Hoe gezond zijn Ali en Fatma? Tien jaar wetenschappelijk onderzoek over gezondheid van en gezondheidszorg voor allochtonen in Vlaanderen (1984–1993). Een kritisch overzicht [How healthy are Ali and Fatma? Ten years of scientific research on health and health care for allochthons in Flanders (1984–1983): A critical review]. Antwerp: Universitaire Instellingen Antwerpen, ESOC-publicatie nr. 33.

Devisch, R. (1985). Symbol and psychosomatic symptom in bodily space–time: The case of the Yaka of Zaïre. *International Journal of Psychology, 20*(4/5), 589–616.

Devisch, R., & Gailly, A. (1985a). Dertleşmek: The sharing of sorrow. A therapeutic self-help group among Turkish women. *Psychiatria e Psicoterapia Analitica, IV*(2), 133–152.

Devisch, R., & Gailly, A. (Eds.). (1985b). Symbol and symptom in bodily space–time. *International Journal of Psychology, 20*(4/5).

Dobbels, P. (1991). Een vergelijking van het klachtenpatroon tussen Turken en Belgen: Een empirische studie op basis van gegevens uit 20 Genkse huisartspraktijken [A comparison of the complaints of Turks and of Belgians: An empirical study based on data from 20 general practices in Genk]. Brussels: Vrije Universiteit.

Fernando, S. (1969). Cultural differences in the hostility of depressed patients. *British Journal of Medical Psychology, 42*, 67–75.

Gailly, A. (1982). Etnogeneeskunde en -psychiatrie bij Turken [Ethnomedicine and ethnopsychiatry among Turks]. *Kultuurleven, 49*, 67–80.

Gailly, A. (1985). Life recedes when exchange fails: Clinical anthropology among Turkish patients. *International Journal of Psychology, 20*, 521–538.

Gailly, A. (1986). Ziekte en gezondheid in Turks kultuursymbolisch perspectief [Sickness and health in a Turkish culture-symbolic perspective]. In *Nationale Vereniging voor Geestelijke Gezondheidszorg* (pp. 79–107). Ghent: Nationale Vereniging voor Geestelijke Gezondheidszorg.

Gailly, A. (1988). Psychische klachten bij Turken en hun benadering [Psychological complaints among Turks and their approach]. Brussels: Cultuur en Migratie.

Gailly, A. (1991a). De gecekondu's en Brusselse Turkse migrantenwijken: Allebei "Arabesk"? [The gecekondus and Brussels Turkish immigrant neighborhoods: Both "arabesque"?] *Opbouwwerk Brussel, 22*, 3–9.

Gailly, A. (1991b). Time perspective of motivational goals of Belgian and Turkish adolescents in Belgium and of Turkish adolescents in Turkey. Paper presented at the IACCP Congress, Liège.

Gailly, A. (in press). Psychopathology of immigrants and across-cultural therapy. In A. Ugalde (Ed.), *International labor migrants.* Houston: University of Texas Press.

Gailly, A., & Devisch, R. (1984). No son for my stifling husband: The "other" in illness. A clinical anthropological study of a Turkish family. *Analytic Psychotherapy and Psychopathology, 1*, 151–163.

Gailly, A., Devisch, R., & Corveleyn, J. (1985). "Etre" aux limites de sa condition: analyses psychodynamique d'un cas de psychose hystérique en milieu Turc immigré en Belgique ["To be" at the limits of one's condition: Psychodynamic analyses of a case of hysterical psychosis in the Turkish immigrant milieu in Belgium]. In E. Jeddi (Ed.), *Psychose, famille et culture* (pp. 356–375). Paris: L'Harmattan.

Kendell, R. (1970). Relationship between apression and depression: Epidemiological implications of a hypothesis. *Archives of General Psychiatry, 22*, 308–318.

Kleinman, A., & Good, B. (Eds.). (1985). *Culture and depression.* Berkeley: University of California Press.

Leman, J., & Gailly, A. (1991). *Thérapies interculturelles* [Intercultural therapies]. Brussels: Editions Universitaires De Boeck.

Manço, A., & Manço, U. (1992). *Turcs de Belgique. Identités et trajectoires d'une minorité* [*Turks in Belgium: Identities and trajectoires of a minority*]. Brussels: Info-Türk.

Phallet, K. (1993). Culturele waarden en persoonlijke keuzen: Groepsloyaliteit en prestatiemotivatie bij Turkse en Belgische jongeren [Cultural values and personal choices: Group loyalty and performance motivation among Turkish and Belgian youth]. Doctoral dissertation, University of Leuven.

Peeters, R., Gailly, A., & De Muynck, A. (1994). De geestelijke gezondheidszorg voor de allochtonen in Vlaanderen: Inventaris en aanzet tot evaluatie [Mental health care for allochthones in Flanders: Inventory and start of an evaluation]. *Diagnostiek-Wijzer, 1–2*, 21–30.

Timmerman, C. (1992–93). Turkish young women and the school system in Turkey and in Belgium. *Migration, 15*, 103–125.

Van De Mieroop, E., Peeters, R. F., & De Muynck, A. (1989). Hoe ziek zijn Ali en Fatma? Onderzoek naar ziekte en gezondheid van vreemdelingen in Vlaanderen en Brussel. Een stand van zaken [How sick are Ali and Fatma? A study of sickness and health of foreigners in Flanders and Brussels: The current situation]. Antwerp: Universitaire Instellingen Antwerpen, ESOC-Publicatie No. 21.

Westermeyer, J. (1989). *Mental health for refugees and other migrants.* Springfield, IL: Charles C Thomas.

IV

Native Peoples

11

The Aboriginal Peoples of Canada

Colonialism and Mental Health

JAMES B. WALDRAM

INTRODUCTION

The original inhabitants of North America have experienced great social upheaval since the arrival of the first Europeans after 1492. While not immigrants per se, they have experienced the negative consequences of the arrival of immigrants, initially from Europe, and have been forced to abandon their traditional territories and ways of life. Some were forcibly removed as entire communities or populations to other regions; some were confined to small parcels of "reserve" lands; some were taken away to residential schools; and some were enticed to move into cities. Throughout these events, government efforts at assimilation proved variably successful. The purpose of this chapter is to describe the current mental health implications of these processes with a particular focus on the aboriginal population of Canada.

THE CULTURAL BACKGROUND

Scientists generally believe that the aboriginal population of North America migrated from Asia across a Bering Strait land bridge somewhere between 12,000 BP and 70,000 BP (although the lower estimate is more widely accepted).

JAMES B. WALDRAM • Department of Native Studies, University of Saskatchewan, Saskatoon, Saskatchewan, Canada S7N 5E6.

Ethnicity, Immigration, and Psychopathology, edited by Ihsan Al-Issa and Michel Tousignant. Plenum Press, New York, 1997.

Furthermore, it is believed that this migration took the form of separate waves of Asian populations, with the Inuit of the arctic arriving most recently. By the time Europeans arrived in what would become known as Canada, there were likely thousands of autonomous aboriginal "bands," as they are referred to in older anthropological literature, or "nations" in the contemporary discourse. Linguists have identified 11 different language families within this diversity. The concept of "culture area," employed by North Americanists to describe the cultural adaptations of the aboriginal populations (e.g., Driver, 1969, p. 17), has resulted in the division of Canada into major categories, each definable by cultural similarities within the category, and dissimilarities between categories. So, for instance, in the arctic culture area we find the Inuit, primarily hunters and fishers with an adaptation to the tundra and sea; in the subarctic boreal forests we find the Athapaskans (or Dene) (e.g., Slave, Hare, Chipewyan) and Algonkians (e.g., Cree, Ojibwa), also primarily hunters and fishers. In the eastern woodlands we find farming peoples, such as the Iroquoian-speaking groups (e.g., Mohawk, Huron), living in settled villages. On the Northwest Coast were the hunting and fishing peoples, such as the Haida and Tsimshian, who exploited the vast resources of the sea and rivers. And on the plains were aboriginal groups, such as the Blackfoot and Plains Cree, who developed a bison-hunting adaptation. The cultural and linguistic diversity was dazzling.

With the arrival of Europeans in the northern part of North America, major population shifts and declines commenced. There has been great debate over the issue of precontact demographics (e.g., Trigger, 1985, p. 354), with North American estimates ranging from 1 to 2 million, all the way up to 18 million (Waldram, Herring, & Young, 1995, pp. 3–6; Dobyns, 1966; Thornton, 1987). Methodological problems are significant, and the debate will likely never be resolved. Nevertheless, we do know that European contact resulted in the spread of new "virgin soil" diseases, such as smallpox, influenza, and cholera, and that mortality certainly increased. It is likely that the social, cultural, and economic changes wrought by European contact played an important synergistic role in decreasing population numbers, since removal from resources was a primary consequence of contact. In the case of Canada, postconfederation (1867) census data lead to the conclusion that the Canadian Indian population reached a nadir in the early 20th century, at 127,000, after which the population began to increase to the point where it may have reachieved its levels at contact by the early 1960s.

A census undertaken in 1991 indicated that 1,002,675 individuals declared themselves to be of "aboriginal" heritage. It is also believed that at least 38,000 aboriginal people did not participate in the census. In essence, the aboriginal population constitutes a small minority within the Canadian population, approximately 4%, but in certain regions (especially the West and North) this proportion can rise dramatically (e.g., in the eastern arctic the Inuit are the majority). In the census, and for purposes of this chapter, the term *aboriginal* is used to collectively encompass all "Indian" cultural groups, plus the Inuit and the mixed-heritage group known as the Metis. The 1991 census indicates that 744,845 identified an Indian origin, 43,000 an Inuit origin, and 174,710 a Metis origin. It is accepted by all analysts that these figures underestimate the aboriginal population.

The inherent artificiality of any general treatment of aboriginal mental health issues should be emphasized. Today, not only are there individuals who are still well integrated in their aboriginal cultures as they currently exist, there are also aboriginal peoples with varying degrees of orientation to the Anglo- and Franco-Canadian cultures (what I will collectively refer to as the "Euro-Canadian culture"). Hence, use of an aboriginal "variable" in comparison to a "nonaboriginal" one, within the context of much psychological and mental health research, is problematic.

CONTEMPORARY EPIDEMIOLOGY

Perhaps surprisingly, there are few data on psychopathology among aboriginal Canadians, despite ever-increasing attention to mental health issues. This section will attempt to address what data are available, but more attention must necessarily be given to end-stage indicators of psychopathology.

National-level mortality data are readily available only for the registered Indian population (i.e., those aboriginal peoples recognized by the federal government as "Indians" for purposes of federal programs). Table 1 summarizes the most comprehensive of these data.

The implications for mental health are pertinent particularly with respect to alcoholism/cirrhosis, motor vehicle accidents, suicide and homicide, and to a lesser extent other causes of accidental death, such as drowning and fires. As I will discuss later, the role of alcohol in particular is striking when examining many of these causes of death.

The data in Table 1, which lists leading causes of mortality for reserve Indians (with the corresponding data for Canada), clearly demonstrate the significance of sudden, traumatic, and accidental or deliberate deaths, particularly in comparison to disease. Indian reserve females experience lower rates in comparison to males, but in all instances for these types of deaths they are higher than for Canadian males and females. Particular attention should be drawn to the alcoholism/cirrhosis and suicide data, as these will form case studies later in this chapter. For females (1979–1983), the alcoholism/cirrhosis rate was over five times higher for reserve Indians than for Canadians, and the suicide rate 2.5 times higher. For Indian reserve males, the mortality rate due to alcoholism/cirrhosis was over twice as high, and that for suicide almost three times as high.

Table 2 presents data on age-specific mortality rates. Mortality ratios for

Table 1. Age-Standardized Mortality Rates for Leading Causes of Death by Gender Ages 0 to 64 on Indian Reserves, 1979–1988, and for Canada, 1979–1983, per 100,000[a]

	Indian reserves			Canada
Cause of death	1979–1983	1984–1988	% change	1979–1983
Females				
Alcoholism/cirrhosis	29.8	17.5	−41.3	5.5
Motor vehicle accidents	29.4	18.3	−37.8	10.4
Coronary heart disease	25.4	26.6	4.7	20.7
Cerebrovascular disease	23.0	12.9	−43.9	8.6
Suicide	16.8	9.5	−43.5	6.6
Diabetes	13.7	12.7	−7.5	2.4
Cancer of uterus/cervix	11.0	8.4	−23.6	3.6
Homicide	10.2	7.6	−25.5	1.6
Pneumonia	9.5	7.4	−22.1	2.3
Fires	6.3	8.0	27.0	1.5
All causes	334.6	276.6	−17.3	173.4
Males				
Coronary heart disease	80.9	60.9	−24.7	82.6
Motor vehicle accidents	75.2	60.2	−19.9	29.9
Suicide	59.9	45.5	−24.0	21.5
Alcoholism/cirrhosis	33.2	33.4	0.6	14.2
Homicide	24.4	17.7	−27.5	3.1
Drowning	21.4	11.9	−44.4	3.8
Lung cancer	15.8	12.8	−19.0	27.7
Cerebrovascular disease	15.3	11.8	−22.9	10.7
Fires	14.2	12.8	−9.9	3.0
Pneumonia	12.9	7.7	−40.3	3.7
All causes	561.0	464.9	−17.1	340.2

[a]From Mao, Moloughney, Semenciw, & Morrison (1992).

Table 2. Age-Specific Mortality Rates, per 100,000, Indian Reserves and Canada, 1977–1982[a]

	Males			Females		
Age	Reserves	Canada	Ratio	Reserves	Canada	Ratio
1–9	118.4	49.8	2.38	91.3	37.2	2.46
10–19	218.1	92.5	2.36	85.1	37.1	2.29
20–29	438.7	158.0	2.78	184.2	52.1	3.53
30–39	517.1	163.9	3.16	276.2	84.2	3.28
40–49	716.4	391.1	1.83	424.8	215.7	1.97
50–59	1131.4	1054.4	1.07	854.4	535.3	1.60
60–69	2507.3	2544.7	0.99	1578.8	1245.7	1.27
70+	5883.6	7943.9	0.75	4228.8	5449.2	0.78

[a]From Mao et al. (1986).

reserve Indians do not begin to approach those of Canadians in general until the more advanced years. A bottleneck appears particularly between the ages of 20 and 39 for both aboriginal males and females. Not surprisingly, it is in these age groupings that mortality from suicide, accidents, and violence are particularly high. For example, data for Saskatchewan Indians between the ages of 25 and 44, in 1986, demonstrate that the highest mortality was recorded for motor vehicle accidents (105 per 100,000), followed by suicide and self-inflicted injury (50 per 100,000), homicide and intentional injury (20 per 100,000), injury with intent undetermined (19 per 100,000), and pneumonia and influenza (19 per 100,000). For the 45 to 64 age group, the mortality rate for motor vehicle accidents had dropped only slightly to 100 per 100,000, but had been overtaken by cancer and coronary heart disease as the leading cause of death (Health Status Research Unit, 1989, pp. 71–72; these data are approximations).

Mortality data for aboriginal peoples varies extensively from region to region, and such data are not always readily available. Age-standardized mortality rates for various provinces are provided in Table 3. These data demonstrate that, for the period 1977 to 1982, Indians living on reserves in Alberta had the highest mortality rates, more than double the Canadian rate and significantly higher than the total Indian reserve rate for both males and females (Mao, Morrison, Semenciw, & Wigle, 1986, p. 264). It is likely that the high Alberta rate for this period reflected the consequences of a rapid influx of money into a small number of communities that benefited from oil and natural gas revenues. Problems with alcohol and drugs, accidents and violent death, and suicide all increased significantly (York, 1989). In more recent years, these communities have gained a greater measure of control over these aspects of their lives, and it is believed the mortality rates have declined significantly.

Statistical data on mortality present a very incomplete picture of the kinds

Table 3. Age-Standardized Mortality Rates (ASMR) per 100,000 for Selected Provinces, 1977–1982, Ages 1 to 69[a]

	ASMR	
Indian reserves	Males	Females
Ontario	581.6	344.0
Manitoba	540.8	332.6
Saskatchewan	573.0	387.4
Alberta	849.2	485.7
All reserves	588.5	350.0
Canada	407.7	200.7

[a]From Mao et al. (1986, p. 264).

of lifestyles led by the deceased prior to death. An ambitious study by Jarvis and Boldt (1982) attempted to provide detailed information on the circumstances surrounding the deaths of aboriginal peoples in Alberta, by going beyond the medical examiner's certificates. These researchers undertook a 12-month prospective study of deaths in 35 aboriginal communities in the late 1970s, by interviewing the survivors concerning the circumstances surrounding the deaths. They concluded that, "Natives [aboriginal peoples] encounter death under very different circumstances and from different causes than do other Canadians and the style of death reflects a style of life that is different from that of the general population" (Jarvis & Boldt, 1982, p. 1347). In particular, they found that these aboriginal peoples tended to die younger than other Canadians and most often in clusters of two or more. That is, "They commonly share their moment of death with their friends," usually outside of the hospital and in "the company of friends" (Jarvis & Boldt, 1982, p. 1347). Deaths were most frequent on weekends, in the early hours of the morning. Some 32% of deaths were due to accidents (compared to only 8.6% for the population as a whole), especially fire and motor vehicle accidents. Suicide claimed almost as many victims as these accident causes. The researchers were able to determine that over 40% of the deaths were directly attributable to alcohol use, and that the majority of victims were legally impaired at the moment of their death. The authors concluded that the physical circumstances of the lives of aboriginal peoples partly explained mortality patterns: geographical isolation, poor transportation infrastructure, and the intense social life of small communities are examples. But they also identified the social conditions under which aboriginal peoples live as more important, including lower educational and employment levels.

ALCOHOL

The paramount role of alcohol in aboriginal mortality was also borne out in a Saskatchewan study (Szabo, 1990), with respect to registered Indians. This study demonstrated that alcohol use was involved in 92% of motor vehicle accidents where the driver was killed and in 45% of suicides in the 15 to 34 age bracket. Some 80% of the deaths due to exposure were also alcohol related.

Alcohol is considered by most health professionals, aboriginal and non-aboriginal alike, to be the most serious social health problem among aboriginal peoples. Despite this fact, and the obvious role that alcohol plays in the high rates of sudden, traumatic death, it is not always recognized that it is a *minority* of aboriginal peoples overall who experience difficulties in their use of alcohol. A study of alcohol and drug use among Indian people in Saskatchewan in 1984 indicated that only 5% of the 900 adults surveyed (on 12 reserves and 5 urban centers) reported using alcohol on a daily basis, and only 6% were categorized as "chronic" alcohol users. Over 62% reported either no consumption or "social" drinking only, leading the researchers to conclude that the alcohol abuse levels were between 35 to 40% of the adult population. The most common consumption pattern was one of periodic consumption of large quantities, as opposed to more frequent use; this type of consumption may explain in part the high rates of injury and sudden death in the population. There were no similar provincial data with which to compare these figures (Federation of Saskatchewan Indian Nations, 1984).

SUICIDE

Suicide rates are strikingly high among the Canadian aboriginal population and have demonstrated a gradual increasing trend over recent years. The 1987, age-standardized registered Indian suicide rate was 38.4, in contrast to only 14.1 for Canadians as a whole (Canada. Medical Services Branch, 1991). Table 4 presents data on suicides by age group, and it is significant to note not only the bottleneck age category of 20 to 29 for registered Indians, but also the fact that suicide rates compare favorably with national rates by age 50, and furthermore that suicide is very rare among elderly Indian peoples. A comparison of males and females indicated that for all age brackets except 50 to 59, the male rate was higher. The overall male suicide rate of 57.8 per 100,000 (compared to the Canadian male rate of 23.8) was almost four times higher than the female rate of 14.5 (compared to the female Canadian rate of 6.3) and 6.5 times higher in the 20 to 29 age bracket.

From a regional perspective, data for 1984–1988 show the Yukon with the

Table 4. Suicide Rate per 100,000, 1984–1988[a]

Age	Registered Indians	Canada	Ratio
0–9	0.3	0.0	—
10–19	38.9	7.0	5.6
20–29	80.8	18.4	4.4
30–39	41.9	17.8	2.4
40–49	35.3	18.1	2.0
50–59	19.1	19.4	1.0
60–69	18.3	17.0	1.1
70–79	4.4	18.9	0.2
80+	0.0	18.5	0.0

[a]From Canada. Medical Services Branch. Steering Committee on Native Mental Health (1991, p. 47).

highest rate (61.9 per 100,000), followed by Alberta (52.1), the Atlantic provinces (43.0), and Saskatchewan (35.1) (Canada. Medical Services Branch, 1991, p. 52). A retrospective study by Garro (1988) for registered Indian suicide deaths between 1973 and 1982 revealed a rate of 40.15 per 100,000. Most Canadian provinces are very large, with substantial "northern" areas as well as southern areas and urban centers. In both Manitoba (Garro, 1988) and Saskatchewan (Fiddler, 1986), considerably higher Indian suicide rates have been identified for the more southerly regions, that is, regions where there is more urbanization and greater access to nonaboriginal society. Similarly, a study of youth suicide in Manitoba suggested that rates were considerably higher in urban areas (Sigurdson et al., 1994). It also has been suggested that aboriginal communities are more likely to experience "cluster" suicide, including parasuicide, than nonaboriginal communities (Shore, 1975; Ward & Fox, 1977; Brant, 1993; Kirmayer, 1994).

Data for Saskatchewan, 1985–1986, demonstrate some patterns to aboriginal suicide that may hold nationally (although there are no comparable national data). In comparing the involvement of alcohol and drugs in suicide, these data demonstrated that 41% of the aboriginal deaths involved alcohol, compared to 25% for nonaboriginal suicides; 23% of aboriginal deaths involved alcohol and drugs, compared to 16% for nonaboriginal victims; and 11% of aboriginal suicides involved drugs only, compared to 23% for nonaboriginals (Health Status Research Unit, 1989, p. 28). The Manitoba youth study showed that alcohol was involved in almost 61% of aboriginal suicides, compared to 43% of nonaboriginal suicides (Sigurdson et al., 1994, p. 400). These data indicate the propensity for aboriginal suicides to engage in alcohol consumption to a greater degree and the nonaboriginal suicides to engage in drug use (Health Status Research Unit, 1989, p. 28).

MORBIDITY

Data on psychopathological morbidity are more problematic for the aboriginal Canadian population. Most data pertain to hospitalization rates. Data for the province of Saskatchewan is particularly useful, because of the efforts of this province to develop reliable health data bases.

Hospitalization due to injury and poisoning for registered Saskatchewan Indians in the 1 to 4 age bracket was about twice that for Saskatchewan residents in general in 1985; it was more than five times higher for the 5 to 14 group and almost six times higher for those aged 15 to 24 (Health Status Research Unit, 1989).

Two studies in the 1970s attempted to measure the prevalence of psychiatric disorders among the Saskatchewan registered Indian and general populations. Roy, Choudhuri, and Irvine (1970) undertook a survey of 18 rural municipalities and 10 Indian reserves and discovered an overall Indian prevalence rate of 273 per 10,000, compared to 152 per 10,000 for the Saskatchewan non-Indian population. Data from this study are presented in Table 5, where it can be seen that in each category the Indian rate was higher. Martens (1973) examined the prevalence of anxiety in 17 rural municipalities and 8 Indian reserves, using a scale developed from the Cornell Medical Index. Her study suggested that 65% of the Indian subjects exhibited symptoms of anxiety, compared to 50% for the residents of the rural municipalities. As Fritz and D'Arcy (1983) point out, both studies suffered from important limitations, including their focus on only one rural area of the province. These authors also note that Roy et al. (1970) used a different method of data collection for the Indian and non-Indian populations, and that Marten's scale "may be as much a reflection of poor physical health or general life stress as it is of a psychiatric disorder" (Fritz & D'Arcy, 1983, p. 71).

Some data are also available on the utilization of mental health services. Hendrie and Hanson (1972), in a Winnipeg study at a psychiatric institute, found that Indian and Metis patients with a personality disorder diagnosis received fewer follow-up outpatient appointments and had shorter hospital stays than nonaboriginals. The researchers suggest that hostility toward psychiatric care was not a factor in this difference, but a possible factor was that the staff tended to believe that Indian and Metis patients were less likely to benefit from outpatient therapy.

Other Saskatchewan utilization data are available for 1969 to 1973 (Fritz & D'Arcy, 1983). Although considerably dated, it remains one of the better bodies of data on this topic. In general, these data indicated that Indians had higher overall admission rates to both public and private psychiatric facilities, the Indian rate being 11% higher for public facilities and 62% higher for private facilities. However, the Indian outpatient treatment rate was 20 and 23% lower in public and private treatment facilities, respectively.

In terms of psychiatric diagnosis, admissions to public sector facilities for

Table 5. Saskatchewan Psychiatric Disorder Prevalence Rate, per 10,000, in 1970[a]

Disorder	Indian	Non-Indian
Psychoses	91	57
Schizophrenia	57	16
Functional	34	30
Neuroses	83	57
Alcoholism	13	6
Mental retardation	66	23
Other disorders	21	9

[a]From Roy et al. (1970) and Fritz & D'Arcy (1983).

treatment of alcoholism, neuroses, and behavior disorders were highest among the Indian group, whereas treatment for schizophrenia and psychoses appeared more common for non-Indians. For private sector treatment, Indian admission rates were higher in all these categories except psychoses. The largest gap in admission rates exists for alcoholism in both the public and private sectors, where Indian rates were over three times higher than non-Indian rates (Fritz & D'Arcy, 1983).

In terms of outpatient rates, the Indian rates were lower in every category except alcoholism and addictions, where Indian rates were more than twice those of non-Indians for public treatment facilities and over five times higher for private facilities.

Overall trends in these data suggest increasing utilization rates for both Indian and non-Indian populations, but that the increase for Indians was generally much greater. Fritz and D'Arcy (1983, p. 82) caution, however, that this may simply reflect an increase in Indian access to these facilities, especially in rural areas where outpatient programs have been developed, as well as greater Indian population increases. The fact that Indian patients had higher admission rates but lower outpatient treatment rates than non-Indians suggests to these authors that Hendrie and Hanson's (1972) assessment may be accurate: The views of treatment staff that Indian communities were more pathological, combined with views that Indians were less compliant, may have led to greater admissions as opposed to outpatient treatment.

DEPRESSION

While it is widely accepted that the high rates of aboriginal alcoholism and suicide suggest significant problems with depression, very little research has been undertaken on this issue. Shore and Manson (1985) have argued that many testing instruments are culturally inappropriate and that certain affective states are misunderstood or misdiagnosed, primarily for cultural reasons. Nevertheless, the published scientific literature demonstrates few attempts to assess and understand the extent to which depression is a problem for aboriginal peoples.

A Manitoba study of the leaders of 57 Indian reserves by Rodgers and Abas (1986) suggested that almost half believed depression to be a serious problem in their communities. Another study done for the First Nations Confederacy in Manitoba, which defined depression as "hopelessness and despair about the future," also indicated that depression was considered a serious problem (Timpson et al., 1988). Studies of the prevalence of clinically defined depression are rare.

Armstrong (1993, p. 224), for one, argues that "the chronic stresses of daily life, rather than diagnosable psychiatric disorders, account for Native

Indians' high rates of arrest, homicide, suicide, incarceration, wife and child abuse, and violent death." Furthermore, while lacking hard data, he also suggests that primary mood disorder (bipolar) is rare among Canadian aboriginals and that unipolar depression is primarily reactive. He continues that "most depressive symptoms appear to be related to the difficulty of coping with an environment that is extremely stressful," and that entire communities can be affected (Armstrong, 1993, p. 224). These conditions include the geographic (long, cold winters that limit exposure to daylight), alcoholism and solvent abuse, lack of recreational programs, sexual abuse, identity confusion, and unemployment. The high sudden-death rate, as documented earlier in this chapter, may also be a factor, since in many communities grieving may appear to be a constant, ongoing process in which virtually everyone has been touched by the tragic death of a loved one.

In a unique study, Timpson and co-workers (1988) examined depression in a small, northwestern Ontario Ojibwa community. Working with community Elders, they learned that within the Nishnawbe (Ojibwa) language, depression referred to "concepts of loneliness and sadness" as well as the implications of the term used by Western medicine (Timpson et al., 1988, p. 6). The Elders believed that depression was not a new phenomenon and that shame was a major cause of depression in the past, sometimes leading to suicide. However, in past years the demands of survival allowed little time to dwell on problems; in recent years this has changed. They viewed the increase in depression as a result of the loss of spirituality (i.e., traditional religious beliefs and practices), with less sharing and a greater emphasis on materialism. In effect, the Elders identified a whole-scale shift in worldview, in which the relationship between people and nature had been disrupted. Timpson and colleagues (1988, p. 6) suggest that "the description of the loss of spirituality is remarkably similar to the concepts of normlessness and anomie."

Timpson et al. (1988, p. 7) have also argued that more traditional symptoms, such as "sensations of spirits of the dead invading a person's body, cursing, and frightening visual hallucinations" are being presented, especially to Native mental health counselors, and that these have often been labeled reactive or psychotic depression. The authors present a case study in which a woman, experiencing disorientation and sensations of turning into a loon and developing cannibalistic urges, was referred to a traditional healer with some success.

EXPLANATIONS

Clearly, there is a link between the major psychological problems experienced by Canadian aboriginal peoples. Depression, alcohol abuse, suicide, and accidental and violent deaths all suggest an underlying social pathology that has resulted in the rates of death from these causes to be among the highest in the world. How is it possible to explain this situation, given that Canada is one of the richest countries?

Researchers have for many years examined the issue of aboriginal alcohol consumption in North America, and the industrial-like generation of studies have been impressive, if only in weight! Some studies have concentrated on the question of aboriginal biological susceptibility to alcohol, but in the end these studies have been largely inconclusive (e.g., Fenna, Mix, Schaefer, & Gilbert, 1971; Leiber, 1972; Wolff, 1973; Bennion & Li, 1976). In some instances, an aboriginal group is seen to metabolize ethanol more quickly, in others more slowly, and in still others no differences between an aboriginal group and a nonaboriginal group are discernible. One apparent problem in these studies has been the establishment of valid population parameters, or "race," if you will, since there has always been intermarriage between aboriginal groups, and after the arrival of Europeans and Africans this trend continued to mix the gene pool. Nevertheless, many people (including aboriginal people) cling to the belief that aboriginal people are biologically susceptible to alcohol.

Many studies have also been carried out to determine how and why aboriginal peoples drink. There have been many competing theories over the years:

- A belief that drinking stemmed from the suppression of hostility in traditional culture, which was released by consumption (Balikci, 1968).
- Alcohol abuse is a reaction to the pressures of acculturation (Graves, 1967; Hamer & Steinbring, 1980).
- Alcohol consumption patterns were taught to aboriginals by non-aboriginals in the "frontier context" (Honigmann, 1980).
- Alcohol consumption is a learned behavior that fits into the existing cultural pattern of the group (Levy & Kunitz, 1974).
- Alcohol consumption is a reflection of "anomie" in the classic Durkheimian sense (Dozier, 1966).

There are many other theoretical explanations as well. This seemingly excessive concentration on alcohol use among aboriginal peoples is likely the product of both historic and contemporary stereotypical images of the "drunken Indian," a stereotype that, despite its pervasiveness, is empirically unjustified and inherently racist. It is important to stress here that all of this theorizing has contributed virtually nothing to our understanding of either the problem or the solutions.

Most explanations of aboriginal suicide link the problem to the poverty and deprivation experienced by aboriginal people in some areas of the country, combined with the negative effects of cultural loss and despiritualization and the more immediate problem of alcohol and substance abuse. Fiddler (1986), for instance, finds the root of the problem in the history of relations between aboriginal and European Canadians, especially the consequences of racism and discrimination. He suggests that racism has negatively affected the development of strong self-identities among some aboriginal people, through such mechanisms as residential schools, missionization, and government programs designed to assimilate. Fiddler also presents the classic paradox of colonized peoples, where they are "caught between two cultures" and not fully adapted to either. Finally, he notes that the relative deprivation of aboriginal people, vis-à-vis Euro-Canadians, is an important explanatory factor. His arguments are supported by data that suggest suicide rates are higher in the more southerly areas, where access to Euro-Canadian communities is greatest and where the aboriginal cultures are less coherent.

A recent study on suicide by the Royal Commission on Aboriginal Peoples (RCAP, 1994) has identified the following explanations for the high suicide rate of aboriginal peoples:

- Psychobiological factors, such as depression and unresolved grief.
- Life history factors, such as extensive family disruption caused by alcohol, removal of family members, and physical and sexual abuse.
- Culture stress, caused by "massive, imposed or uncontrollable change," such as loss of land, suppression of religion, and racism.

Issues of self-identity are also important, and the RCAP (1994) suggests that the legacy of colonialism has been to severely damage aboriginal people's sense of their own self-worth and that of their cultures.

The notion of a "residential school syndrome" has emerged in recent years to explain the psychological and social consequences of this educational system. Beginning in the early 1800s, many aboriginal peoples were placed in residential schools to promote their education and assimilation. These schools operated up to 10 months of the year, during which the children had very little or no contact with their families and communities. During these periods, they were instructed in English and punished if they spoke their own languages; likewise, they were forced to adopt Western style clothing, food and eating habits, and manners and customs. Corporal punishment, unfamiliar to aboriginal cultures, was used to enforce conformity with assimilationist goals. Recently, it has emerged that the sexual abuse of some children also occurred in some schools. The effect was to greatly deculturalize many individuals, such that they could no longer fit into their aboriginal cultures, and to contribute to many psychological problems (Haig-Brown, 1988; Bull, 1991).

The separation of children from their families had a profound effect on the nurturing of parenting skills in subsequent generations. In effect, there has been a breakdown of traditional child-rearing patterns; those who went through the residential school system learned only the abusive, military-style "parenting" of the missionaries and school staff (Ing, 1991). Included in these learned behaviors were inappropriate attitudes toward members of the opposite sex and toward sexuality. Children were taught that their aboriginal cultures were inferior and that their languages were primitive. As a result, respect for the community Elders began to wane, leading to problems in the transmission of cultural and parental knowledge. Loss of language and culture also contributed to the development of self-esteem problems.

Residential school syndrome is not yet recognized as a psychological disorder, but rather pertains to the psychological, sociological, and cultural consequences of the residential experience.[1] These include the development of self-esteem and identity problems, lack of parenting skills (and therefore the development of problems with children, such as solvent abuse and criminality), alcoholism, and sexual abuse. There is no scientific literature on this syndrome; rather, community-based workshops and healing initiatives are emerging to deal with these issues. Recent years have seen the emergence of such workshops with an emphasis on admitting the existence of problems in communities and the need to begin healing. Indeed, when the leader of one major aboriginal organization in Canada went public with the admission that he, too, had been sexually abused in a residential school, the door opened for others to step forward as well. This process is particularly interesting in the manner in which the aboriginal people themselves are handling it in their own way, in the absence of input from mental health professionals.

RECENT TREATMENT INITIATIVES

Aboriginal peoples in Canada have moved effectively to gain control of the treatment and recovery process in recent years. The "healing" movement has gained strength and international recognition, through its marriage of the biopsychosocial model of Western biomedicine to traditional healing approaches. Alcohol and substance abuse problems have proved particularly amenable to this integrative approach.

The most influential, aboriginally controlled treatment facility in Canada is Poundmaker's Lodge, located just north of Edmonton, Alberta. Poundmaker's Lodge operates a residential alcohol and substance abuse program that is based on the premise that a culturally sensitive environment must be created so that "holistic" healing of the mind, body, and spirit can ensue. The loss of cultural identity is seen to be at the root of substance abuse problems, and hence much of their program entails cultural reeducation, combined

[1]Some analysts of aboriginal mental health have begun to view residential school syndrome as one component of a more generalized posttraumatic stress disorder. In this formulation, both the people as individuals and the people as cultures have undergone intense trauma and violence as a result of colonization. This is a promising area of investigation (Duran & Duran, 1995).

with traditional healing and spirituality. Sweet grass and sweat lodge ceremonies are important components of this healing approach, led by aboriginal Elders and healers who serve also as counseling staff. However, the 12-Step Alcoholics Anonymous program, as well as parallel programs such as Narcotics Anonymous, have also been included, with only minor modifications.

Associated with Poundmaker's Lodge is the Nechi Institute, a facility for training aboriginal alcohol and substance abuse counselors. Graduates from the Nechi Institute come from all aboriginal areas of Canada and often return to their home communities to work in similar treatment programs.

The integration of traditional aboriginal approaches in the healing movement has become a Canada-wide phenomenon. Jilek (1982), for instance, has documented his collaboration with traditional healers from the Coast Salish people in the psychiatric treatment of aboriginal alcoholics. In northern Ontario, the traditional Algonquian ceremony known as the "shaking tent" is being used in the diagnosis and treatment of substance abusers (Anishinaabeg, 1993). Many hospitals in Canada have begun to allow traditional healers to participate in the treatment of aboriginal patients, led by the Lake of the Woods Hospital in Kenora where a healer was hired within the hospital's Department of Psychiatry (Young & Smith, 1991).

Beginning in the 1970s, the Correctional Service of Canada began to allow traditional aboriginal ceremonies within federal prisons. While these programs developed slowly, and Elders often experienced harassment and desecration of sacred objects, the programs persevered. Today, involvement with the Elders, learning about aboriginal cultures and spirituality, and undertaking sweat lodge ceremonies and fasts have become important components of the forensic treatment process (Waldram, 1993, 1994, 1997).

There are many other initiatives that are emerging, but which are as yet not widely documented. The community sobriety movement, for instance, best exemplified in the extraordinary story of Alkali Lake, British Columbia (Johnson & Johnson, 1993), is gathering steam. "Healing circles," ad hoc groups of aboriginal individuals, are springing up, allowing an avenue for the collective expression of the distresses brought about by racism, oppression, and marginality. "Bush therapy" is also occurring, particularly in the treatment of young people, wherein an Elder takes the individual into the bush for an extended period of time to teach him or her about survival as a means of building self-esteem.

Programs aimed specifically at suicide prevention are not well documented. Many of the programs designed for alcohol and substance abuse treatment also deal with the issue of suicide, since these problems are related. The RCAP (1994) provided some sketches of successful suicide prevention and intervention programs in its report. The common thread that binds these programs is described by the RCAP (1994, p. 42):

> there is evidence in research and in Aboriginal experience that a clear and positive sense of cultural identity and institutions that allow for collective self-control, along with strong bonds of love and mutual support in family and community, can act as protective forces against despair, self-destructiveness and suicide.

Programs in communities such as Wikwemikong, Ontario and Big Cove, New Brunswick combine the biopsychosocial approaches of biomedicine with traditional healing and spirituality and work to strengthen self-respect within the communities. Across Canada, crisis intervention teams have been developed, consisting primarily of aboriginal professional people, who work to intervene with potential suicides or else work with communities to prevent cluster suicides subsequent to a successful one. Some communities have also adopted the use of hot line telephone counseling and intervention services. However, as the RCAP (1994) suggests, there is little information available on what truly works with respect to suicide prevention; nevertheless, the aboriginal approach appears in contrast to the biopsychosocial model in that it attempts broader community involvement, as well as the reintegration of the individual into the culture (often through the use of traditional healing approaches and spirituality).

CONCLUSION

The available evidence suggests that aboriginal peoples as a category within Canada experience significantly higher rates of mortality due to sudden, traumatic causes and higher rates of alcohol abuse and suicide. With respect to other psychopathological data, little is available that allows for comparative discussion. Concentrating on selective psychopathological data can lead to a misrepresentation of the aboriginal health picture, however, contributing to the stereotypical image of the inherent pathological state of aboriginal peoples and communities. It is essential to emphasize here that the problems discussed in this chapter affect only a minority of aboriginal peoples, as they do Canadians in general.

The current state of affairs can be clearly linked to the traumatic effects of colonialism, including geographic and economic marginalization, and attempts at forced assimilation. Aboriginal communities and organizations, recognizing that any programs emanating from the federal and provincial governments are not the answer, have reacted to this colonialism by developing their own initiatives. These aboriginal programs typically select from the best of the biopsychosocial approaches, adapt them if necessary to local cultures, and combine them with programs to revitalize the cultures and traditions through the use of spirituality and traditional healing. These initiatives suggest that the root of the problem, as seen in these communities, lies with the damage done to the cultures as a result of colonialism, and that it is only through the strengthening of these cultures that the problems will be addressed.

REFERENCES

Anishinaabeg. Medical Professionals. (1993). *Okunongegayin.* A community-driven initiative for successfully intervening with Anishinaabeg children, teens and young adults in distress. Final report to the Health Innovation Fund, Premier's Council on Health, Well-being and Social Justice, Ontario Ministry of Health.

Armstrong, H. (1993). Depression in Canadian Native Indians. In P. Cappeliez & R. J. Flyn (Eds.), *Depression and the social environment: Research and intervention with neglected populations* (pp. 218–234). Montreal and Kingston: McGill-Queen's University Press.

Balikci, A. (1968). Bad friends. *Human Organization, 27,* 191–199.

Bennion, L., & Li, T. K. (1976). Alcohol metabolism in American Indians and whites. *New England Journal of Medicine, 294,* 9–13.

Brant, C. (1993). Suicide in Canadian aboriginal peoples: Causes and prevention. In *The Path to Healing* (pp. 55–71). Report of the National Roundtable on Aboriginal Health and Social Issues. Ottawa: Royal Commission on Aboriginal Peoples.

Bull, L. R. (1991). Indian residential schooling: The Native perspective. *Canadian Journal of Native Education, 18,* 1–63.

Canada. Medical Services Branch. Steering Committee on Native Mental Health. (1991). *Statistical profile on native mental health.* Background Report No. 1. Ottawa: National Health and Welfare.

Dobyns, H. (1966). An appraisal of techniques for estimating aboriginal American population with a new hemispheric estimate. *Current Anthropology, 7,* 395–416.

Dozier, E. P. (1966). Problem drinking among American Indians: The role of sociocultural deprivation. *Quarterly Journal of Studies on Alcohol, 27,* 72–87.

Driver, H. (1969). *Indians of North America* (2nd ed.). Chicago: University of Chicago Press.

Duran, E., & Duran, B. (1995). *Native American postcolonial psychology.* Albany: State University of New York Press.

Federation of Saskatchewan Indian Nations. (1984). *Alcohol and drug abuse among treaty Indians in Saskatchewan.* Regina: Federation of Saskatchewan Indian Nations.

Fenna, D., Mix, L., Schaefer, O., & Gilbert, J. (1971). Ethanol metabolism in various racial groups. *Canadian Medical Association Journal, 105,* 472–475.

Fiddler, S. (1986). *Suicides, violent and accidental deaths among treaty Indians in Saskatchewan.* Regina: Federation of Saskatchewan Indian Nations.

Fritz, W., & D'Arcy, C. (1983). Comparisons: Indian and non-Indian use of psychiatric services. In P. Li & B. S. Bolaria (Eds.). *Racial minorities in multicultural Canada* (pp. 68–85). Toronto: Garamond.

Garro, L. C. (1988). Suicides by status Indians in Manitoba. *Arctic Medical Research, 47*(Suppl. 1), 590–592.

Graves, T. (1967). Acculturation, access, and alcohol in a tri-ethnic community. *American Anthropologist, 69,* 306–321.

Haig-Brown, C. (1988). *Resistance and renewal: Surviving the Indian residential school.* Vancouver: Tillacum.

Hamer, J., & Steinbring, J. (1980). Alcohol and the North American Indian: Examples from the subarctic. In J. Hamer & J. Steinbring (Eds.). *Alcohol and native peoples of the North* (pp. 1–29). Washington, DC: University Press of America.

Health Status Research Unit. (1989). *Health status of the Saskatchewan population: Risk factors and health promotion priorities.* Saskatoon: University of Saskatchewan, Department of Community Health and Epidemiology.

Hendrie, H., & Hanson, D. (1972). A comparative study of the psychiatric care of Indians and Metis. *American Journal of Orthopsychiatry, 42*(3), 480–489.

Honigmann, J. (1980). Perspectives on alcohol behavior. In J. Hamer & J. Steinbring (Eds.), *Alcohol and native peoples of the North* (pp. 267–285). Washington, DC: University Press of America.

Ing, N. R. (1991). The effects of residential schools on native child-rearing practices. *Canadian Journal of Education, 18,* 65–118.

Jarvis, G. K., & Boldt, M. (1982). Death styles among Canada's Indians. *Social Science and Medicine, 16,* 1345–1352.

Jilek, W. G. (1982). *Indian healing: Shamanic ceremonialism in the Pacific Northwest.* Surrey, BC: Hancock House.

Johnson, J., & Johnson, F. (1993). Community development, sobriety and after-care at Alkali Lake Band. In Royal Commission on Aboriginal Peoples (Eds.). *The path to healing* (pp. 227–230). Ottawa: Royal Commission on Aboriginal Peoples.

Kirmayer, L. J. (1994). Suicide among Canadian aboriginal peoples. *Transcultural Psychiatric Research Review, 31,* 3–58.

Leiber, C. S. (1972). Metabolism of ethanol and alcoholism: Racial and acquired factors. *Annals of Internal Medicine, 76,* 326–327.

Levy, J., & Kunitz, S. (1974). *Indian drinking: Navajo practices and Anglo-American theories.* New York: Wiley.

Mao, Y., Moloughney, B. W., Semenciw, R., & Morrison, H. I. (1992). Indian reserve and registered Indian mortality in Canada. *Canadian Journal of Public Health, 83,* 350–353.

Mao, Y., Morrison, H., Semenciw, R., & Wigle, D. (1986). Mortality on Canadian Indian reserves 1977–1982. *Canadian Journal of Public Health, 77,* 263–268.

Martens, E. (1973). *Utilization of medical care by Saskatchewan Indians in the North Battleford area.* Masters thesis, Department of Social and Preventive Medicine, University of Saskatchewan.

Rodgers, D. D., & Abas, N. (1986). A survey of native mental health needs in Manitoba. In *Depression in the North American Indian: Causes and treatment* (pp. 9–31). Proceedings of the 1986 annual meeting of the Canadian Psychiatric Association, Section on Native Mental Health, Ottawa.

Roy, C., Choudhuri, A., & Irvine, D. (1970). The prevalence of psychiatric disorders among Saskatchewan Indians. *Journal of Cross-Cultural Psychiatry, 1*(4), 383–392.

Royal Commission on Aboriginal Peoples (RCAP). (1994). *Choosing life: Special report on suicide among aboriginal people.* Ottawa: Supply and Services.

Shore, J. H. (1975). American Indian suicide—Fact and fantasy. *Psychiatry, 38,* 86–91.

Shore, J. H., & Manson, S. M. (1985). Cross-cultural studies of depression among American Indians and Alaska natives. *White Cloud Journal, 2*(2), 5–11.

Sigurdson, E., Staley, D., Matas, M., Hildahl, K., & Squair, K. (1994). A five year review of youth suicide in Manitoba. *Canadian Journal of Psychiatry, 38*(8), 397–403.

Szabo, E. L. (1990). *Mortality related to alcohol use among the status Indian population of Saskatchewan.* Ottawa: Indian and Northern Health Services, Medical Services Branch, Health and Welfare Canada.

Thornton, R. (1987). *American Indian holocaust and survival: A population history since 1492.* Norman: University of Oklahoma Press.

Timpson, J., McKay, S., Kakegamic, S., Roundhead, D., Cohen, C., & Matewapit, G. (1988). Depression in a Native Canadian in Northwestern Ontario: Sadness, grief or spiritual illness. *Canada's Mental Health, 36*(2–3), 5–8.

Trigger, B. G. (1985). *Natives and newcomers: Canada's "Heroic age" reconsidered.* Montreal: McGill-Queen's University Press.

Waldram, J. B. (1993). Aboriginal spirituality: Symbolic healing in Canadian prisons. *Culture, Medicine and Psychiatry, 17,* 345–362.

Waldram, J. B. (1994). Aboriginal spirituality in corrections: A Canadian case study in religion and therapy. *American Indian Quarterly, 18*(2), 197–214.

Waldram, J. B. (1997). *The Way of the Pipe: Aboriginal spirituality and symbolic healing in Canadian prisons.* Peterborough: Broadview.

Waldram, J. B., Herring, A., & Young, T. K. (1995). *Aboriginal health in Canada: Historical, cultural and epidemiological perspectives.* Toronto: University of Toronto Press.

Ward, J. A., & Fox, J. A. (1977). A suicide epidemic on an Indian reserve. *Canadian Psychiatric Association Journal, 22*(8), 423–426.

Wolff, P. H. (1973). Vasomotor sensitivity to alcohol in diverse Mongoloid populations. *American Journal of Human Genetics, 25,* 193–199.

York, G. (1989). *The dispossessed: Life and death in native Canada.* London: Vintage UK.

Young, D. E., & Smith, L. L. (1991). *Native community involvement in health care in Canada since the 1970s: A review of the literature.* Edmonton: Canadian Circumpolar Institute, University of Alberta.

12

The Maori of New Zealand

PERMINDER SACHDEV

E tipu, e rea, mo nga ra o tou ao,
Ko to ringa ki nga rakau a te pakeha, hei ora mo to tinana,
Ko to ngakau ki nga taonga a o tipuna, hei tikitiki no to mahunga,
Ko to wairua ki te Atua, nana nei nga mea katoa.

Grow up, O tender plant, for the days of your world,
Your hand to the tools of the *Pakeha* for the welfare of your body,
Your heart to the treasured possessions of your ancestors, as a crown for your head,
Your spirit to God, the Creator of all things.

Sir Apirana Ngata,
in the autograph book of a young Maori girl

INTRODUCTION

The Maori are the indigenous Polynesian people of New Zealand, or *Aotearoa* (the land of the long white cloud), who are said to have arrived in that country in the early part of this millennium. The traditional Maori society was agricultural and had a tribal organization. The Maori had a highly developed system of warfare and, at the time of the arrival of the European, had reached a high point in the arts of canoe construction, weaving, and building. A detailed account of Maori society before and since colonization can be obtained from classic texts by Best (1924), Buck (1950), Firth (1959), and Metge (1976).

The British naval officer, James Cook, who paved the way for the colon-

---

PERMINDER SACHDEV • School of Psychiatry, University of New South Wales, and Neuropsychiatric Institute, The Prince Henry Hospital, Sydney, Australia.

Ethnicity, Immigration, and Psychopathology, edited by Ihsan Al-Issa and Michel Tousignant. Plenum Press, New York, 1997.

ization of the country, estimated the Maori population at between 100,000 and 300,000 toward the end of the 18th century (Schwimmer, 1974). A century later, the possibility was seriously being considered that the Maori race might not survive. The 1906 census estimated the Maori population at about 42,000. The latter half of the 20th century has witnessed a major turnaround, with the Maori being 15.1% (511,278) of the total population of New Zealand at the 1991 census and recording a higher total fertility rate (2.28) than the *Pakeha* (New Zealander of European descent) (2.10). As would be expected from a higher birth rate, the population is youthful, with 71% under the age of 30 years and only 2% above 65 years (Census, 1986). The life expectancy of the Maori is 7–8 years lower than that of the *Pakeha.* The population has become progressively urbanized, with the proportion of urban individuals rising from 17.7% in 1951 to 78.6% in 1981.

Most indicators suggest that the Maori are a socially disadvantaged group. About two thirds of Maori people are located in the two lowest socioeconomic classes, a proportion that is double that of the non-Maori group. Their unemployment rate is about twice as high as that of the non-Maori, and the average Maori family has a lower income and is less likely to own its home. About 60% of Maori school-leavers have no formal qualifications (Pomare & de Boer, 1988). The Maori are markedly overrepresented in prison statistics and fare poorly on statistics of social stability such as domestic violence, broken marriages, court appearances, and dependence on social welfare (Department of Statistics, 1993).

GENERAL COMMENTS ON RESEARCH IN MAORI MENTAL HEALTH

Although the anthropological and ethnographic literature on the Maori is extensive (Hanson & Hanson, 1983), the psychiatric literature is sadly deficient. No epidemiological work on psychiatric illness in the Maori has been published. The literature is also largely deficient in an integrative psychological analysis of the Maori and their society and culture, although some commendable efforts have been made by anthropologists (e.g., Salmond, 1978; Hanson & Hanson, 1983; Metge, 1986) and theologians (Johansen, 1954; Smith, 1974). An oral debate on Maori health practices has gone on for a long time and many prominent Maori leaders have been physicians, but it is relatively recently that Maori perspectives on health have appeared in the published literature (Durie, 1985, 1994; *Hui Whakaoranga,* 1984; Rolleston, 1989). An overview of Maori mental health must, therefore, draw upon a somewhat small volume of published work.

Who Is a Maori?

Researchers of Maori issues have often struggled with the difficult task of "defining" a Maori. Different definitions have been used by government departments, legislative bodies, social scientists, health researchers, and educationists, and Hunn (1961) identified ten statutory definitions. The major thrust in the past was to define a Maori by the "degree of biological descent," with the census considering anyone with "more than half Maori blood" as being Maori. There has been a recent shift from this biological grouping to a more sociological one. Sociologists, and the Maori community itself, argued that the more appropriate method of identifying a Maori was by "self-categorization" by the individual, so that anyone who claimed to be a Maori was categorized as one. It was presumed that the subjects used cultural descent as the criterion, although one could not dismiss the possibility that some might still use biological descent as a major factor. This definition is more egalitarian than the previous one, and may also be more appropriate for the study of behavioral patterns. However, it leads to difficulties in situations in which ethnic identification is uncertain, variable, or dual, and may be inappropriate for genetic studies.

Another method that has sometimes been applied is to assess the degree of "Maoriness" and to categorize individuals on the basis of an arbitrarily defined cutoff (Ritchie, 1963). While it may be possible to quantify an individual's degree of affiliation with some core cultural values of a group, the problem of deciding a cutoff has been difficult to resolve, and most researchers do have to resort of some form of self-categorization as a starting point in the delineation of the population for study.

Maoritanga

There is, quite understandably, a lack of agreement on what constitute the core values of Maori culture, but some attempts have been made in this regard. A highly respected Maori leader, the late Sir Apirana Ngata, identified the following eight components as being central to *Maoritanga* (traditional Maori culture): the Maori language; the sayings of the ancestors; traditional chant songs; posture dances; decorative art; the traditional house and *marae* (meeting place); the body of *marae* customs, particularly those pertaining to the *tangi* (death) and the traditional welcome; and the retention of the prestige and nobility of the Maori people (Ritchie, 1963, p. 37). Some attempts have been made by researchers to quantify Maoriness (Ritchie, 1963; Harker, 1971) but these have been considered inadequate and have not been widely accepted. They can be criticized (Metge, 1958) for treating Maori culture as being on a kind of continuum, with traditional values and practices being at one end and European culture at the other, with an implicit assumption that movement toward the *Pakeha* culture was progress or upward mobility. This approach also neglects the relational aspects of culture.

It is useful, nevertheless, to identify factors that the Maori regard as being salient to being a Maori, and my own understanding is that these are: (1) an ineffable emotional and spiritual attachment to the land; (2) sharing of a myth of the origin of the world (from *Rangi* and *Papa*) and of the tribe (migration from the mythical *Hawaiki*), as well as an extensive shared mythology; (3) a well-developed kinship system with strong links with the ancestors providing a continuity with the past; (4) the Maori *aroha* (love), with obligations toward kinsfolk being met even at personal cost; (5) participation in the formal and ritualistic aspects of the culture, the most important being the *hui* (ceremonial gathering); (6) interest in *whakapapa* (genealogy) and Maori history; and (7) the use of Maori language.

PSYCHIATRIC ILLNESS IN THE MAORI: AN ETIC PERSPECTIVE

The Health Experience

Since the Maori and *Pakeha* share the same political, economic, and health systems, but differ markedly on a number of cultural characteristics, they offer an excellent opportunity to compare the illness experience of two ethnic groups (Sachdev, 1989a). A number of aspects of Maori health have been reviewed recently (Awatere, Casswell, & Cullen, 1984; Murchie, 1984; Mackay, 1985; Pomare & de Boer, 1988). Most reviewers agree that the Maori have a pattern of morbidity different from the *Pakeha*, with the Maori performing poorly on many important health statistics. Infant mortality rates are higher for the Maori, and cot-deaths occur twice as frequently in the Maori as the non-Maori. Respiratory diseases cause two to three times more deaths in Maori people at all ages, and the Maori also die more frequently from cancer (except bowel), renal disease, rheumatic and hypertensive heart disease, and diabetes (Pomare & de Boer, 1988). Maori children have an eight times greater morbidity from rheumatic fever, nine times from ear infections and deafness, and are eight times more likely to die from accidents (Durie, 1987). Hepatitis B infections and chronic carriage of the virus, leading to the development of chronic hepatic disease, are extremely high in the Maori. Although there has been a marked improvement in the mortality statistics of the Maori population since the 1970s, particularly in the areas of respiratory, heart, and cerebrovascular disease, the rates of hospitalization for most major causes still is about twice as high for the Maori (Pomare & de Boer, 1988). A significant proportion of this excess physical morbidity is attributable to behavioral factors, in particular, that relating to smoking, alcohol use, obesity, and accidents, and this will be discussed later.

Psychiatric Morbidity Data

The available data on mental illness in the Maori are largely limited to the official Department of Health statistics collected from psychiatric inpatient units and published annually from 1953. The first major survey of Maori patients in mental hospitals was published in 1962 (Foster, 1962), and further surveys have been published periodically. All these data are hospital based, and no population-based surveys have been conducted with the exception of surveys of alcohol abuse (Awatere et al., 1984) and women's health (Murchie, 1984), both of which were limited in their aims. Such data have been called "second-hand information" (Plunkett & Gordon, 1960), and have significant limitations. They do not provide prevalence rates but rather rates-under-treatment or utilization rates, since they exclude the untreated mental illness in the community. The patients seeking hospitalization are a selected group, with multiple factors determining this selection. Furthermore, they are largely a reflection of severe mental illness, usually the psychoses, which constitutes only the tip of the iceberg of total mental illness in the community.

The issue of the appropriateness of applying the Western psychiatric diagnostic classification to the Maori population has never been systematically examined, and it remains an unspoken assumption in all the available data that at least the major psychiatric disorders can be reliably diagnosed irrespective of the ethnic origin of the patient. The author's clinical experience of Maori patients suggests that this assumption may be largely true, but needs a rigorous examination. The data on neurotic and personality disorders, however, should be treated with considerable skepticism because of possible diagnostic difficulties.

Overall Psychiatric Morbidity

Using rates of first psychiatric admissions as indices of visible psychiatric morbidity, the Maori populations shows an increase in morbidity rates since the 1950s, with especially rapid increases in the early 1960s and 1980s (Figure 1). Whether this progression has now ceased is uncertain. For the group as a whole, the average Maori does less well than the non-Maori in his or her risk of psychiatric hospitalization, but the difference is not very marked. The morbidity risk is particularly greater for the young Maori in the age group 20–40 years (Figure 2), and this group has shown a marked worsening over the years. The elderly Maori get admitted less often, but the historical trend in this age group is toward parity with their *Pakeha* counterparts. Children under 10 years have figures comparable with the non-Maori. Surveys of patients in psychiatric hospitals give rates comparable with the first admission rates by ethnicity (Sachdev, 1989a).

The proportion of Maori admitted involuntarily to hospital under the Mental Health Act is similar to that of the *Pakeha*, but relatively more Maori are admitted involuntarily to psychiatric hospitals under the Criminal Justice Act. The readmission rate for the Maori is higher (2.4 readmissions for each admission, compared with 1.8 for the non-Maori).

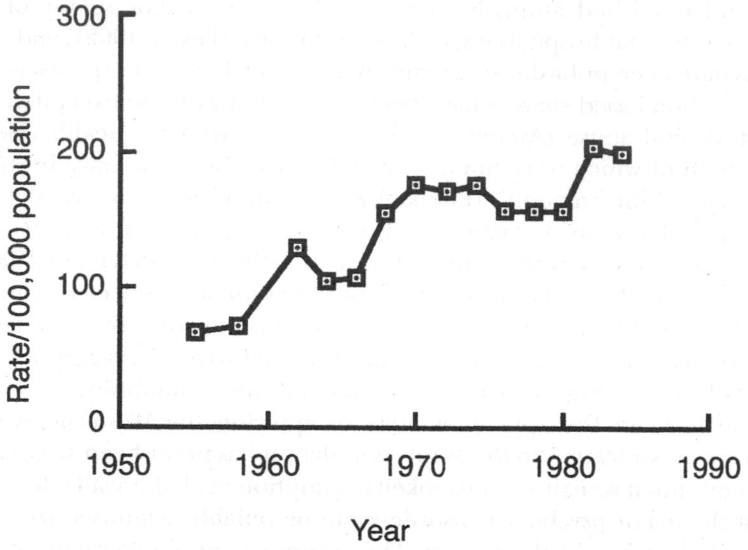

Figure 1. Nonstandardized first psychiatric admission rates for the Maori: historical trend (Department of Health, Wellington). (Reprinted from Sachdev, 1989a, with permission.)

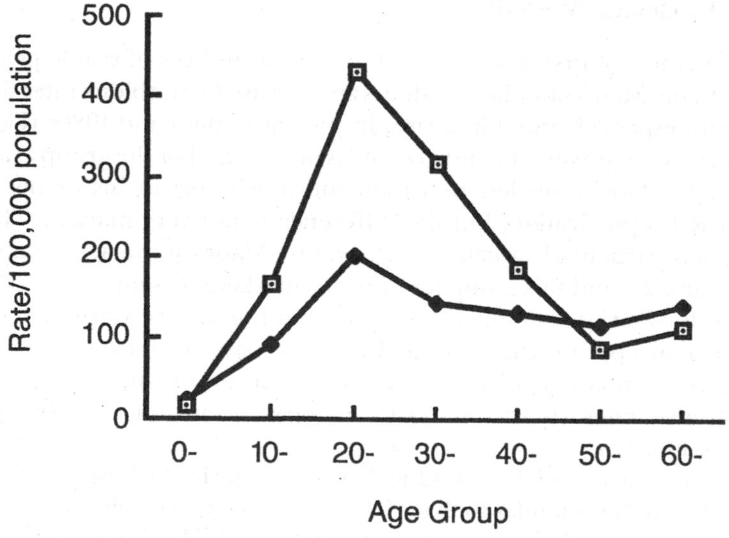

Figure 2. Age-specific rates for 1984 for first psychiatric admissions of Maori (open squares) and non-Maori (Department of Health, Wellington). (Reprinted from Sachdev, 1989a, with permission.)

Psychiatric Morbidity by Diagnosis

When specific psychiatric disorders are examined, schizophrenia and alcohol dependence are overrepresented in the Maori, whereas neurotic depression is less and dementia markedly less.

Schizophrenia. The first admission rates per 100,000 for schizophrenia was 23.7 (adjusted rate 17.1) in 1983, much higher than the 11 per 100,000 for the overall population. Rates of readmission for schizophrenia are also higher. The phenomenology of schizophrenia in the Maori has not been systematically examined, and preliminary data suggest that there may be considerable cultural content in the symptoms (Sachdev, 1989a). Although Maori elders are frequently, and the *tohunga* (Maori priest) occasionally, involved in the management of these patients in many centers, antipsychotic medication is usually accepted and no significant differences in the pharmacodynamics have been noted.

Depressive Disorders. The hospital utilization for manic–depressive illness is not markedly different in the two communities, but relatively fewer Maori are admitted with a diagnosis of neurotic depression. The spectrum of depressive disorders in the Maori has not been examined, and it is not known whether somatic symptoms or absence of guilt characterize depression in the Maori as in many non-Western cultures (Leff, 1981). A significant feature of Maori mental health has been the relatively lower rates of suicide, especially among Maori women. Upon reviewing the 1974–1978 data, Smith and Pearce (1984) concluded that when corrected for age and social class, the relative risk of death from suicide was 0.5 in the case of the Maori male in the age group 15–64 years and 0.4 in the case of Maori women. In the mid-1980s, the suicide rate was 7.9 per 100,000 for the Maori and 12.7 for the non-Maori. The possible reasons for the lower suicide rates have not been examined, but the following have been speculated upon: a negative cultural sanction (Hui Whakaoranga, 1984); group orientation in problem solving, thereby reducing the onus on the individual (Ritchie, 1963); and "outward" psychological orientation, which diminishes guilt and self-blame (Sachdev, 1990c). Another important aspect of Maori culture is the presence of elaborate rituals related to death (*tangihanga*), which are likely to have a positive impact on the psychological response to bereavement (Oppenheim, 1973).

Alcohol Abuse and Dependence. The alcohol-related morbidity and mortality is much higher in the Maori. First admissions for alcohol abuse and dependence have increased steadily since the 1950s, and the increase in the 1980s has been especially marked (Sachdev, 1989a). Because many Maori with alcohol-related problems end up in prison, the hospital figures may underestimate the extent of the problem. Smith and Pearce (1984) calculated that Maori males were 1.9 times as likely as non-Maori to have their deaths recorded as being due to cirrhosis of the liver. The Maori are also more likely to have fatal roads accidents attributable to alcohol intoxication and to be charged with driving under the influence of alcohol. Even though alcohol appears to have a greater impact on Maori health, the Awatere et al. (1984) study suggested that the daily alcohol consumption was about the same for both Maori and non-Maori of either sex. The pattern of drinking, however, was different for the Maori. They drank less often but consumed more on each occasion; the high consumption did not fall with age; and they had more than their share of excessive drinkers.

Comment

The psychiatric hospital utilization rates by the Maori are significantly different from the non-Maori and have shown a major change in the last three decades. If one examines this change by diagnosis (Sachdev, 1989a), it becomes clear that it is accounted for largely by increased number of admissions for alcohol abuse and dependence and personality disorders, and first admissions for schizophrenia and depressive disorders have not changed significantly in this period. This suggests that the change is unlikely to be solely due to a shift in attitude to psychiatric hospitalization or an increasing awareness of psychiatric illness in the Maori community. This historical trend is not dissimilar to that described in other societies at a time of change (Jarvis, 1866; Goldhamer & Marshall, 1949), with psychotic disorders remaining relatively stable and non-psychotic disorders showing an increase during times of stress and socio-cultural change (Krapf, 1963; Spradley & Phillips, 1972). This leads one to consider the hypothesis that the changes in psychiatric morbidity rates reflect the sociocultural change the Maori community has undergone in this period, the most striking being the rapid urbanization. That urbanization has a significant impact on mental health has been adequately documented in the past (Schwab & Schwab, 1978). The change due to urbanization is quite fundamental even when not associated with a cultural change. In the case of the Maori, the move to a city also involves a move into a *Pakeha*-dominated culture. The traditional fabric of society, with the extended family (*Whanau*) as the basic unit, is broken, taking away the support system and the controls on behavior that are so important for the young Maori. Maori from different tribes are thrown together by chance, and the role of the *tangata whenua* (people of the land) becomes quite different. Because of the separation from the kin, traditional child-rearing practices are disrupted. The city, being modeled on a European society, demands a much greater acceptance of the *Pakeha* culture than that necessary in the countryside. To this demanding environment, the Maori brings a relatively poor education and job skills, thereby compounding the disadvantage. The 1960s were the period when rapid urbanization first occurred, and the impact was seen on the mental health of the first generation of Maori urban dwellers. The 1980s were the period when the children of that generation grew into young adulthood and bolstered the psychiatric hospital and prison populations.

A comment must also be made on the use of alcohol by the Maori. One must examine the role of cultural and social factors in attempting to understand the pattern of alcohol use. It can be argued that alcohol is not an integral part of Maori society. Alcohol is not an accepted part of the Maori ceremonial, and is not allowed on the *marae*. The pattern of drinking by the Maori is more akin to that in "dry" societies where the introduction of alcohol has been recent. Negrete (1973) suggested that the negative associations with alcohol, such as unemployment, marital adjustment, and criminality, were more marked in the dry societies. The other major factors are poverty and sociocultural stress (Horton, 1943). It has also been suggested that in the urban setting, the public bar may function as a substitute *marae* (meeting place).

BEHAVIORAL FACTORS AFFECTING PHYSICAL HEALTH OF THE MAORI

As stated above, the Maori have been shown to be at a greater risk of illness and death than the non-Maori. It is estimated that a significant proportion of this excess morbidity and mortality can be attributed to at least four behavioral factors: smoking, obesity, alcohol use, and accidents (Pomare, 1980; Smith & Pearce, 1984). Proportions of excess Maori mortality that could be attributed to behavioral factors were: obesity, 5% for both sexes; smoking, 15% for males and 16% for females; alcohol (excluding alcohol-related accidents), 10% for males and 2% for females; accidents, 17% for males and 8% for females (Smith & Pearce, 1984). These approximate figures serve to highlight the important role played by behavioral factors. In addition, there is a reported excess, not related to social class, of five times or more for Maori mortality due to rheumatic and hypertensive heart disease, nephritis, bronchiectasis, diabetes, and tuberculosis, all diseases for which effective treatment is available, thereby suggesting an inadequate utilization of health services by the Maori or a lack of appropriate services.

For a detailed discussion of the contributions of the individual behavioral factors, the reader is referred to other sources (Smith & Pearce, 1984; Durie, 1987; Pomare & de Boer, 1988; Sachdev, 1990a). The census data as well as two research studies (Stanhope & Prior, 1975; Flight, McKenzie-Pollock, Hamilton, Salmond, & Stokes, 1984) suggest that the Maori have a higher rate of smoking, tend to start smoking earlier, and more Maori women smoke, which they more often tend to continue in pregnancy than the *Pakeha*. There is no evidence to suggest that the psychological or social function of smoking is different in the Maori than in any other ethnic group.

The Maori have a higher prevalence of obesity for both sexes in all age groups in the range 20 to 50 years (Birkbeck, 1979). The majority of the women who participated in the Maori Women's Welfare League Survey (Murchie, 1984) considered themselves to be overweight, and one in eight very overweight. The 1977 National Diet Survey (Birkbeck, 1979) showed that the Maori people ate proportionately more fat (which was usually saturated) and less carbohydrate than the non-Maori. It is difficult to disentangle the various constitutional, environmental, cultural, and personality factors in the etiology of obesity. Some authors have attributed the obesity to changed dietary habits as a result of "Westernization and urbanization" without the changes in behavior that seemingly provide a greater balance in the *Pakeha.* It has been stated that the Maori attitude to obesity is different from the non-Maori, with a greater degree of tolerance of obesity and relatively less preoccupation with thinness (Wakely, 1977). A positive consequence is a lower incidence of anorexia nervosa in the Maori (Hall, 1978). Another possible explanation is based on the externality theory according to which the eating behavior of obese people is determined by external cues rather than internal ones (Schachter & Rodin, 1974). This externality is considered to be a general personality characteristic not restricted to food consumption and ties in to some degree with a largely social and kinship orientation of the Maori (Ritchie, 1963). The contribution of alcohol abuse to obesity must also be considered.

The excess of alcohol-related morbidity and the possible causes of increased alcohol abuse have already been discussed. Death rates from accidents are higher in the Maori after correction for social class. Alcohol may explain a part of this excess, but one must speculate on a greater risk-taking behavior in the Maori, empirical evidence for which is lacking.

The health services-seeking behavior of the Maori and their interaction with the health system have received much recent attention, and these will be discussed later in this chapter.

MENTAL HEALTH OF THE MAORI: AN EMIC PERSPECTIVE

Maori Concepts of Health and Illness

In traditional Maori society, the healthy person was *ora* (well, and in health) and held his *manawa ora* (divine gift of health) dearly. He was *tupu* (growing and unfolding his nature) and imbued with strength, courage, honor, and repute. He held his honor and that of his family and tribe in high regard and had no unavenged insults. Ideally, he was born of a high lineage, and thus had the potential for great *mana* (spiritual power or authority) and *tapu* (under sacred influence). By his accomplishments in warfare, the arts, knowledge of rituals and genealogy, oratory and/or food gathering/fishing, he had furthered his *mana.* He exercised his authority with care and compassion and observed the restrictions imposed by the community. In other words, a healthy Maori person functioned well in the physical (*te taha tinana*), spiritual (*te taha wairua*), psychic (*te taha hinengaro*), and family (*te taha whanau*) dimensions, and each aspect was important for the well-being of the individual. The Maori had a holistic approach to health, with a strong spiritual emphasis.

The two Maori words used to denote sickness and death are *mate* and *aitua*. *Mate* ("to be weakened" or "in want of") denotes deficiency in whatever it describes, and when applied to man, it may mean sickness or injury. The word *aitua* means "of ill omen or unlucky" or "misfortune, trouble, disaster, accident," but it is not commonly used in contemporary references.

The contemporary Maori broadly divide illnesses into two categories: *mate Maori* and *mate Pakeha*. They best understand the former as being caused by supernatural influences described by Maori cosmology, with the latter being explained by the natural causation theories of Western medicine. The Maori also often attribute supernatural causes to an illness and call it *mate Maori* after a trial of Western medicine has failed by their assessment. Much of mental illness falls in the category of *mate Maori*, and therefore strictly falls outside the domain of the doctor trained in Western medicine.

Maori Concepts of Causation of Illness

The role of natural causes in the etiology of illness in Maori society prior to European contact was relatively minor. Most illness was conceptualized in supernatural terms. The most common mechanism of illness causation was the attack and possession by a malevolent *atua* (minor god or supernatural being). The direct cause of an attack by a malevolent spirit was usually an infringement of the law of *tapu* (religious prohibition). The contemporary Maori continues to attribute illnesses to this cause, and the common *tapu* violations are the profane handling of genealogies, improper observance of *marae* etiquette, and improper conduct on burial grounds. A patient of the author saw a Maori Elder who attributed his mental illness to having taken alcohol on to the *marae*. Another patient was said to be ill because she had eaten in a spot that was possibly an ancestral grave.

Illness was also attributed to the covert action of an envious, affronted, or malicious human being who used magic to injure his victim. The most important form was *makutu* (sorcery) in which a magical technique was used by the person himself or with the help of a *tohunga* (priest or expert in spiritual matters). Subsequent to the contact with the European and conversion to Christianity, the belief in this form of illness causation gradually waned, and its hold in contemporary society, while not absent, is weak.

Most contemporary Maori accept Western theories of natural causation of illness, and this has been reinforced by some prominent Maori physicians trained in Western medicine. Some aspects of the traditional beliefs, often in an attenuated form, however, have persisted and may even be unconscious. Furthermore, many Maori attribute psychiatric illness to be a consequence of becoming too "*Pakeha*-like," i.e., because of losing Maori identity and, more importantly Maori "spirituality." The illness is seen as God's punishment, somewhat in a Christian sense but perhaps involving the Maori gods, although this is rarely stated explicitly.

Healing in Traditional Maori Society

All ill Maori traditionally consulted a *tohunga* (priest or expert in spirituality) who first arrived at a hypothesis regarding the cause of the problem, much like diagnosing a disease. The usual procedure after diagnosing the problem was to direct the attention of the offending spirit, and great efforts were made to appease its anger by means of expiatory rites. The *tohunga* had an exalted place in Maori society, and they acted as intermediaries between *mena* and the *atua*. They performed religious ceremonies, explained omens and unusual phenomena, settled tribal disputes, and received important guests. European contact, the work of Christian missionaries who rejected the "heathen" practices of some of the *tohunga*, and the introduction of Western medicine altered the status and role of the *tohunga* markedly. The *Tohunga* Suppression Act of 1907 started the final decline of the Maori priest in the traditional mold (Lange, 1968). Although the act was repealed in 1963, the damage to traditional Maori healing had been done.

To some extent, the knowledge and skill associated with being a *tohunga* have been passed down the generations to the present day in many isolated pockets of Maori society. The topic is rarely discussed openly, but someone in the community is generally aware of how and where to contact the *tohunga* when the need arises. As the knowledge used by the *tohunga* is tribal, the effectiveness of rituals and prescriptions is usually restricted to the members of the tribe, and this poses some problems for the urbanized Maori who has often moved away from the tribal area. With the recent resurgence of Maori culture in New Zealand society, the role of the *tohunga* in dealing with Maori patients is increasingly being recognized, and doctors are not averse to their involvement (Rolleston, 1989).

Some Ethnopsychological Maori Concepts

Mana, Tapu, and Noa. These three concepts lie at the heart of Maori culture, and an understanding of these has implications for the etiology and management of illness. Although the belief in these concepts exists in only an attenuated form in modern Maori society, their importance becomes obvious to any psychiatrist or physician working with Maori patients (Sachdev, 1989b).

Mana refers to "power, authority, or prestige" that is spiritual, originating from the *atua*, and spoken of in relation to persons, spirits, or inanimate objects and never in isolation. Individuals build their *mana* from several sources. Every Maori inherits some *mana* from his or her ancestors. Whether this is more or less depends on seniority of descent or birth order (the firstborn having the greatest), sex (the male having the traditional right to higher *mana*), and the *mana* of the ancestors. Although *mana* was a gift from the gods, it had to be endorsed by others for it to be meaningful. A person could increase this endorsement, and thereby increase the *mana*, by great achievement in traditional spheres such as warfare, oratory, carving, and tattooing; by being a charismatic healer; by marrying someone genealogically senior; by acquiring large amounts of land; and by other similar means. High *mana* could therefore be inherited or acquired, and its maintenance required the continued endorsement by others. It could be lost by failing to live up to others' expectations, by greed or covetousness, or by defeat or humiliation. Presence of high *mana* implied high functioning in all spheres of health listed previously. A physician is, to a Maori, a person with high *mana*, and his healing activities and medicines similarly have *mana*. The *mana* of the medicines, however, depends on their demonstrable efficacy, and an ineffective drug loses its *mana*. Furthermore, the *mana* of the doctor ensures that the Maori patient treats him with respect and indeed awe, and this may at times lead to problems in the doctor–patient interaction (Tipene-Leach, 1978).

Tapu refers to that "under religious or superstitious prohibition" and in common usage, it is in the sense of "sacred" but without the ethical connotations of "moral righteousness" implied in the New Testament (Marsden, 1981). It is a state of being imbued with the power of the gods and of being removed from the influence of the profane or common, and it can be applied to a person, place, thing, or action. It generally has positive effects, implying growth or knowledge or victory, but is also used to characterize objects of situations usually considered unclean such as illnesses, corpses, and so on. Most important functions in traditional Maori society, such as illness and healing, war, death, religion, food, and procreation, were greatly regulated by the laws of *tapu*. As discussed earlier, a breach of such a law was the most common cause attributed to the development of illness.

The obverse of *tapu* is *noa*, and it connotes a state of a person or thing in which the sacred influence has been removed. The *noa* state is common and lacking in spiritual influence, but is desirable in many situations because of the lack of restrictions that accompany being *tapu*. The agents most commonly used to remove *tapu* and make an object *noa* are water, the latrine, female genitalia, and cooked food (Hanson & Hanson, 1983).

One can conclude from this discussion that *tapu* and *mana* were important in Maori society for both social control and the explanation of illness. This gave a common basis for both care (medicine) and control in the society. The principles of causation of illness are clearly important in increasing the power of the sanctions and prohibitions and of the individuals who by birth or accomplishment can explain or embody these sanctions. Were it not for the ever-looming threat of illness, much of the *tapu* would lose its potency and the *tohunga* his power. Illness is a powerful force used to make individuals and groups conform to societal regulations. This common ground for medicine and law (control) is not peculiar to Maori society. Turner (1964) observed a similar synthesis in tribal Rhodesia. Cawte (1974) in fact titled his book on the psychological anthropology of the Australian aborigines *Medicine Is the Law.*

Whakama. *Whakama* is a psychosocial and behavioral construct in Maori society that does not have any exact equivalents in Western societies, although shame, self-abasement, feeling inferior, inadequate, and with self-doubt, shyness, excessive modesty, and withdrawal describe some aspects of the concept (Metge, 1986; Sachdev, 1990b). It represents the feeling state in a person when he or she has felt dishonored in the eyes of others because of having failed to honor obligations to kinsfolk or friends, or because of an insult or fall in self-esteem, or the exposure of a sin or other such violation of group rules. It is important to understand the interpersonal context of the concept. Although *whakama* generally refers to individuals, groups may also be *whakama* because of being put in a weak, disadvantaged, or embarrassing position. The manifestations of *whakama* vary widely from being mild and hardly noticeable to others, to serious and catastrophic, being likened to a fire that scorches everything inside (Sachdev, 1990b).

It is perhaps inappropriate to regard *whakama* as a culture-bound syndrome (Simon & Hughes, 1985). The large behavioral repertoire of *whakama* may include depression, withdrawal, aggressiveness, or adjustment disorder from an etic perspective. It does not have the status of an illness within Maori society. An individual with *whakama* may sometimes be advised to consult a psychiatrist, but this is usually due to an inappropriate construction by individuals from a different culture. The common thread in the phenomena that comprise *whakama* is the explanatory model used by the culture with which it has its unique relationship. It must be mentioned that *whakama* is not unique to the New Zealand Maori but is common in the rest of Polynesia. Similar behaviors have been described in the Cook Island Maori, Samoans, and Niueans (McEwen, 1974, p. 13). The Samoan counterpart is called *musu* in which individuals become withdrawn and sometimes sulky and morose (Gluckman, 1977).

THE MAORI AND THE CONTEMPORARY HEALTH SYSTEM

New Zealand has a health system in the Western, scientific tradition, and can be described as a "dual" system comprising state-funded public provisions and state-subsidized private or voluntary provisions. General practice and other primary care belongs to the latter category. The general (or family) physicians are the point of first medical contact except in emergency situations. Eighty percent of hospitals are state hospitals, which are free, and the remaining 20% subsidized by the state. Psychiatric patients occupy nearly 40% of all hospital beds, although this situation is changing because of a move toward deinstitutionalization. The country spends approximately 8% of the gross national product on health.

Until recently, it was taken for granted that the Maori had accepted the health system and were served well by it. In the last two decades, this belief has been progressively challenged (Durie, 1977, 1984, 1987; Older, 1978; Jacobsen, 1983; Broughton, 1984; *Hui Wahkaoranga*, 1984; Pomare, 1986). The relatively poor health status of the Maori, even after accounting for the socioeconomic status, is one argument to suggest that the Maori have not benefited from modern medicine as much as the *Pakeha*. Most of the differences in the health indices between the two communities can be accounted for by sociocultural and environmental rather than genetic factors (Pomare, 1980; Smith & Pearce, 1984). Lifestyle and behavioral factors, as discussed above, account for much of the variance. In addition, Maori attitudes to Western medicine, problems in the communication between *Pakeha* health professionals and Maori patients, the inflexibility of the health system to accommodate the cultural differences of the Maori, and the relics of traditional Maori beliefs and practices have all contributed to some degree.

Health professionals are predominantly *Pakeha*, with less than 1% medical practitioners, 4% nurses, and 2% social workers being Maori (Durie, 1987). Cultural barriers to communication, therefore, have attracted frequent comment from both Maori patients and the professionals themselves. Even though the Maori speak English, often as their primary language, their command of the language and their use of metaphor and sophisticated nuance have been demonstrated to be poorer than the *Pakeha* (Bray & Hill, 1974). They are more likely to misunderstand indirect expressions and double negatives (Metge & Kinloch, 1979). Durie (1984), a Maori psychiatrist, reported that about half of his Maori psychiatric patients felt inadequate in their usage of English, even though they seemed fluent to the staff members. This can have a detrimental effect on doctor–patient relationship, diagnostic precision, and patient compliance. The Maori emphasize the "body language" more and verbalization less than the *Pakeha* (Metge & Kinloch, 1979), and there is a cross-cultural difference in the interpretation of some signs, which can further compromise effective communication.

Problems in communication that arise when the *Pakeha* professional is ignorant or unsympathetic to the differences in communication style are often exacerbated by attitudinal differences. The Maori patient generally holds the health professional in high esteem, as he or she would hold someone with high *mana.* This can lead to excessive responsibility being placed on the professional and a passive role by the Maori patient during the therapeutic encounter, as well as a reluctance to report adverse effects or lack of efficacy of treatment. The decisions may be left to the "expert" rather than the patient participating in a one-to-one encounter (Tipene-Leach, 1978). The patient also wishes for the *whanau* (family) to be involved, and they usually do so in a manner that may be considered intrusive by *Pakeha* norms.

The Maori utilization of the contemporary health system is also affected by a number of Maori traditions that have persisted, albeit in an attenuated form. While the hold of *tapu* on the modern Maori is limited, it still influences attitudes and behavior, sometimes without reaching awareness. While accepting Western treatment, the Maori may simultaneously be exploring his own or his family's circumstances to find the "real cause," which usually involves the breach of some *tapu* law. Other *tapu* rules may make some of the practices in hospitals unacceptable to some Maori. One of these is the mixing of *tapu* and *noa* things. The most common example given is the mixing of things connected with food or cooking (*noa*) with things connected with the body, especially the head (*tapu*). Sometimes, the Maori family may seek the services of *tohunga* alongside the acceptance of modern medicine (Sachdev, 1989c).

The Maori Response to the Deficiencies of the Health System

Modern Maori leaders realize that to improve the health of the Maori community there needs to be a response from the community itself, such that Western medical technology can be adapted to Maori cultural needs (*Hui Wahakaoranga,* 1984). In the last few years, a number of efforts have been made in this direction, which have been discussed in detail elsewhere (Durie, 1987, 1994; Sachdev, in press). The Maori perspective on health has been repeatedly enunciated, with the emphasis being on health as a holistic concept, involvement of the family, and giving priority to preventative strategies. The Maori leaders have tried to convey this to the decision makers within the health administration, often by inviting members of hospital boards and departments of health to experience *taha* Maori firsthand by visiting the *marae* and listening to Maori concerns. Tribal councils, which have been recently revitalized, have given health a high priority in their new agenda.

One major task was to educate *Pakeha* health professionals in those aspects of *Maoritanga* that are likely to impinge upon the diagnosis and management of Maori patients. The Maori have been willing to educate the *Pakeha* about their culture, and the *Pakeha* has in general been responsive, with most professions now including some such learning as a formal part of the curriculum. There has also been an attempt to increase the number of Maori health professionals, and a system of positive discrimination has been set up in many disciplines to achieve this. The results have been slow but encouraging.

There has been an attempt to enlist the services of Maori individuals with stature in the community who are also versed in *Pakeha* culture to act as cultural interpreters for the *Pakeha* health professionals and the Maori patients. In addition, there is an attempt to train Maori paraprofessionals who would take Western medical practices to their people, either in the hospitals or the community. A number of psychiatric hospitals have enlisted the support of Maori *kaumatua* or *pukenga* (those steeped in Maori culture) to act as counselors for Maori patients and assist and advise the staff in regard to management. Maori ministers, especially those from the Ratana Church, have been particularly involved. The psychiatric hospitals in Auckland have lists of local *tohunga* who can be approached for consultation and referral.

The *marae* has a central place in Maori culture; a place to which the Maori belongs, a place he visits regularly and feels at home in, and a place that has high *mana*. It was for this reason that the suggestion that health clinics and other activities be based at the *marae* had a receptive audience. It was considered the best way to combine the Maori and Western traditions, i.e., to take the best from Western medicine and to deliver it to the Maori in a manner that would be readily accepted. A number of such activities now take place. There is governmental support for the development of *marae* health clinics as part of the distribution of the health resources into Maori hands. The clinic is usually set up with a grant from the Department of Health (about $100,000 in some cases), which is distributed through the Area Health Board. The purpose of the clinic is to complement the community health services already in place. Other health programs have been developed that are based on the *marae* and attempt to train young people, often those with a history of a psychiatric disorder.

The trend of increasing psychiatric hospitalization and rehospitalization of the Maori led to a push toward the development of special psychiatric units that were truly bicultural, i.e., they followed Maori *kaupapa* (value systems), had Maori staff, were bilingual in their communication, but were designed to provide Western psychiatric care. The first such unit was set up in Tokanui Hospital situated in Te Awamutu, about 30 km from Hamilton in the heart of the rich dairy country of Waikato, and was called *Whai Ora* (Maori health unit). A 20-bed ward was used for this purpose, staff members steeped in *Maoritanga* and involved with the Maori community were employed, and a nurse with high *mana* was appointed as the unit manager. The daily routine was run strictly according to Maori *kawa*. Each patient was encouraged to become familiar with his or her Maori roots and identify himself or herself in reference to the ancestors. Instruction was imparted in the Maori language. Egalitarianism was identified as a strong guiding principle, in part as a reaction to the perceived hierarchical structure of the usual psychiatric ward. There was, therefore, a greater tolerance of differences. Following the example of the above unit, many other psychiatric hospitals across the country set up bicultural units, with similar aims but sometimes with different structures. Some of the units, for example, the ones set up in Carrington Hospital in Auckland (*whare paia* and *whare hui*), attempted to move a bit too far out of mainstream psychiatry, thereby causing a great deal of political debate. Most units, however, were successfully able to function within the constraints of modern psychiatry.

The *Hui Whakaoranga* (1984) argued for the training of *Ringa Awhina* (cultural interpreters). A number of forums (see Mackay, 1985) have recommended the training of Maori community health workers. One of the models offered is that of the Aboriginal Health Worker Training Program (Cawte, 1987), successfully used in Australia, and other models are available. The Maori Women's Welfare League advocated the training of what it called Maori Community Health Assistants, with a certificate and a salary. A community-based health education scheme in Auckland, called *Te Koputu Taonga*, trains community health workers who educate Maori families on Health matters. Groups like the *Te Ropu Rapu Oranga* (group holding out good health) have sprung up all over the country. An attempt to deal with the problem of "street kids" and solvent abuse was made by setting up *whare manaaki* (houses of caring), often run by a caring couple with community support. The success of many of these ventures, along with sociocultural and educational projects such as *Rapu Mahi*, *Kokiri*, *Kohanga Reo*, and *Matua Whangai*, has been acclaimed (see New Zealand Official Year Book 1986–87).

The Response from Health Institutions

The political system of the country and the health bureaucracy have also become sensitive to the needs of the Maori community. The Department of Health has progressively supported Maori health initiatives and helped develop programs that are appropriate to their needs. In a major policy statement (Partnership Response, 1988) (*Te Urupare Rangapu*), the government reaffirmed its major objectives with a view to the interests of the Maori: honor the principles of the *Treaty of Waitangi*; eliminate the gaps that exist between the educational, social, economic, and cultural well-being of Maori people; provide for Maori language and culture to receive an equitable allocation of resources and a fair opportunity to develop; and promote decision making in the machinery of government in areas of importance to Maori communities. A number of proposals were made to restore and strengthen the operational base of *iwi* (tribe) by moving toward the development of the *Iwi* Authorities by 1994, based on Maori self-reliance on their own terms and to develop a new Ministry of Maori Affairs (1989), with a role to review and comment on all governmental proposals where it believed a Maori perspective was essential. The above proposals were revolutionary in that the Maori had been given much power to determine their own strategies to deal with their problems and to incorporate the Maori perspective into legislative activities. It will not be until the latter 1990s that the success or failure of these initiatives will be judged.

Resurgence of Other Maori Health Institutions

Maori leaders recognize three principal institutions traditionally regarded as critical determinants of good mental health: *whenua* (land), *whanau* (family), and *reo* (language) (Durie, 1985). The importance of land to the Maori has been recognized by the Waitangi Tribunal, with an increased emphasis on honoring some aspects of the Treaty of Waitangi, the original treaty between the British and some Maori tribes that formally established the British in New Zealand. The importance of *whanau* to the Maori has previously been alluded to. The third aspect, that of *reo*, is now receiving increased recognition and resurgence. One initiative that is of particular importance in this regard is that of *Kohanga Reo.* Under this scheme, a number of day centers have been established for preschoolers that exclusively use the Maori language for everyday communication. The intention is to create truly bilingual people who retain a pride in their own language.

In summary, one would tend to agree with Pomare (1986, p. 411) that "Maoris wish to have a greater say in decisions affecting their health—there is disquiet with existing health services.... These community health initiatives are not intended to replace existing health systems, but rather to provide an alternative where deficiencies exist." These measures, in general, reflect the new cultural consciousness and national pride in the Maori of the early 1990s.

THE FUTURE OF MAORI ETHNOPSYCHIATRY

The examination of the mental health issues of the Maori is rewarding for a number of reasons. It highlights the struggle of a Fourth World people to adapt to a Western capitalist economy and a Western health system and provides some strategies for possible success in such a struggle. The mere promise of First World medicine is not enough for a traditional society to incorporate it. While there has been a superficial acceptance of the health system by the Maori, this has been slow and uneven, and many traditional beliefs and practices have impacted on the adaptation. This has been made more difficult by the rapid sociocultural change that the Maori community has undergone in the last three decades.

The Maori experience suggests that for a health delivery system to be effective, it must take into consideration the cultural background of the community it serves. The recent changes in the health administration of New Zealand is a response to this awareness. Much of the initiative has initially come from the Maori community itself, after the recognition that its needs were not being served. The presence of leadership in the community and the role of spokespersons must also be emphasized. The new initiatives do not mean that the principles of modern medicine must be compromised. In fact, they employ the important principles of community medicine, with a strong basis in preventative strategies. The Maori perspective therefore emphasizes a dimension that has been sadly ignored by medicine in general and can be usefully applied to the entire population.

It is unlikely that the Maori will ever return to the health practices of the precolonial period. The continued study of Maori health, physical and psychiatric, is therefore a study of the dynamic interaction of two systems. Both systems are currently robust, and their future development must therefore be watched with interest. It would be of interest to observe if the Maori disadvantage on many health indicators can be reversed by the new initiatives.

The ethnopsychological concepts of the Maori and their traditional concepts regarding disease and health should continue to be studied. There are many areas that have received little scholarly comment or empirical investigation. Psychiatric epidemiology in the Maori has not been formally examined. No structured instruments for psychiatric diagnosis have been standardized in the Maori population. The phenomenology of psychiatric disorders and their longitudinal course have also been investigated. The influence of Maori culture on personality development was studied in the 1960s (Ritchie, 1963; see Sachdev, 1990c, for an analysis), but much has changed in the society to warrant a further assessment. The lexicon of emotions in the Maori has not been systematically examined. Many Maori individuals have migrated, especially to Australia, and their migration experiences would be insightful.

Research involving the Maori is a sensitive subject in that many Maori feel resentful about misrepresentation or exploitation by *Pakeha* researchers. Should research into the Maori be left, then, to the Maori themselves? There is a long list of Maori scholars and researchers who would accomplish this with competence. I would argue, however, that ethnopsychiatric research should be a joint enterprise between the Maori and the *Pakeha*. A Maori may feel resentful if an outsider comes with a bias or a patronizing attitude, but should have no objections if the culturally different researchers provide a unique perspective or attempt a genuine understanding. A Maori researcher may, on the other hand, be unable to resist the urge to become personally involved in the affairs of the community. Future research into Maori health issues should be a partnership between the Maori and the non-Maori.

Acknowledgments. The author is grateful to the many Maori informants, patients, and friends for the material included in this chapter. Debbie-Maree Bargallie assisted with editing and typing. The figures were prepared by the Medical Illustration Unit of the University of New South Wales, and permission to reprint them was granted by the *Australian and New Zealand Journal of Psychiatry*.

REFERENCES

Awatere, D., Casswell, S., & Cullen, H. S. (Eds.). (1984). *Alcohol and the Maori people.* Auckland: Alcohol Research Unit, School of Medicine University of Auckland.

Best, E. (1924). *Maori religion and mythology.* Dominion Museum Bulletin No. 10. Wellington: Government Printer. (Reprinted in 1976)

Birkbeck, J. A. (1979). *New Zealanders and their diet.* Auckland: National Heart Foundation.

Bray, D. H., & Hill, C. G. N. (1974). *Polynesian and Pakeha in new Zealand education.* Auckland: Heinemann Educational Books.

Broughton, H. R. (1984). A viewpoint on Maori health. *New Zealand Medical Journal, 97,* 290–291.

Buck, P. (Te Rangi Hiroa). (1950). *The coming of the Maori.* Wellington: Maori Purposes Welfare Board & Whitcoulls Ltd. (Latest print 1982).

Cawte, J. (1974). *Medicine is the law.* Honolulu: University of Hawaii Press.

Cawte, J. (1987). Aboriginal mental health. *Australian Aboriginal Studies, 1,* 100–109.

Census. (1986). *New Zealand census of populations and dwellings, 1986.* Wellington: Department of Statistics.

Department of Statistics. (1993). *1991 census of population and dwellings:* Wellington: Department of Statistics.

Durie, M. (1977). Maori attitudes to sickness, doctors and hospitals. *New Zealand Medical Journal, 86,* 483–485.

Durie, M. (1984). Maori referrals to a general hospital psychiatric unit. Presented to the RANZCP 9th Annual Symposium, Social and Cultural Section, Royal Australian and New Zealand College of Psychiatrists, Rotorua, New Zealand.

Durie, M. H. (1985). A Maori perspective of health. *Social Science and Medicine, 20,* 483–486.

Durie, M. H. (1987). Implications of policy and management decisions on Maori health: Contemporary issues and responses. In M. W. Raffel & N. K. Raffel (Eds.), *Perspectives on health policy. Australia, New Zealand and United States* (pp. 201–214). New York: Wiley.

Durie, M. (1994). *Whaiora: Maori health development.* Auckland: Oxford University Press.

Firth, R. (1959). *Economics of the New Zealand Maori* (2nd ed.). Wellington: Government Printer.

Flight, R. J., McKenzie-Pollock, M., Hamilton, M. A., Salmond, C. E., & Stokes, Y. M. (1984). The health status of fourth form students in Northland. *New Zealand Medical Journal, 97,* 1–5.

Foster, F. H. (Ed.). (1962). *Maori patients in mental hospitals.* Special Report No. 8. Medical Statistics Branch, Department of Health, Wellington.

Gluckman, L. K. (1977). Clinical experience with Samoans in Auckland, New Zealand. *Australian and New Zealand Journal of Psychiatry, 11,* 101–107.

Goldhamer, H., & Marshall, A. M. (1949). *Psychosis and civilization: Two studies in the frequency of mental illness.* Glenco, IL: Free Press.

Hall, A. (1978). Family structure and relationships for 50 anorexia nervosa patients. *Australian and New Zealand Journal of Psychiatry, 12,* 263–268.

Hanson, F. A., & Hanson, L. (1983). *Counterpoint in Maori culture.* London: Routledge & Kegan Paul.

Harker, R. K. (1971). Socio-economic and cultural factors in Maori academic achievement. *Journal of the Polynesian Society, 80*(1), 20–41.

Horton, D. (1943). The functions of alcohol in primitive societies: A cross-cultural study. *Quarterly Journal of Studies on Alcohol, 4,* 200–210.

Hui Whakaoranga. (1984). *Maori health planning workshop.* Wellington: Department of Health.

Hunn, J. K. (1961). *Report on department of Maori affairs, 1960.* Wellington: Government Printer.

Jacobsen, C. T. (1983). Family medicine in a Maori community. *New Zealand Family Physician, 10,* 182–185.

Jarvis, E. (1866). Influence of distance from and nearness to an insane hospital on its use by people. *American Journal of Insanity, 22,* 361–366.

Johansen, J. P. (1954). *The Maori and his religion in its non-ritualistic aspects.* Copenhagen: Ejnar Munksgaard.
Krapf, E. E. (1963). Social change in the genesis of mental disorder and health. In H. P. David (Ed.), *Population and mental health* (pp. 97–103). Berne: Hans Huber.
Lange, R. T. (1968). *The Tohunga and the government in the 20th century.* Auckland: Auckland Historical Society.
Leff, J. (1981). *Psychiatry around the globe: A transcultural view.* New York: Marcel Dekker.
Mackay, P. (1985). *The health of the Maori people.* Whangarei: Northland Community College, New Zealand.
Marsden, M. (1981). God, man and universe: A Maori view. In M. King (Ed.), *Te Ao Hurihuri: The world moves on* (pp. 143–164). Auckland: Longman Paul.
McEwen, J. M. (1974). Understanding Polynesians. In D. H. Bray & C. G. N. Hill (Eds.), *Polynesian and Pakeha in New Zealand education.* Vol. II, *Ethnic difference and the school* (pp. 6–15). Auckland: Heinemann Educational Books.
Metge, A. J. (1958). The Rakau studies: A critique. *Journal of the Polynesian Society, 67,* 352–371.
Metge, J. (1976). *The Maoris of New Zealand: Rautahi.* London: Routledge & Kegan Paul.
Metge, J. (1986). *In and out of touch: Whakamaa in cross cultural context.* Wellington: Victoria University Press.
Metge, J., & Kinlock, P. (1979). *Talking past each other.* Wellington: Victoria University Press.
Murchie, E. (Ed.). (1984). *Rapuora—Health and Maori women.* Wellington: The Maori Women's Welfare League.
Negrete, J. C. (1973). Cultural influences on the social performance of alcoholics: A comparative study. *Quarterly Journal on the Study of Alcoholism, 34,* 905–916.
Older, J. (1978). *The Pakeha papers.* Dunedin: John McIndoe.
Oppenheim, R. S. (1973). *Maori death customs.* Wellington: Reed.
Partnership Response. (1988). *Policy statement from the Office of the Minister of Maori Affairs, New Zealand.* Wellington: Government Printer.
Plunkett, R. J., Gordon, J. E. (1960). *Epidemiology and mental illness.* Joint Commission on Mental Illness and Health Monograph Series No. 6. New York: Basic Books.
Pomare, E. W. (1980). *Maori standards of health: A study of the 20 year period 1955–1975.* MRC Special Report series No. 7. Auckland: Medical Research Council of New Zealand.
Pomare, E. W. (1986). Maori health: New concepts and initiatives. *New Zealand Medical Journal, 99,* 410–411.
Pomare, E. W., & de Boer, G. M. (1988). *Hauora—Maori standards of health.* Special Report Series 78. Wellington: Department of Health.
Ritchie, J. (1963). *The making of a Maori.* Wellington: Reed.
Rolleston, S. (1989). *He Kohikohinga: A Maori health knowledge base.* Wellington: Department of Health.
Sachdev, P. (1989a). Psychiatric illness in the New Zealand Maori. *Australian and New Zealand Journal of Psychiatry, 23,* 529–541.
Sachdev, P. (1989b). *Mana, Tapu, Noa:* Maori cultural constructs with medical and psychosocial relevance. *Psychological Medicine, 19,* 959–970.
Sachdev, P. (1989c). Maori elder–patient relationship as a therapeutic paradigm. *Psychiatry, 53,* 393–403.
Sachdev, P. (1990a). Behavioural factors affecting physical health of the Maori. *Social Science and Medicine, 30,* 431–440.
Sachdev, P. (1990b). Whakama: Culturally determined behaviour in the New Zealand Maori. *Psychological Medicine, 20,* 433–444.
Sachdev, P. (1990c). Personality development in traditional Maori society and the impact of modernization. *Psychiatry, 53,* 289–303.
Sachdev, P. (in press). The New Zealand Maori and the contemporary health system: The response

of an indigenous people to mainstream medicine. In S. Okpaku (Ed.), *Clinical methods in transcultural psychiatry.* Washington, DC: American Psychiatric Press.

Salmond, A. (1978). *Te Ao Tawhito:* A semantic approach to the traditional Maori cosmos. *Journal of the Polynesian Society, 87,* 5–28.

Schachter, S., & Rodin, J. (1974). *Obese humans and rats.* Potomac, MD: Lawrence Erlbaum.

Schwab, J. J., & Schwab, M. E. (1978). *Sociocultural roots of mental illness: An epidemiological survey.* New York: Plenum Press.

Schwimmer, E. (1974). *The world of the Maori.* Wellington: Reed.

Simon, R. C., & Hughes, C. C. (1985). *The culture bound syndromes.* Dordrecht: Reidel.

Smith, A. H., & Pearce, N. E. (1984). Determinants of differences in mortality between New Zealand Maoris and non-Maoris aged 15–64. *New Zealand Medical Journal, 97,* 101–108.

Smith, J. (1974). *Tapu removal in Maori religion.* Memoir No. 40. Wellington: Polynesian Society.

Spradley, J. P., & Phillips, M. (1972). Culture and stress: A quantitative analysis. *American Anthropologist, 74*(3), 518–529.

Stanhope, J. M., & Prior, I. A. M. (1975). Smoking behaviour and the respiratory health in a teenage sample: The Rotorua Lakes Study. *New Zealand Medical Journal, 82,* 71–76.

Tipene-Leach, D. (1978, November). *Maoris—Their feelings about the medical profession.* Auckland: Community Forum.

Turner, V. W. (1964). A Ndembu doctor in practice. In A. Kiev (Ed.), *Magic, faith and healing* (pp. 230–263). New York: Free Press.

Wakely, G. (1977). Obesity or authority? Cultural aspects of patient care. *New Zealand Medical Record, 2*(2), 72–79.

V

Jamaicans, Jews, and Gypsies as Minorities or Immigrants

13

Migration, Ethnicity, and Adaptation

Mental Health in Jamaican Children and Adolescents in Jamaica, Britain, and Canada

CHRISTOPHER BAGLEY

INTRODUCTION

Migration is a stressful experience, even for those who are ethnically similar to the host culture and share many of the same values, as research by Murphy (1973) and Eisenstadt (1952) has shown. Thus, the Jewish immigrants to Israel studied by Eisenstadt experienced considerable stress (sometimes manifesting itself as mental illness in the migrant). In Murphy's work, migrants from England to Canada had higher rates of mental illness if they had settled in Francophone Quebec, rather than in Anglophone Ontario.

In examining the psychosocial adaptation of migrants, the concept of *ethnicity* is preferable to that of race, since it defines a set of cultural, linguistic, and religious codes that the ethnic group (which is also often endogamous) uses as markers of identity in terms of values and practices passed between generations. Ethnic groups sometimes, but certainly not always, have physical characteristics (e.g., skin color) that makes them easily distinguishable, in the language of Canadian multiculturalism, as "visible minorities."

CHRISTOPHER BAGLEY • Department of Social Work Studies, University of Southampton, Southampton, England SO17 1BJ, United Kingdom.

Ethnicity, Immigration, and Psychopathology, edited by Ihsan Al-Issa and Michel Tousignant. Plenum Press, New York, 1997.

Newly migrant ethnic groups (and individuals in these groups) may choose between two opposite ideal types of relationship with the host culture: *assimilation* and *integration.* Successful assimilation usually means that many of the markers of identity that have distinguished an ethnic group are rapidly abandoned as the group seeks to merge with the host society. This, it will be argued, is especially easy in Canada (in contrast to Britain), which is a country founded and sustained by immigrants. Some individuals will seek unique ways of adapting to the host culture, and it is a measure of the maturity of a democratic plural society that these individual modes of adaptation can be tolerated (Campfens, 1980). It is this latter concept that sociologists have addressed as integration.

Traditionally, research has shown that immigrants have higher rates of diagnosed mental illness compared with those who did not migrate and with long-settled members of the host community (Bagley, 1971a). There are two distinct reasons for this. The first is the migration of individuals who are maladapted (and may have early signs of mental illness) prior to migration. The easier the process of migration, the more likely this is to occur. This may account for the very high rate of psychiatric hospital admissions in immigrants from Ireland to Britain (Bagley & Binitie, 1970; Cochrane, 1995).

Canada has traditionally maintained strict checks on the health of immigrants, who must be prescreened in the country of origin before being allowed to leave for permanent settlement in Canada.[1] This may account, for example, for the low rates of mental illness in elderly Chinese (aged 60 to 74) migrating from Hong Kong to Canada to join adult children already settled in Canada (Bagley, 1993)

When the aspirations of immigrants for assimilation or integration are thwarted by strong racist forces in society, then various outcomes are possible. Individuals or groups may withdraw into highly traditional cultural patterns (e.g., Pakistanis in Britain: Verma, Mallick, Neasham, Ashworth, & Bagley, 1986), or into rebellious groups (e.g., religious sects such as Rastafarianism in Britain, and its loosely affiliated black youth culture: Bagley, 1975). Some may become political radicals, seeking to change aspects of social structure that restrict their legitimate aspirations. Others, who have naively accepted the symbolic goals of the host society, may retreat into depression or despair and anger against themselves and others, which may become manifest as mental illness (Bagley, 1971b).

[1]The Canada Immigration Act allows for health screening in the country of origin and the rejection of immigrants considered undesirable on grounds of health or political and moral character. This writer (C.B.) emigrated from Britain to Canada in 1980 and had to submit to the most thorough medical examination of his life. He was then subjected to political scrutiny by an immigration counselor (sic) in London who advised: "You may have a job to go to, but we want to know if you're the kind of person we want in Canada."

CANADIAN STUDIES

The work outlined below aims to illuminate the pattern of adaptation of young Jamaicans in Canadian society in terms of identity, self-perception, and ways of perceiving the external world. In children aged 4 to 6, the measures used have been the Pre-School Racial Attitudes Measure (Williams & Morland, 1976) and the self-esteem measure devised by Ziller (1972). In children aged 9 to 11, the instruments used have been a measure of cognitive style, the Children's Embedded Figures Test designed by Witkin, Oltman, Ruskin, and Karp (1971). In children aged 13 to 18, we have used the Coopersmith self-esteem measure (Coopersmith, 1967) as well as the Canadian test of basic skills (King, 1981) in some Canadian and British groups. The usual methodologies of cross-cultural research have been employed, including the methods of back-translation of instruments, establishment of local validity studies where possible, and the use of ethnically appropriate interviewers.

Children in one or more of the three age groups have been studied in Britain, Canada, and Jamaica. The Canadian children studied include those of Anglo-Celtic settlers; children of the Blackfoot nation; and children of Jamaican, Italian, and Japanese settlers (Bagley, 1988a). In addition, comparisons have been made (in terms of self-concept) of adolescents in Britain, Canada (Calgary and Toronto), and other countries (Bagley & Mallick, 1995). These studies, while using methodologies drawn from psychology, have employed the perspective of anthropology in trying to identify culturally specific and culturally universal aspects of human perception, motivation, and behavior that are relevant for the understanding of mental health and adaptation. The purpose of these various research programs, besides undertaking basic work in the fields of culture, cognition, and personality, has been to examine the extent to which the experience of migration and other aspects of social change modifies the basic psychological orientation of children and adolescents and the degree to which particular patterns of psychological orientation are functional or dysfunctional in terms of adapting to a new culture.

JAMAICAN SOCIAL STRUCTURE

Jamaica is a culturally divided, plural society with several layers of ethnicity, power, social stratification, and region (urban versus rural) that are often in conflict (Smith, 1960). Clarke's (1974) model depicting ethnic pluralism in the island shows the similarities of ethnic stratification in 1800 (during slavery), in 1850 (shortly after the emancipation of slaves), and in 1970 (soon after independence from British colonial rule). Jamaica's segmented society is depicted in terms of a color–class pyramid. At the base of each pyramid (in each of the three periods) is a large mass of people, over two thirds of the population, who are black (slaves in 1800, plantation workers in 1860, and a black proletariat in 1970). This black population, descended from African slaves with little admixture with other ethnic groups, remains in poverty: Economic oppression has replaced the bonds of slavery. Higher in the pyramid are the middle and upper classes who are rarely black: They are "brown" (people of mixed race) and a commercial class of Lebanese, Chinese, or Sephardic Jews (usually of Portuguese origin). In 1962, when Jamaica received its independence from colonial rule, whites were at the apex of the pyramid (as they were in the days of slavery), forming a small but powerful ruling class. Only with the election of the Manley government in the 1970s was very much progress made in altering this traditional social structure and power balance.

The old plantation houses still stand, and sugar cane and bananas are still grown and cut. Until the 1970s, some of these plantations were still owned by white families, descendants of the English families who owned these same plantations in the time of slavery. The memory of slavery remains, though it is not often talked about (Segal, 1995). The reasons for this are complex. The folk memory of the experience of slavery is one of pain, suffering, and a deep and abiding anger (Segal, 1995). Life in rural Jamaica is full of African words, customs, and systems of social organization. English culture and language have been imposed on these African cultural roots, and Jamaicans have integrated many European values, feelings, and attitudes into their identity. This has been particularly fostered by an educational system imported from England, with high school achievement examined until the 1980s by examinations imported from England.

The regime of public schools is strict and authoritarian, with large classes and frequent use of corporal punishment. The occupational system is in many ways ascriptive, and there remains evidence of placement of children from poorer families (inevitably, black) in nonacademic classes that do not enable the students to complete high school leaving certificates (Bagley, 1979).

Despite a ritualistic faith in education (particularly among the religious lower classes), alienation from school values seems to be widespread among many black students. A frequently heard cry at the end of a school year is "Free paper come," a poignant echo from the days of slavery. "Free paper come" was the declaration of the masses who carried out a revolt against the British occupation forces and the slave owners in 1832, a revolt based on false rumors of emancipation.

African language forms survive in Jamaican speech; so do family norms, but in ways curiously modified by slavery. The patriarchal, polygynous system of West Africa survives in ways changed by slavery. A common pattern in rural Jamaica is for a man to have married only his first wife according to Christian tradition and to have at least one other wife attached by customary law, who takes the same surname as the senior wife. First and subsequent wives meet one another daily and are usually friends, although there is a clear hierarchy of prestige. Children of wives by the same father may spend long periods of their life in one another's homes, "adopted" by one wife or another when there is a need for a child of particular age and sex in that household. The parties in this polygynous arrangement do not usually see much contradiction between polygamy and fundamentalist Christian practice.[2]

Many African customs, folkways, religious rituals, and family systems survived in various degrees of modification, beneath the surface of a culture that embodies many elements of the culture of the slave-owning and colonial class (Henriques, 1968). The most salient of these is cultural expression through music, but many other forms, including the polygynous tradition of marriage outlined above, remain (see also Barrett, 1976, for an account of many other African survivals in Jamaican culture). Other survivals include the practice of burying family members inside the family compound (a reflection of the tradition of obtaining guidance from the spirits of ancestors).

Cultural and personal evaluations of color, ethnicity, and blackness are an ambiguous and emotional part of Jamaican identity. To be black is to be the descendant of a slave; to have been a slave (or to be similar to one's great grandparents who were slaves) is an emotional fact often cloaked with ambiguity (Segal, 1995). Although slavery was formally abolished in 1834, British rule maintained a harsh colonial regime for at least another 100 years, during which social conditions were only a little above those of slavery and any independent political aspirations of the black population were suppressed.

Jamaica has a set of economic and population problems that are common to many Caribbean countries. These problems stem directly from the economics of slavery: A large African population was brought to these plantation societies to work in a labor-intensive economy. Emancipation was not simply a function of liberal enlightenment; it occurred primarily for economic reasons, when the profit from sugar cane and associated products no longer justified the investment in slaves. Emancipation left a huge population of former slaves that was out of balance with the ecological base of Jamaica; the choice was between emigration and chronic poverty.

Jamaicans have emigrated in large numbers in the present century, to Cuba, Central America, Britain, the United States, and Canada. Remittance from overseas provides a significant part of income for Jamaicans who have not migrated.

The principal aspiration of those who migrate is to increase educational and occupational opportunities and achievement for themselves and their children (Thomas-Hope, 1982). Maintenance of the "private identity"—the

[2]My father-in-law, Owen Young of Clarendon, Jamaica, has 25 children by his four concurrent wives. He and his family have provided many of the cultural insights in this chapter on the enduring Africanness of Jamaican life.

hidden world of African speech forms, rituals, and family practices—remains a covert form of identity, which is liberated or celebrated briefly in holidays in the migrants' country of adoption.

Jamaicans leave their country armed with the legacies of the British colonial regime: English-based educational qualifications and motivations and, often, an excellent command of the Queen's English. These acquisitions put them at an advantage in competition with other immigrant Canadians, other factors being equal, such as the absence of discrimination based on skin color. Blockage of legitimate aspirations of a migrant group by a racist social structure could lead (as in Britain) to various kinds of maladaptive responses, including extreme alienation from the goals of the major society, retreat into subcultures, and deviant behavior of various kinds, including aggression and resistance toward majority institutions (Bagley, 1975). Educationally (in Britain at least) this can lead to maladaptation in school (Rutter, Yule, Berger, Yule, & Bagley, 1974) and early dropout (Bagley, 1982).

Jamaicans in the early years of postwar migration to Britain had a singular faith in both the cultural ascendancy and the fairness of the metropolitan culture: London was seen as the seat of justice as well as the center of the Commonwealth. The expectations of these Jamaican immigrants to Britain of nondiscrimination were quickly disappointed (Bagley & Verma, 1979; Cross & Entzinger, 1988). In contrast, these same aspirations in Jamaican migrants in Canada and the United States were met with a much greater degree of acceptance (Bagley, 1988b). One reason is that Canada, unlike Britain, is a country geared to the acceptance of immigrants who have been carefully selected to fill certain economic roles.

PERCEPTIONS OF COLOR AND ETHNICITY BY JAMAICAN CHILDREN

The evidence on the salience of skin color and blackness in Jamaican society indicates that there is much ambiguity about the meaning and importance of being black, ranging from an extreme and aggressive expression of an African identity (as in Rastafarianism) to an emphasis (by black people) on having "fair" skin and white hair texture and style (Young & Bagley, 1982).

We explored this issue in psychometric terms using the Pre-School Racial Attitudes Measure (PRAM) and the Color Meanings Test (CMT) devised by Williams and Morland (1976). There is a long history of using photographs of black and white individuals in an attempt to assess how children from different ethnic groups perceive and evaluate people whose skin color and general appearance is similar to themselves and their parents; however, the instruments devised and validated by Williams and Morland were the first attempt at standardization of such measures.

The CMT elicits choices from young children between pictures of objects, toys, and animals on the basis of evaluative descriptors (e.g., "nice" versus "nasty" in relation to a white horse and a black horse). The theory underlying this test is that young children aged between 4 and 6 will evaluate the colors black and white in ethnocentric terms: It would be perfectly natural for a young white child to evaluate the color white in positive terms and for a black child to evaluate black positively. The CMT measures young children's color preferences (usually, black vs. white). The PRAM extends the color preferences of the child to evaluations of different colored individuals (black or white), including children, someone like the child, and adults like the child's parents. Using probability theory, Williams and Morland (1976) were able to assess scores on the CMT and PRAM in three ranges: "white bias," "no bias" (random responses), and "black bias." However, their young American subjects, both black and white, showed a strong bias in evaluating the color white over black, frequently expressing dislike of children who looked like them, and parents who were black.

We found that children's evaluations of black and white people were based on their evaluation of the colors black and white (the correlations between the CMT and the PRAM are in excess of 0.60). Again, in the normative group of American children, black preschoolers preferred white figures, as did their white peers (Bagley & Young, 1983). We replicated this work in England with black Jamaican and white children, and obtained quite similar results to the US researchers (Bagley & Young, 1988).

We also administered the CMT and the PRAM to black children in rural Jamaica[3] and found that these children had the highest levels of negative perception of black people of all the groups tested; this was despite the fact that the tester was black and the large majority of these rural children lived in a region (Clarendon) far from the tourist areas and had rarely seen a white person, except on TV. Jamaican children who had migrated with their parents to Britain had a more favorable perception of black people than did children who had not migrated. One possible reason for this was the that experiencing competition with and racism from whites for the first time heightened the ethnic consciousness of these migrants and their children.

What should we expect, then, of Jamaican children who have migrated to Canada? In this society, which appears to be less racist than is Britain (Thomas-Hope, 1982), will children view themselves more positively than Jamaican children in Britain? We first replicated previous work in Britain and Jamaica (carried out in 1977) in 1983 with a fresh sample of children of the same age in rural Jamaica (Bagley & Young, 1988). We found that there had been some positive movement, but still the majority of black children in rural Jamaica preferred the color white and white figures in forced choice responses to the CMT and the PRAM.

In this study we also obtained data on these tests with samples of black

[3]The tester in all of these studies was a black female (Loretta Young).

children ($n = 44$) and white children ($n = 58$) living in urban Toronto, Canada. All of the black children were children of migrants from Clarendon, the rural area of Jamaica where the previous sample had been collected. These black children had significantly more positive perceptions of other black people than did children in any of the previous studies in Britain, Jamaica, or the United States. These results do support the idea (expressed by previous writers such as Henriques, 1968, and Foner, 1973) that the meaning and status of skin color is a psychological struggle for many Jamaicans. Chronically negative self-evaluations may underlie both the development of deviant behaviors (Kaplan, 1980) and vulnerability to stressors, which lead to mental illnesses (Bagley, Mallick, & Verma, 1979; Bagley & Young, 1990). Our data do indicate that children of Jamaican migrants in Toronto seem to change their perception of color quite rapidly, losing many of the negative stereotypes of blackness that seem to have been so deeply rooted in Jamaican culture, being another of the psychological wounds inflicted by slavery (Henriques, 1968).

It is worth noting that we administered the same tests (the CMT and the PRAM) to children in urban Ghana (Bagley & Young, 1988) and found that these children had the most positive perception of blackness of any of the groups we tested. For these children, evaluation of their skin color was a nonissue. They *were* black, and this was a part of their identity that was entirely noncontroversial, without evaluative significance or logical alternative. The colonial enterprise had hardly influenced their country in this respect; but in those unfortunate enough to be captured, enslaved, and transported to the West Indies, being black became synonymous with slavery and shamefulness. Becoming lighter in skin (through the process of concubinage) was the only possibility that most slaves had for upward mobility for many centuries, and a significant color bias emerged.

COGNITIVE STYLES: PERCEIVING AND EVALUATING ONESELF IN SPATIAL CONTEXT

Parallel to work on perceptions of color in different cultural groups, we tested children aged 9 through 11 (often the older siblings of the preschoolers tested with the PRAM) in a variety of cultural settings and under a variety of migrant conditions. The test used, the Children's Embedded Figures Test (CEFT), was devised by Witkin and colleagues (1971) and requires the child to locate shapes embedded in increasingly complex backgrounds. Ability on this task has been shown to vary according to ecological context, social values, and family systems, and is also predictive of some types of psychopathology (Berry, 1976, 1991; Demick, 1991; Santostefano, 1991; Wapner & Demick, 1991; Witkin, 1978; Witkin et al., 1974). Agricultural peoples were shown to be highly field dependent; that is, they found perceiving shapes independently of familiar perceptual and social clues a very difficult task. However, research in China and Japan could not replicate this finding (Bagley, 1995).

Cultures with a strong family tradition that retained even adult children within the folds of family influence fostered highly field-dependent perceptual styles (Berry, 1976). In all cultures, women (who are retained more closely within families) tend to be more field dependent (Witkin et al., 1971). Highly field-dependent individuals tend to be disoriented and highly anxious when separated from traditional spatial and social orientation points, for example, following migration from traditional life in a rural area to a modern urban culture (Bagley, 1983a).

Modernization—the movement from peasant societies based on subsistence agriculture toward degrees of technological modernization and urbanization—has been shown to be associated with the movement toward perceptual field independence (Berry, 1991). A key research question is the time it takes (weeks, months, or years) for a highly field-dependent person to develop a field-independent cognitive style in a new environment. The ultimate expression of field independence is found in the only child of busy, urban middle-class parents, as we found in a study of children in a middle-class commuter suburb in England (Bagley & Wong, 1983).

We hypothesized, based on studies of peasant peoples in Central America (Berry, 1976), that children in rural Jamaica would be highly field dependent (Bagley & Young, 1983). Data bore out this idea, with Jamaican children having levels of field dependence as high as any of the rural groups in developing countries studied by cross-cultural psychologists (Berry, 1991). The question to be asked, in terms of migration, is whether movement from a traditional rural culture to a busy metropolitan area such as London or Toronto is associated with a change in perceptual style, and over what period of time such change takes place. Put another way, how soon will the multiple stimuli of a large city change the perceptual style of children who previously lived in rural Jamaica?

Our argument was that Jamaican students in England, in course of time, would also assimilate English cognitive styles. Our English data supported that idea (Bagley & Young, 1983). Other things being equal, the ability to develop environmentally appropriate cognitive styles is a reflection of an individual's ability to handle stress (Demick, 1991). Rigid, field-dependent cognitive styles in the face of stressors in modern society are associated with higher levels of alcoholism, psychosomatic disorders, hysterical defenses, shame and guilt, paranoia, and obsessive–compulsive disorders (Korchin, 1986).

In a Canadian study in replication of previous work (Bagley, 1985) we showed that children from rural Jamaica rapidly acquired cognitive styles that were similar to those of their Canadian peers in the Toronto schools they attended. These levels of perceptual differentiation were achieved despite the fact that many of the Jamaican children returned to rural Jamaica for summer holidays and retained strong cultural links with their country of origin. As a generalization, we suggested that it took the same time (2 years or less) for a Jamaican child to acquire the perceptual skills and behavioral style necessary for urban survival as it took him or her to acquire another essential Canadian skill, that of the ability to ice skate.

SELF-ESTEEM AND SELF-CONCEPT

The evaluation of self and the external world as it relates to oneself is an aspect of personal functioning and a well-established correlate of psychopathology, such as depression (Roberts & Monroe, 1994). There are competing and perhaps complementary models of how low self-esteem is linked to depression, but one well-supported model suggests that poor self-esteem reflects developmental trauma, adverse family factors, loss of significant others (including the loss of one's culture and close kin through migration), and the stigmatized position of certain ethnic minority groups (a position in Canada chiefly held by Native Indian people: Bagley, 1988a). Poor self-esteem is associated with vulnerability to new stressors, so that the individual is particularly likely to develop depressive illness (Bagley & Young, 1990).

Membership in a particular ethnic group may involve a particular self-conception, especially if that ethnic group has a differential or disadvantaged position in society (Bagley et al., 1979; Louden, 1983). The relationship of Jamaican ethnic identity to self-concept is complex, in part because the issue has become politicized. Black advocates in Britain and America complain bitterly when members of their group are characterized in research studies as having low self-esteem, claiming that this often becomes yet another self-fulfilling prophecy (Stone, 1980). In Canada, we have been able to link ethnicity directly to self-esteem in the case of the preschool children in the study of evaluation of color and ethnicity, using Ziller's (1972) measure of self-esteem (this test requires young children to locate stick figures depicting themselves in relation to "bad" or "good" figures on a felt board). It should be stressed that in young children, self-esteem is a very fluid construct and is frequently rooted in specific situations rather than in personality, so that the child may have high self-esteem in one task or situation and low self-esteem in another. Global measures of self-esteem in young children are likely to have relatively poor validity. Given these measurement difficulties, we have been able to show some links between nonverbal self-esteem and positive evaluation of one's own color in the Toronto children studied (Bagley & Young, 1988). These data indicated no differences in self-esteem between black and white groups.

A comparative study was undertaken between London, England, and Calgary, Canada, examining levels of scholastic achievement and self-esteem (Bagley, 1989). This study showed that by the time they are 13, Canadian students are about a year behind the average British student (from any ethnic group) of this age on standardized scholastic tests (King, 1981). The differences in achievement increase so that by the time of high school graduation there is about a 2-year difference in achievement between British and Canadian students: The average 16-year-old in Britain will achieve at the same level as an average 18-year-old in Canada. Yet this stress on achievement in Britain has its price. We found that the British students had significantly poorer self-esteem than their Canadian counterparts. Moreover, poor scholastic achievement was related to poorer self-esteem in the British students, but not in the Canadians. We speculated that the emphasis in Canadian schools on social participation and personal development (in other areas than the purely scholastic) might be particularly functional for the absorption and adaptation of immigrant groups.

What appears to happen in the process of adaptation is that the major folkways of Canadian culture are rapidly learned, particularly for groups exposed to the inclusive and easygoing nature of the Canadian school system. Such rapid inclusion of aspects of Canadianness into one's personal identity is quite compatible with the retention of a cultural style, which is expressed mainly within the folds of the family or in ethnic organizations. Immigrants in Canada acquire a public culture and present a public face, but often they also retain a private culture that to a greater or lesser extent resembles the old culture in ways that are functional for living in Canada (Bagley & Young, 1991).

This is a hypothesis rather than a conclusion, but it is certainly compatible with our observations and evidence. Suffice it to say that the adaptation of immigrants in Canada is an area neglected by government and academics, perhaps because of the Canadian view of minority adaptation as an easy and straightforward process.

COMMUNITY MENTAL HEALTH STUDIES AND SCHOOL-BASED STUDIES OF MINORITY GROUP ADAPTATION IN CANADA

While hospital-based studies linking diagnoses of formal mental illness are available in Britain (e.g., Cochrane, 1995), similar studies appear to be unavailable in Canada. Wedenoja (1995), in a review of psychiatric studies of Jamaican emigrants, located over 100 studies of Caribbean emigrants in Britain but only five brief, clinical studies in Canada. This is, on the face of things, another indication that ethnicity and race have low salience in Canadian government statistics; immigrants are accepted as newcomers, not as members of racial minorities with marginalized status, to be studied and worried over.

Thomas-Hope (1982) has shown that immigrants from the Caribbean to Ontario in the 1970s were largely satisfied that they had achieved or were achieving their principal goals, acquiring occupational and educational status for themselves and their children. The comparative study in England found that Caribbean immigrants were profoundly dissatisfied and often faced major hurdles of racial discrimination in achieving basic goals of occupational and educational advancement (Bagley & Verma, 1979). Discrimination brings profound stresses. Experiencing discrimination (including the internalized self-evaluation at supposed failure, which should actually be laid at the door of a racist social structure) may actually lead, in some immigrants, to a *social* etiology of schizophreniform psychoses (Bagley, 1971b).

In Canada, because of the absence of hospital-based data on mental illness in immigrants, special studies have to be carried out (e.g., Beiser & Fleming, 1986). The alternative to hospital statistics is the community mental health survey, which randomly samples members of the general population, asking them to complete standardized mental health measures and to give information of any past hospitalizations or consultations for psychiatric illness. Demographic information collected can include a respondent's identification of his or her ethnicity or national origin and heritage. A survey of 679 adults in Calgary (Bagley & Ramsay, 1985) indicated that those with national origin in the United Kingdom had significantly better mental health than those born in Canada, but those born in the United States had significantly poorer mental health. (No other group had elevated profiles for impaired mental health; Native peoples were not included in this urban survey.)

When social class was controlled, the difference between the Canadians of British origin and other immigrants ceased to be significant. The British immigrants were well-educated, professional people, and higher educational and occupational status were both variables associated with better mental health. In addition, immigrants from the United Kingdom are carefully screened on health grounds. However, when education and occupation were controlled, the mental health of the American immigrants remained significantly poorer than that of the native-born Canadians. We speculated, without direct evidence, that the ease with which Americans can cross the border into Canada and obtain permanent residence means that some marginalized Americans (including those with incipient or actual mental disorder) may find their way into Canada. If this is the case, the situation may parallel the British situation in which Irish immigrants are known to have much higher levels of mental illness (Cochrane, 1995). Further community mental health surveys of 1500 men and women aged 18 to 27, randomly selected from the Calgary population, however, could not replicate the earlier finding of poorer mental health in those born in America (Bagley, 1991; Bagley, Wood, & Young, 1994).[4]

[4]One ethnic group in Canada experiences both considerable racial discrimination, high levels of substance abuse, and suicidal behavior: the aboriginal peoples of Canada. We have argued that much of the energy of Canadian racism is directed toward this scapegoated group, allowing immigrants and their descendants to be tolerant toward one another (Bagley & Verma, 1979). An examination of the Alberta Medical Examiner's records on death in suspicious circumstances indicated very high rates of "careless death" (usually associated with alcoholism) and suicide in aboriginal people, in comparison with those from other ethnic groups (Bagley, Woods, & Khumar, 1990).

The small group of Afro-Caribbeans ($n = 17$) in this survey had good mental health levels. All but two of these men and women were professional "secondary migrants" who had spent several years in Toronto before migrating to Calgary to take professional posts.

A 1993 survey of 2120 Alberta high school students, based on stratified random sampling of schools in urban, small town, and rural areas, asked students to complete a questionnaire that included a measure of self-esteem (Kaplan–Rosenberg scale) and Sanford, Offord, Boyle, and Pearce's (1992) measures of mental health, validated in a large community survey in Ontario. Students were also asked to complete a measure of ethnic origins. Few significant variations of five mental health indicators of clinical disorder (emotional disorder, conduct disorder, somatic disorder, hyperactivity, and suicidal ideas and behavior) were found across ethnic groups. Post hoc analysis indicated that the 33 individuals in this survey of Afro-Caribbean descent (including five Jamaicans) had mental health and self-esteem levels similar to those of their peers, but the 177 Native Indian and Metis students had significantly poorer scores on all of the five mental health indicators and on the measure of self-esteem.

Results of this study (some of which are presented in Table 1) indicate similarities of adjustment across ethnic groups. Our findings are essentially

Table 1. Proportions of Visible Minorities Falling into Clinical Categories in 2102 Canadian High School Students

		Percentage in clinical category[b]	
Ethnic group[a]	*N*	Emotional disorder	Conduct disorder
Aboriginal	177	29.9	19.2
Chinese	110	13.7	4.5
Indian subcontinent	88	17.0	7.0
Other Asian	25	20.0	12.0
Afro-Caribbean	33	15.1	9.1
White European	1669	15.3	7.5

[a]Eighteen students with ethnicity based on origins in Central and South America or the Middle East not included in the above table. "Aboriginal" includes 65 Metis, descended from aboriginal unions with early French settlers. Scheffe posthoc analysis of scores on measures of emotional and conduct disorder: Aboriginal $p < 0.01$ on measures of emotional and conduct disorder. "Other Asian" (mainly Vietnamese) $p < 0.05$ on measures of emotional and conduct disorder. No other group comparison significant.

[b]"Clinical categories" based on Ontario norms established by Sanford et al. (1992).

similar to those of Monroe-Blum, Boyle, Offord, and Kates (1989), which found that immigrant children in the Ontario Child Health Study had similar levels of adjustment when compared with children born in Canada. The measures used in that study (described by Sanford et al., 1992) were also those used in our Alberta study (Bagley, Bolitho, & Bertrand, 1995).

CONCLUSIONS

Migrant groups bring various psychological styles and ethnic values and practices into new cultures. Particularly in children these psychological patterns are altered and changed in ways that should facilitate adaptation in an accepting culture; or (if the immigrants are rejected on grounds of appearance or cultural customs) alienation and anger may result, as in Britain and to some extent in other European countries (Cross & Entzinger, 1988). Provided that the host country is not racist and does not reject the race or culture of the migrants and is relatively tolerant of most new migrants, adaptation will be successful and rates of mental illness will be no higher than rates recorded for long-settled immigrants. The school system in Canada provides a kind of openness that is powerfully acculturative, in terms of the public presentation of ethnicity. Canadian multicultural policy nevertheless allows migrants to retain a private ethnic identity in which traditional religion, language, and folkways may still be practiced.

Jamaica, like other Caribbean slave societies, is a synthetic rather than a naturally developed culture: Segmentation and conflict were built in from the very beginning (Van Lier, 1950). In Jamaican society, deep dissatisfactions and conflicts remain. The memory of slavery is strong, but is not often spoken of. The evidence examined in this chapter is consistent with (but does not prove) the idea that in Canada many young Jamaicans experience positive identity changes and can achieve their primary goals of occupational and educational advancement, an aspiration largely thwarted by Britain's racist social structure (Thomas-Hope, 1982).[5] This tentative conclusion must be tempered by the fact that good empirical studies on the extent and nature of racism in Canadian society are generally unavailable.

Multicultural policy in Canada has succeeded by default rather than by design in allowing landed immigrants from Jamaica an upwardly mobile lifestyle, usually unchecked by racial discrimination (Campfens, 1980). A secondary effect of this may be that psychopathology in a formal sense appears to have a low incidence among Jamaican immigrants in Canada. This tentative conclusion must be qualified by the fact that there are no official statistics available on

[5]This is not meant to imply that Canada is free of racism. Discrimination against black people does exist, but it is not of the pervasive and systemic nature of British racism (see Henry & Ginzburg, 1985; Henry & Tator, 1985).

rates of psychiatric illness in Jamaicans in Canada. This probability has to be considered in the context of the fact that vulnerable or mentally ill relatives are left behind in Jamaica and those who do develop mental illness in Canada are sent home. The evidence for this is most clearly established for repatriates from Britain (Wedenoja, 1995), and it is estimated that one in seven of readmissions to Jamaica's principal psychiatric hospital returned from Britain following psychiatric illness (usually schizophrenia). The rate of schizophrenia in West Indian immigrants from Britain has been characterized as "amongst the highest reported in the world literature" (Harrison, 1990). There is no parallel evidence of high rates of schizophrenia in the 100,000 Jamaicans who have settled in Canada or of the potential impact of racism (or the general absence of racism) on mental health in these immigrants. In contrast, British studies (reviewed by Burke, 1984) have identified racism as a factor in high rates of diagnosed psychiatric illness in Afro-Caribbean immigrants in Britain.[6]

My general thesis is that there is a vulnerability in the Jamaican national psyche that is reflected in its citizens who still feel the scars of slavery. When in a racist country like Britain, the whip of racism is raised once again, the reaction is retreat, anger, struggle, and sometimes despair and psychopathology. But a *relatively* less racist country like Canada (which discriminates against indigenous peoples more than against black immigrants) allows the ordinary ambitions of Jamaicans accepted as immigrants to be achieved.

This thesis is advanced tentatively, but is consistent with the evidence we have offered on the evaluation of personal color, the development of a field-independent cognitive style, the development of good self-esteem, and the absence of higher rates of psychopathology in Afro-Caribbeans. This hypothesis is based on surveys and research studies in western Canada, Toronto, and Ontario. The studies have identified, in community mental health and school-based surveys, mental health profiles of Afro-Caribbean migrants that are no different from those of settled white immigrants and their descendants, in contrast to earlier British surveys that showed very high rates of conduct and other disorders in children of Caribbean immigrants (Rutter et al., 1974) and high rates of diagnosed mental illness (Cochrane, 1995).

Research on the psychopathology of immigrants must address a number of methodologically difficult issues: the issue of selection (requiring comparative work with a nonmigrant population from the country of origin); the social psychological issues of identity formation and ways of handling stress in the new

[6]Burke's (1984) argument is that in generally racist societies (Britain, South Africa, Southern United States, Australia, and New Zealand in their treatment of indigenous peoples) racism is a form of profound stress that may cause the emergence of psychiatric illnesses. In Canada, such profound racism appears to be reserved for Native Indian people. While no formal epidemiological studies of psychosis in Native peoples are available, it has been established that they have very high rates of suicidal behavior (Bagley et al., 1990).

culture; the degree to which the new culture accepts the aspirations for assimilation or cultural retention of the immigrant groups; how the host society regards and accepts these aspirations at both government and community levels; how the second generation of immigrants views the compromises and accommodations of their parents; the degree of acculturation of the children of immigrants; and the complex issue of cultural uniqueness in the presentation of signs of mental distress and the possible biases in diagnostic systems.

REFERENCES

Bagley, C. (1971a). Migration, race and mental health. In H. Bleibreu & J. Downs (Eds.), *Human variations: Readings in physical anthropology* (pp. 100–112). Beverly Hills, CA: Glencoe Press.

Bagley, C. (1971b). The social aetiology of schizophrenia in immigrant groups. *International Journal of Social Psychiatry, 17,* 292–304.

Bagley, C. (1975). Sequels of alienation: A social psychological view of the adaptation of West Indian migrants to Britain. In K. Glasser (Ed.), *Case studies on human rights and fundamental freedoms* (pp. 252–285). The Hague: Nijhoff.

Bagley, C. (1979). A comparative perspective on the education of black children in Britain. *Comparative Education, 15,* 62–81.

Bagley, C. (1982). Achievement, behaviour disorder and social circumstances in West Indian and other immigrant groups. In G. Verma & C. Bagley (Eds.), *Self-concept, achievement and multicultural education* (pp. 107–148). London: Macmillan.

Bagley, C. (1983a). Cultural diversity, migration and cognitive styles. In J. Berry & R. Samuda (Eds.), *Multicultural education in Canada* (pp. 355–364). Toronto: Allyn and Bacon.

Bagley, C. (1983b). Cognitive styles, ethnicity, social class and socialization in cross-cultural perspective. In C. Bagley & G. Verma (Eds.), *Multicultural childhood: Education, ethnicity and cognitive styles* (pp. 3–15). Aldershot, UK: Gower Press.

Bagley, C. (1985). Education, ethnicity and racism: A European–Canadian comparison. In S. Modgill (Ed.), *Multicultural education: The interminable debate* (pp. 10–19). Falmer, UK: Falmer Press.

Bagley, C. (1988a). Cognitive style and cultural adaptation in Blackfoot, Japanese, Jamaican, Italian and Anglo-Celtic children in Canada. In G. Verma & C. Bagley (Eds.), *Cross-cultural studies of personality, attitudes and cognition* (pp. 120–143). London: Macmillan.

Bagley, C. (1988b). Education for all: The Canadian dimension. In G. Verma (Ed.), *Education for all: A multicultural perspective* (pp. 98–117). Falmer, UK: Falmer Press.

Bagley, C. (1989). Self-concept and achievement in British and Anglo-Canadian high school students. *Canadian and International Education, 18,* 77–78.

Bagley, C. (1991). The prevalence and mental health sequels of child sexual abuse in a community sample of women aged 18 to 27. *Canadian Journal of Community Mental Health, 10,* 103–116.

Bagley, C. (1993). Mental health and social adjustment in elderly Chinese immigrants in Canada. *Canada's Mental Health, 41,* 6–10.

Bagley, C. (1995). Field independence in children in group-oriented cultures: Comparisons from China, Japan and North America. *Journal of Social Psychology, 135,* 523–525.

Bagley, C., & Binitie, A. (1970). Schizophrenia and alcoholism in Irishmen in London. *British Journal of Addictions, 65,* 3–7.

Bagley, C., Bolitho, L., & Bertrand, L. (1995). Ethnicity and mental health in Canadian high school students. Unpublished paper, University of Calgary.

Bagley, C., & Mallick, K. (1995). Negative self-perception and the structure of adolescent stress in Canadian, British and Hong Kong students. *Perceptual and Motor Skills, 81,* 123–127.

Bagley, C., Mallick, K., & Verma, G. (1979). Pupil self-esteem: A study of black and white teenagers in British schools. In G. Verma & C. Bagley (Eds.), *Race, education and identity* (pp. 176–191). London: Macmillan.

Bagley, C., & Ramsay, L. (1985). The prevalence of suicidal behaviors, attitudes and associated social experiences in an urban population. *Suicide and Life-Threatening Behavior, 15,* 151–160.

Bagley, C., & Verma, G. (1979). *Racism, the individual and society.* Farnborough, UK: Saxon House.

Bagley, C., & Wong, L. (1983). Cognitive style and group independence in English 10-year-olds. In C. Bagley & G. Verma (Eds.), *Multicultural childhood: Education, ethnicity and cognitive styles* (pp. 63–80). Aldershot, UK: Gower Press.

Bagley, C., Wood, M., & Khumar, H. (1990). Suicide and careless death in an aboriginal population. *Canadian Journal of Community Mental Health, 29,* 127–142.

Bagley, C., Wood, M., & Young, L. (1994). Victim to abuser: Mental health and behavioral sequels of the sexual abuse of males in childhood. *Child Abuse and Neglect, 18,* 683–697.

Bagley, C., & Young, L. (1983). Class, socialization and cultural change: Antecedents of cognitive style in Jamaica and England. In C. Bagley & G. Verma (Eds.), *Multicultural childhood: Education, ethnicity and cognitive styles* (pp. 16–26). Aldershot, UK: Gower Press.

Bagley, C., & Young, L. (1988). Evaluation of color and ethnicity in young children in Jamaica, Ghana, and Canada. *International Journal of Intercultural Relations, 12,* 45–60.

Bagley, C., & Young, L. (1990). Depression, self-esteem and suicidal behavior as sequels of sexual abuse in childhood. In M. Rothery & G. Cameron (Eds.), *Child maltreatment: Expanding our concepts of helping* (pp. 183–219). Hillsdale, NJ: Lawrence Erlbaum.

Bagley, C., & Young, L. (1991). The rights and duties of immigrants. *Policy Options, 12,* 17–18.

Barrett, L. (1976). *The Sun and the drum.* London: Heinemann.

Beiser, M., & Fleming, J. (1986). Measuring psychiatric disorder in Southeast Asian refugees. *Psychological Medicine, 16,* 627–639.

Berry, J. (1976). *Human ecology and cognitive style.* Beverly Hills, CA: Sage.

Berry, J. (1991). Cultural variations in field dependence-independence. In S. Wapner & J. Demick (Eds.), *Field dependence–independence: Cognitive styles across the life span* (pp. 289–308). Hillsdale, NJ: Lawrence Erlbaum.

Burke, A. (1984). Racism and psychological disturbance among West Indians in Britain. *International Journal of Social Psychiatry, 30,* 50–68.

Campfens, H. (1980). *The integration of ethno-cultural minorities in the Netherlands and in Canada.* The Hague: The Government Publishing Office for the Ministry of Cultural Affairs.

Clarke, C. (1974). *Jamaica in maps.* London: University of London Press.

Cochrane, W. (1995). Mental health minorities and immigrants in Britain. In I. Al-Issa (Ed.), *Handbook of cultural and mental illness: An international perspective* (pp. 347–360). Madison, CT: International Universities Press.

Coopersmith, S. (1967). *The antecedents of self-esteem.* San Francisco: Freeman.

Cross, M., & Entzinger, H. (1988). *Lost illusions: Caribbean minorities in Britain and the Netherlands.* London: Routledge.

Demick, J. (1991). Organismic factors in field dependence–independence: Gender, personality and psychopathology. In S. Wapner & J. Demick (Eds.), *Field dependence–independence: Cognitive styles across the life span* (pp. 209–244). Hillsdale, NJ: Lawrence Erlbaum.

Eisenstadt, S. (1952). The process of absorption of new immigrants in Israel. *Human Relations, 5,* 1–20.

Foner, N. (1973). *Status and power in rural Jamaica: A study of educational change.* New York: Teacher's College Press.

Harrison, G. (1990). Searching for the causes of schizophrenia: The role of migrant studies. *Schizophrenia Bulletin, 16,* 663–671.

Henriques, F. (1968). *Family and colour in Jamaica.* London: McGibbon and Kee.

Henry, F., & Ginzburg, E. (1985). *Who gets the work? A test of social discrimination in employment.* Toronto: Urban Alliance on Race Relations.

Henry, F., & Tator, C. (1985). Racism in Canada: Social myths and strategies for change. In R. Bienvenue & J. Goldstein (Eds.), *Ethnicity and ethnic relations in Canada: A book of readings* (pp. 40–59). Toronto: Butterworth.

Kaplan, H. (1990). *Deviant behavior in defence of the self.* Palisades, CA: Goodyear.

King, E. (1981). *The Canadian Test of Basic Skills.* Toronto: Nelson.

Korchin, S. (1986). Field dependence, personality theory, and clinical research. In M. Bertini, L. Pizzamiglio, & S. Wapner (Eds.), *Field dependence in psychological theory, research and application* (pp. 45–56). Hillsdale, NJ: Lawrence Erlbaum.

Louden, D. (1983). Self-esteem and cultural identity in black adolescents in Britain. In C. Bagley & G. Verma (Eds.), *Multicultural childhood: Education, ethnicity and cognitive styles* (pp. 124–149). Aldershot, UK: Gower Press.

Monroe-Blum, H., Boyle, M., Offord, D., & Kates, N. (1989). Immigrant children: Psychiatric disorder, school performance, and service utilization. *American Journal of Orthopsychiatry, 59,* 510–519.

Murphy, H. (1973). Migration and the major mental disorders. In C. Zwingman & M. Pfister-Ammende (Eds.), *Uprooting and after* (pp. 100–115). Heidelberg: Springer-Verlag.

Roberts, J., & Monroe, S. (1994). A multidimensional model of self-esteem and depression. *Clinical Psychology Review, 14,* 161–181.

Rutter, M., Yule, B., Berger, M., Yule, N., & Bagley, C. (1974). Children of West Indian immigrants: Rates of behavioural deviance and psychiatric disorder. *Journal of Child Psychology and Psychiatry, 15,* 241–262.

Sanford, M., Offord, D., Boyle, M., & Pearce, A. (1992). Ontario Child Health Study: Social and school impairments in children aged 6 to 16 years. *Journal of the American Academy of Child and Adolescent Psychiatry, 199,* 60–67.

Santostefano, S. (1991). Cognitive style as a process coordinating outer space with inner self: Lessons from the past. In S. Wapner & J. Demick (Eds.), *Field independence–dependence: Cognitive styles across the life span* (pp. 269–288). Hillsdale, NJ: Lawrence Erlbaum.

Segal, R. (1995). *The black diaspora.* London: Faber & Faber.

Smith, M. (1960). Social and cultural pluralism in Jamaica. *Annals of the New York Academy of Sciences, 83,* 763–777.

Stone, M. (1980). *The education of the black child in Britain: The myth of multiracial education.* London: Fontana Books.

Thomas-Hope, E. (1982). Identity and adaptation of migrants from the English-Caribbean in Britain and North America. In G. Verma & C. Bagley (Eds.), *Self-concept, achievement and multicultural education* (pp. 227–239). London: Macmillan.

Van Lier, R. (1950). *The development and nature of society in the West Indies.* Amsterdam: Royal Institute of the Indies.

Verma, G., Mallick, K., Neasham, T., Ashworth, B., & Bagley, C. (1986). *Education and ethnicity.* London: Macmillan.

Wapner, S., & Demick, J. (Eds.). (1991). *Field dependence–independence across the life span.* Hillsdale, NJ: Lawrence Erlbaum.

Wedenoja, W. (1995). Social and cultural psychiatry of Jamaicans at home and abroad. In I. Al-Issah (Ed.), *Handbook of culture and mental illness: An international perspective* (pp. 215–230). Madison, CT: International Universities Press.

Williams, J., & Morland, K. (1976). *Race, color and the young child.* Chapel Hill: University of North Carolina Press.

Witkin, H. (1978). *Cognitive styles in personal and cultural adaptation.* Worcester, MA: Clark University Press.

Witkin, H., Oltman, R., Ruskin, E., & Karp, S. (1971). *A manual for the Embedded Figures Test.* Palo Alto, CA: Consulting Psychologists' Press.

Witkin, H., Price-Williams, D., Bertin, D., Christiansen, B., Oltman, P., Ramirez, P., Van Meel, M., & Van Meel, J. (1974). Social conformity and psychological differentiation. *International Journal of Psychology, 9,* 11–29.

Young, L., & Bagley, C. (1982). Self-esteem, self-concept and the development of black identity. In G. Verma & C. Bagley (Eds.), *Self-concept, achievement and multicultural education* (pp. 191–211). London: Macmillan.

Ziller, R. (1972). *Manual for the self–other orientation inventories.* Delaware, NJ: University of Delaware Press.

14

The Mental Health of Jews Outside and Inside Israel

YORAM BILU and ELIEZER WITZTUM

INTRODUCTION: THE QUESTION OF JEWISH PREDISPOSITION TO MENTAL ILLNESS

Since they emerged on the world scene in the second millennium BCE, the Jews have been, in terms of historical continuity and impact on human civilization, one the most visible groups on the globe. The unique fusion of a pioneering religious monotheism and peoplehood in Judaism created a strong sense of group consciousness; but this sentiment could only seldom be translated into a political suzerainty in the contested territory where Jewish collective identity had been crystallized. Between the destruction of the Temple in Jerusalem by the Romans in the first century CE and the establishment of the State of Israel in 1948, most of the Jews had lived in scattered communities among other peoples. As an ethnically, culturally, and religiously distinct minority they were subject to oppression and persecution to an extent hardly matched in human history, but they managed to survive despite their anomalous and endangered existence in the Diaspora. This dialectic of persecution and survival gave rise to polar views regarding the mental health of the Jews. While their resilience and adaptability, together with their intellectual and cultural achievements, were

---

YORAM BILU • Department of Psychology, and Department of Sociology and Anthropology, The Hebrew University of Jerusalem, Jerusalem 91905, Israel. **ELIEZER WITZTUM** • Mental Health Center, Ben-Gurion University of the Negev, Beer-Sheva 84170, Israel.

Ethnicity, Immigration, and Psychopathology, edited by Ihsan Al-Issa and Michel Tousignant. Plenum Press, New York, 1997.

taken as an indication of exceptionally good mental health, even more attention was focused on the psychic toll on existence of prolonged duress.

The notion of the inherent susceptibility of the Jews to specific forms of mental illness was part of the received wisdom of the Western medical and psychiatric establishment throughout the 19th and the early 20th centuries. Well-known figures like Charcot, Kraft-Ebbing, and Lombroso subscribed to and propagated this notion, though they accounted for it differently. Charcot attributed the fact that "nervous illnesses of all types are innumerably more frequent among Jews than among other groups" (quoted in Gilman, 1993, p. 94) to the inbred weakening of the nervous system. Kraft-Ebbing expressed the view that the Jew was liable to neurasthenia because he was "an overachiever in the arena of commerce or politics" (quoted in Gilman, 1993, p. 95). Lombroso, himself a Jew, discarded the concept of "degeneration" when he discussed his own people and he saw Jewish proneness to mental illness as stemming from a "residual effect of persecution" (quoted in Gilman, 1993, p. 101).

In the fin de siècle medical discourse, these accounts represented paradigmatic views about the mental health of the Jews. Charcot's stance is congruent with a host of biological–racial views that emphasized hereditary factors intensified by excessive inbreeding as directly affecting Jewish constitution. Kraft-Ebbing's formulation echoes a wide array of explanations focusing on "typical" Jewish dispositions and practices, from "the restless striving for profit" (which puts excessive pressure on the brain) and extreme cosmopolitanism to preoccupation with mysticism and enhanced sensuality. While these two lines of reasoning were cloaked with the dignified scientific terminology of Western medicine and psychiatry of the time, from a present-day perspective they sometimes appear as informed by antisemitic stereotypes created in the pagan world and disseminated in the Christian orbit throughout the centuries (Heinemann, 1939–40).

The third, more empathic view, encompasses a wide variety of environmental–historical explanations that highlighted various adverse conditions characteristic of Jewish life as a marginal minority as distress-enhancing factors. The exponents of this view, many of whom were Jewish physicians, typically put the blame on the crippling yoke of "a 2000-year Diaspora" and "a struggle for mere existence up to emancipation" (Gilman, 1993, p. 100). In premodern Europe it was the oppression and persecution of the Jews as the emblematic Other, religiously hated, culturally despised, and socially rejected, that were deemed the main reason for their susceptibility to psychopathology. But these psychic scars from the past were now augmented by the giant leap from traditional to modern life, enabled by the Emancipation, which exposed the Jews, ill-prepared and marginal, to the pressures and adversities of civilization and made them an easy prey to mental illness. Since the malevolent effects of this transition were most strongly felt by East European Jewish males coming out from the closed world of orthodoxy, the analysis marked them as a population at a particular risk. This view, most blatantly expressed in the argument that "(T)he Jewish population (of Warsaw) alone is almost exclusively the inexhaustible source of the supply of specimens of hysterical humanity, particularly the hysteria in the male, for all the clinics of Europe" (Fishberg, 1911, p. 6), became the standard view in European psychiatry.

From the mid-19th century up to the first decades of the 20th century, statistical studies have documented the higher incidence of mental illness among European Jews in comparison with the populations around them (Gilman, 1993, p. 103; Murphy, 1982). The gap was particularly noted for the affective disorders, which emerged, like hysteria and neurasthenia before them, as maladies predominated by Jews. The association of depression with Jews of East European extraction, still consistently being reported in the psychiatric literature (see below), gave rise to the colloquial diagnostic label *melancholia agitata Hebraica* (Hollingshead & Redlich, 1958).

As Gilman (1993) and Murphy (1982) cogently contend, the aforementioned statistics were probably inflated by the disproportionate concentration of the Jews in urban areas, which are less tolerant than rural areas to the presence of mentally ill in society. It is also possible that urban Jews had developed a better network for the identification and treatment of illness. Nevertheless, the overrepresentation of Jews in specific types of mental illness was too recurrent to be explained away by methodological considerations alone. Gilman (1993) identifies the psychic pain instigated by overt social pressures and specifically the predicament of displacement and immigration as an important trigger to mental instability. Murphy (1982), while doubting the immediate association between acute grief reaction following persecution and *melancholia Hebraica*, highlights the sociocultural variables of geographic mobility and the severance of earlier communal ties as the mediating link underlying the differential statistics.

What can a contemporary student learn from the case of East European Jewry in the late 19th and the early 20th centuries? First, the debate demonstrates how difficult it is to disentangle myth from reality in a field of study strongly pervaded by emotion and social stereotypes. Second, it highlights the futility of approaching the issue at hand with global, context-free conceptualizations focusing indiscriminantly on "the Jewish race." The susceptibility of East European Jewry to certain types of psychopathology appears historically situated. It was influenced by a particular constellation of political and sociocultural factors that were not the lot of Jewish populations in other places and in other times. A genetic factor underlying this susceptibility is made unlikely by the fact that in New York, for example, Jews of the same extraction did not have higher admission rates for affective psychosis than other immigrants in the 1920s (Malzberg, 1931). Differential findings like this also exclude a pancultural factor stemming from a "common Jewish heritage." Note, for example, that in Amsterdam between the two world wars an excess of affective disorders was evident among Ashkenazim (Jews of East and Central European extraction) but not among Sephardim (the descendants of the Jews expelled from the Iberian peninsula at the end of the 15th century) (see Grewel in Kohn & Levav, 1994). In line with current views of "race" and "ethnicity" as cultural constructions more than purely physical, biologically based essences, Jewish reality appears highly complex and diversified. The differentiating impact of a millennia-long diasporic existence in a wide variety of geographically removed and culturally distinct settings, augmented by increasing (but differential) processes of secularization and assimilation that corroded the importance of Jewish religion as a unifying factor, has constituted the Jewish universe as sharply divided communities that sometime appear more akin, in appearance and lifestyle, to the indigenous populations around them than to each other. This picture has been only partially changed by the establishment of Israel, as we shall soon see.

Third, the notion that European Jews were predisposed to psychopathology had political implications with direct bearings on the question of the mental health of contemporary Jewry. As mentioned before, Jewish medical practitioners, rather than denying the stigma of mental instability, attributed it to the degenerating effects of the Jewish anomalous and precarious existence in the Diaspora. The Zionist movement offered the most radical solution to the Jewish problem. In its utopian vision, the "new Jew" who would grow up as a sovereign citizen in his own homeland would be entirely exempt from the psychic complexes that characterized his kin and ancestors under the oppressive conditions of life in exile (Levav & Bilu, 1980). Needless to say, this naive expectation could not be fully realized. The establishment of Israel may have liberated the Jews living there from the crippling yoke of a "2000-year Diaspora," but at the same time it created new foci of stress, stemming from the multiple military, political, economic, and sociocultural problems that the young country had to withstand from its inception. On the other hand, the contemporary Jewish communities in the Western world, where most of the studies on the mental health of Jews outside Israel have been conducted, live today under relatively auspicious conditions to which the classic Zionist arguments of the "negation of the Diaspora" do not apply. The Zionist reply would be that political freedom and economic welfare do not guarantee psychological stability. The task of forging and maintaining a Jewish identity outside Israel, in a shrinking Jewish world characterized by secularization and assimilation, may be particularly vexatious. In the last analysis, a comparison of Jewish life in Israel and in the Diaspora in terms of psychological well-being appears complicated and equivocal.

The radically divergent modes of Jewish existence that evolved in Israel and abroad call for a comparative discussion. We start with a very brief survey of the mental health of Jews outside Israel, based on Sanua's (1989) comprehensive review on contemporary Jewry. Then we move to Israeli Jewry (Bilu, 1995), which constitutes the main focus of this chapter.

THE MENTAL HEALTH OF JEWS OUTSIDE ISRAEL

Since most of the studies on the mental health of non-Israeli Jews were conducted in North America, the conclusions derived from them should not be overgeneralized. American Jewry constitutes the largest Jewish community in the world and also the strongest in terms of economic power and social status, but it certainly cannot be taken to represent the entire gamut of contemporary Jewish existence in terms of ethnocultural variability.

Epidemiological studies have found that, in comparison with Protestants and Catholics, Jews were concentrated more in the mild or moderate categories of impairment and less in the serious categories. In terms of specific categories, Jews tended to have more cases of psychoneuroses (and correspondingly had the highest rate of ambulatory treatment) and affective disorders, but they had less schizophrenia, disorders related to advanced age, alcoholism, and drug addiction (Cooklin, Ravindram, & Carney, 1983; Hollingshead & Redlich, 1958; Malzberg, 1962, 1963; Strole, Langer, Michael, Opler, & Rennie, 1962). Higher rates of major depression and dysthymia and lower rates of alcohol abuse were also found among American Jews in recently collected data from the National Institute of Mental Health (NIMH) Epidemiological Catchment Area Study (Yeung & Greenwald, 1992; Levav & Kohn, 1995).

Most of the clinical studies that compared Jewish and non-Jewish patients dealt with schizophrenic and affective disorders. More than in other ethnic groups, the family dynamics of Jewish psychotics and schizophrenics have been characterized by pathological mother–child relationship fraught with overprotectiveness and ambivalence (Sanua, 1963, 1989). In terms of subtypes of schizophrenia, Breen (1968) found that American Jews tended to have higher rates of hebephrenic, catatonic, and simple types and lower rates of paranoid type as compared to African Americans. He suggested that this pattern was the result of emphasis in Jewish families on strong ties, the withholding of aggressive expression, and the development of dependency.

The vulnerability of Jews to depression, indicated in the epidemiological studies discussed above, is strongly supported by clinical research dealing with psychiatric samples and cases. The challenge is how to account for "one hundred years of psychiatric literature (that) have made reference to Jews being at a higher risk to affective disorders" (Levav & Kohn, 1995, p. 3) without resorting to genetic explanations based on the problematic notion of the "Jewish race." One major explanation is the aggression internalization hypothesis (Sanua, 1989). The fact that Jews tend to be underrepresented in mental disturbances characterized by the loosening of inhibitions, such as alcoholism, drug abuse, and antisocial behaviors (see below), may be taken as an indirect corroboration of this hypothesis. One may wonder whether this postulated inhibition has been informed by moral values and cultural ideals inscribed in Jewish religion or by a collective defense mechanism stemming from a centuries-long existence as a threatened minority. Another explanation highlights the marginal position of Jews in society as a key factor (Fernando, 1975).

As Sanua (1989) has suggested, the social and cultural explanations for the higher incidence of depression among Jews should not be viewed as mutually exclusive:

> The tensions developing from an achievement-seeking and highly ethically oriented system, which does not permit release through acting out or alcohol abuse, together with some sense of alienation caused by marginality, may both be factors having cumulative effects. (p. 195)

The low prevalence of alcoholism among Jews in the Western world is well documented (Calahan, 1970; Monteiro & Schuckit, 1989; Schmidt & Popham, 1976; Skolnick, 1958). Since excessive drinking among Jews was found to be related to alienation from Jewish culture and religious orthodoxy and weakening of family ties (Glassner & Berg, 1984; Glatt, 1975), "the great Jewish drink mystery" (Keller, 1973) appears to be associated with the internalization of Jewish cultural mores and values (Snyder, 1962; Skolnick, 1958; Singer, 1958).

THE MENTAL HEALTH OF JEWS IN ISRAEL

As aforementioned, the Zionist ideology envisioned the establishment of a Jewish homeland as a panacea to the multitudinous ills of the Jews' anomalous existence in the Diaspora. In demographic terms, Israel, with a fast-growing Jewish population of over 4.5 million, appears more viable than the Jewish communities in the West; and in psychological terms, Israeli Jews appear more secure in their Jewish identity than most Jews abroad. On the other hand, Israel faces the cumbersome task of developing and maintaining a modern democracy under continuous disruption by emergency conditions. These conditions, particularly the persistent military and terrorist threats and the need to absorb the massive waves of Jewish immigrants (to whom Israel is committed ideologically), exert considerable pressures that are likely to enhance mental distress.

After reviewing general epidemiological data, we will focus on some major sociocultural and politicohistorical variables that appear to have bearing on the mental health of Israelis: intra-Jewish ethnocultural diversity, immigration (focusing on the recent exodus of Jews from the ex-Soviet Union and from Ethiopia), the Holocaust, and war-related trauma (focusing on the recent wars in Lebanon and in the Persian Gulf).

Epidemiological Data on Mental Health among Israeli Jews

Community studies reviewed by Aviram and Levav (1981), though barely comparable methodologically, produced fairly consistent findings. In all of them, psychoses and neuroses were higher among women than men, but the gap was reversed for personality disorders. Higher rates of emotional disorders were also noted among Israeli of lower socioeconomic status and immigrants when compared to Israelis of higher socioeconomic status and native-born, respectively. These patterns were reestablished in more recent studies (e.g., Levav & Arnon, 1976; Levav & Abramson, 1984).

Ethnicity appears only tenuously related to psychopathology In Jewish Israeli society. It is true that Sephardim or Mizra'him ("Easterners") have been usually overrepresented on various scales of emotional distress (e.g., Maoz, Levy, Brand, & Halevi, 1966), but when social class was effectively controlled, this effect immediately subsided. It appears that the higher morbidity rates of Sephardim are more strongly associated with socioeconomic disadvantages, given their general underprivileged position in Israeli society, rather than with ethnicity per se (Eaton, Lasry, & Sigal, 1979; Levav & Abramson, 1984).

Research based on the national register data encompassing all admissions to inpatient psychiatric facilities since the early 1950s (Rahav, Popper, & Nahon, 1981) portrayed mental disorder in Israel as a relatively stable and persistent phenomenon, in which groups of different residential locations, ethnic origin, cultural background, and immigration cohorts are represented in roughly equal proportions. This picture is at odds with other epidemiological studies based on hospital admissions that have reasserted the contribution of variables such as immigration and social class to differential rates of psychopathology (e.g., Gershon & Leibowitz, 1975; Halevi, 1963). In common with community studies, however, it has been found that the association between ethnicity and mental disorders is intricate and defies generalizations. This intricacy calls for a closer look at the ethnic factor and its effect on psychopathology among Israeli Jews.

Ethnicity and Mental Health among Israeli Jews

It should be noted that the Ashkenazi–Sephardic dichotomy is far from representing two monolithic blocks of contrasting cultural worlds. It is true that upon immigrating to Israel Ashkenazi communities usually had been more exposed to modernization processes than their counterparts from Africa and Asia. But in view of the wide cultural differences between, say, Jews of Morocco, Yemen, Iran, and India, it appears that in lumping them together researchers have created a rich but near-vacuous ethnic amalgam.

Ethnic origin appears to be associated with differential prevalence rates of specific forms of psychopathology. Particularly, higher rates of schizophrenia were found among Sephardim, while Ashkenazim were overrepresented in affective disorders (e.g., Gershon & Leibowitz, 1975; Miller, 1979). We discussed the well-documented association of Ashkenazi Jews with depression consistently found in studies in Europe and in America. But the Israeli data must be evaluated with caution, since most of the studies that yielded it did not control for social class variables (cf. Eaton & Levav, 1982). Kohn and Levav (1994) found severe methodological problems in all ten studies that found that Ashkenazim had higher rates of affective disorders than Sephardim.

Sephardim appear to have higher rates of personality disorders, alcoholism, and drug addiction (Aviram & Levav, 1981; Snyder & Palgi, 1982). Since these disorders may be taken as indicators of "social pathology," it is reasonable to assume once again that socioeconomic factors play a more decisive role here than ethnicity per se. In accounting for the fact that Sephardim have higher rates of criminal behavior and prostitution, Eaton and co-workers (1979) have emphasized that they constitute a socially disadvantaged group, exposed to more stressful life events and less equipped to cope with crisis situation than Ashkenazim. The dire consequences of this underprivileged status are likely to be lower self-esteem and increased hostility against socially advantaged groups. In this vein, Landau (1975) has found that the homicide rate among Sephardim was twice as high as among Ashkenazim. By contrast, Ashkenazim showed higher levels of inward-oriented hostility. Miller (1976) has demonstrated that suicides rates were higher among Ashkenazim, though Sephardim have higher rates of attempted suicide.

While in most epidemiological studies the broad ethnic categories of Ashkenazim versus Sephardim seem to prevail, culturally oriented psychiatrists, psychologists, and medical anthropologists have collected rich data on specific mental configurations common in ethnocultural groups defined by country of origin. The review of this material is beyond the scope of this chapter (see Bilu, 1995, and Levav & Bilu, 1980, for discussions of psychiatric syndromes in various Jewish groups in Israel), but in the following section, ethnicity will be discussed in the context of the mental health of two recently arrived immigrant groups.

Immigrants at the Door: Russian and Ethiopian Jews in Israel

"The ingathering of the exiles" of the scattered Jewish people in its historical homeland has been the ultimate Zionist reason for Israel's establishment and existence. The cardinal importance accorded to immigration in Israel is reflected on many levels: It is inscribed in Israeli state legislation, as the "Law of Return" unconditionally entitles every Jew to become an Israeli citizen; it is encapsulated in the positive meaning ascribed to the word "immigration" in Hebrew—*aliya* or "ascent"; and it is reflected in the coordinated efforts invested by the state to facilitate the absorption of the newcomers. The history of Israeli society can be portrayed as a succession of immigration waves, from the first, prestate *aliyot* (pl.) of idealist "pioneers," who shaped the social and political infrastructure of the future state and provided it with a once-potent socialist Zionist ethos, to the poststate nonselective *aliyot* of Holocaust survivors from Europe in the late 1940s and the Sephardic or Mizrahi Jews from the Muslim orbit in the 1950s and the 1960s. The *aliyot* of Jews from the ex-Soviet

Union and from Ethiopia, started in the 1970s and the 1980s, are the most recent layers in the immigrant society of Israel.

As a stressful event, the dire consequences of immigration—culture shock, status loss, low self-esteem, and a growing sense of marginality and alienation (e.g., Shuval, 1982)—might have direct bearings on the emotional well-being of the newcomers. In Israel, however, the ideological climate is very favorable to immigrants, and the resources invested in absorption are supposed to mitigate the predicaments of homecoming. In addition, the culturally oppressive "melting pot" ideology of the early postindependence years gave way to a more tolerant policy of ethnocultural pluralism.

These stress-alleviating factors notwithstanding, from a mental health perspective most immigrant groups to Israel should be viewed as populations at risk. This is particularly true when the newcomers' Jewish identity or Zionist convictions are not strong enough to inoculate them ideologically against inevitable hardships; when the cultural gap between their native society and Israeli culture is wide and disorienting; when they cultivate unrealistically high expectations of "homecoming," which later, when shattered, exacerbate a sense of frustration and despair; when they are exposed to the painful gap between a welcoming ideology and a cold, sometimes hostile, stereotypically based responses of old-timers; and when they were exposed to considerable stress and trauma before and during immigration. As we shall show, most of these risk factors are relevant to the recent immigrations from the ex-Soviet Union and Ethiopia.

Mental Health Problems of Russian Immigrants. The first massive wave of immigrants from the Soviet Union took place in the 1970s and included some 150,000 newcomers. The second, bigger wave, precipitated by the collapse of the Soviet Union, has encompassed thus far more than 400,000 newcomers. This recent influx has made Russian Jews the largest Jewish group in Israel today. Both populations share a similar demographic and occupational background, which makes them one of the most highly educated and professionally trained *aliyot,* but they differed in their motivation for immigration. While the first wave was fairly ideological, propelled by a massive Jewish and Zionist revival, most people in the second wave were pushed to emigrate from the former Soviet Union because of adverse life conditions.

The "cultural character" of the immigrants conveys the imprint of "Homo Sovieticus" (Goldstein, 1984), the product of an oppressive social system that emphasized restraint, obedience to authority, and conformity with the collective at the expense of emotional expressivity and individuality, but at the same time inadvertently propagated dogmatism, mistrust, and cynicism. This background, exacerbated by tenuous links to Jewish heritage (in the more recent immigrants) and cultural ethnocentrism, has made the absorption of many of the recent newcomers a difficult task, posing a potential threat to their emotional well-being. We base our discussion of the current research on the mental health of these immigrants in Israel on a recent review by Lerner, Mirsky, and Barasch (1994).

A nationwide survey of recently arrived immigrants found that they were significantly more demoralized than a matched Israeli representative sample (Lerner et al., 1994). The same demoralization scale was used in an earlier study to compare Soviet Jews who immigrated to Israel and the United States in the 1970s (Flaherty, Kohn, Levav, & Birz, 1988). While the immigrants to the United State indicated more improvement in their standards of living, the Americans were also significantly more demoralized, and hence at higher risk for developing a psychiatric disorder. The difference is explained by the more welcoming ambiance and stronger social support experienced by the immigrants to Israel, as well as by the higher saliency of a common Jewish identity (presumably stronger in the first place among those who chose to immigrate to Israel). In line with this explanation, it was found that recent immigrants from the former Soviet Union who had a stronger Jewish identity were less susceptible to depression and other symptoms (Epstein, 1992). Aside from a strong Jewish identification, a subjective feeling of having social support was also found to be a distress-mitigating factor (Lerner et al., 1994). In contrast, enhanced demoralization was associated with former residence in areas in the Ukraine, Belorussia, and Southern Russia exposed to increased radiation following the Chernobyl disaster, as well as in the former Central Asian Soviet republics. Radiation anxiety and a particularly noted cultural distance from Israeli society are likely to be the respective mediating factors.

Since one of the peaks of the recent immigration from the ex-Soviet Union in 1990–1991 coincided with the Persian Gulf crisis and the Gulf War, it was possible to examine the impact of these potentially stress-enhancing events on the well-being of the newcomers (Lerner et al., 1994). Contrary to expectation, it was found that demoralization among the immigrants had *decreased* following the war. Probably the common experience of war had a unifying effect on all Israelis, facilitating a feeling of belongingness in the newcomers and temporarily abating the ongoing predicaments of absorption. Even high-risk immigrants—single parents, the handicapped, and the elderly—were only modestly affected by the Gulf War. Mirsky, Barasch, and Goldberg (1992) have found that their complaints during and after the war were primarily related to everyday objective difficulties of absorption rather than to the war as stress-enhancing event.

Although immigrants from the former Soviet Union tend to suffer from increased levels of demoralization, they are more reluctant than Israelis to refer to psychiatric and psychological facilities for help (Levav, Kohn, Flaherty, Lerner, & Eisenberg, 1990). Nevertheless, given the higher rates of nonspecific distress (demoralization) among immigrants, it is not surprising that they are overrepresented in psychiatric admissions (reported in the central psychiatric case register). Popper and Horowitz (1992) have found that in 1990–1992 the admission rate among immigrants was about 35% higher than in the general population and the proportion of those who remained hospitalized more than 1 year was 50% higher. Half of the admissions occurred within the first 3 months after *aliya.* More hospitalized immigrants than Israelis were diagnosed as suffering from depression, a psychiatric label strongly associated with demoralization. These high rates of morbidity presumably stem from the stress of transition and the lack of social support to which certain at risk groups—physically or mentally handicapped, the elderly, people migrating on their own, and one-parent families—are particularly exposed. Due to the nonselective character of the immigration to Israel and to the peculiar sociological and demographic features of ex-Soviet Jewry, these groups constitute a considerable portion of the immigrant population (Lerner et al., 1994).

In addition to the groups just specified, adolescent immigrants are at a particular risk since in their case, age-related emotional instability may be superimposed on and exacerbate the agony and pain of "ordinary" absorption. Studies summarized by Lerner et al. (1994) show how ill-equipped are these adolescents (being less autonomous, more dependent, and more morally rigid than their Israeli peers) to function in a democratic ambiance that valorizes personal freedom and personal responsibility. Many of them, exposed to the drastic changes in the ex-Soviet Republics following the collapse of the Communist regime, had suffered from symptoms of disorientation already prior to *aliya.* Given that their emotional attachment to Judaism and their motivation to immigrate to the Jewish state were meager in the first place, it is not surprising that many of them display hostility toward everything Israeli and tend to seclude themselves in "cultural enclaves" of their peers (Mirsky & Kaushinsky, 1988, 1989; Mirsky, Ginat, Perl, & Ritzner, 1992).

In order to meet the psychiatric needs documented above, a community mental health approach has been applied to the newcomers, with a special emphasis on outreach and prevention. Aside from assigning positions of mental health professionals to that end, the program includes retraining immigrant psychologists and psychiatrists in Western mental health approaches, acquainting Israeli practitioners with the cultural background of the newcomers and providing them with culturally sensitive tools, and promoting veteran immigrants as mediators in self-help programs (Lerner et al., 1994).

Mental Health Problems of Ethiopian Immigrants. For many centuries Jews have been living in tiny communities in northern Ethiopia, making their living through simple agriculture and craftsmanship. Although devotedly observant, their religious traditions, limited to biblical law, were quite distinct from mainstream Judaism from which they were effectively cut off until the modern era. Only in 1973 were they officially recognized as Jews by the rabbinical establishment in Israel, and this recognition paved the way for their *aliya.* Two dramatic peaks in the immigration of Ethiopian Jews were Operation Moses (1984–1985), in which thousands of Jews who had fled to refugee camps in the Sudan were secretly transferred to Israel, and Operation Solomon (1991), which brought to Israel the remnants of Ethiopian Jewry, concentrated in Addis Ababa, in a special airlift (Budowski, David, & Eran, 1994; Lerner et al., 1994). Following this exodus, the Jewish Ethiopian community in Israel ("Beta Yisrael") presently numbers over 55,000.

A convergence of stress factors makes the immigrants from Ethiopia susceptible to emotional problems. First, the enormous gap between Ethiopian and Israeli society and culture is very difficult to bridge. Coming from a rural, technologically simple background, marked by an authoritative atmosphere, rigidly defined social roles, religious devotion, focus on the extended family, and little formal education, Ethiopian Jewry is probably the most traditional group of newcomers ever to stake a claim in the "Israeli dream." In contrast to the modern Israeli ethos, which emphasizes equality, assertiveness, openness, initiative, and direct speech, Ethiopian Jews' social codes value hierarchical ranking, humbleness and politeness, emotional restraint, patience, and indirect speech. This discrepancy, aggravated by high visibility due to skin color distinctiveness and lingering doubts regarding the newcomers' Jewish origin, is a fertile ground for cross-cultural misunderstandings that might lead to distress and demoralization.

Second, many of the immigrants who came to Israel during Operation Moses underwent an arduous odyssey, replete with traumas (severe malnutrition, attacks by soldiers and bandits, death of close relatives, illnesses in the camps), which taxed them physically and emotionally. Many of the newcomers, particularly youngsters, separated from their kin on the way, had to withstand the predicaments of homecoming without the support of their extended families. To help them accommodate to the new country under these inauspicious preconditions, Ethiopian Jews were housed for long periods of time in special absorption centers where they enjoyed extra social and material support. While these centers mitigated to some extent the culture shock of the newcomers, they also promoted their dependence on the absorbing authorities and secluded them from Israeli reality (Ben-Ezer, 1992).

Clinical and ethnographic studies have documented the adverse emotional effects of traumatization and culture loss on the newcomers (Arieli, 1988; Arieli & Aycheh, 1993; Minuchin-Itzighson & Hanegbi, 1988). Grief and mourning reactions were particularly noted, but they often found expression through somaticized idioms of distress (Ben-Ezer, 1990; Ratzoni, Apter, Blumensohn, & Tiano, 1988) and culture-specific syndromes (Durst, Minuchin-Itzighson, & Jabotinsky-Rubin, 1993; Schreiber, 1995). A mental health survey of adult Ethiopian Jews living in one urban community (Arieli, 1992; Arieli & Aycheh, 1993) found that more than one quarter of them suffered from moderate to severe symptoms of anxiety, depression, somatization, and sleep disorders. The severity of psychopathology was correlated with the severity of trauma on the way to Israel, as well as with age, low level of education, difficulties in language acquisition, and concern over the lack of religious observance in Israel. While psychopathology usually declined with the length of residence in Israel, it was judged to be quite high even 5 years after *aliya.*

The high rate of suicide among Ethiopian Jews is a tragic indication of the sense of hopelessness that many of them experience in face of the difficulties of absorption. Ratzoni, Blumensohn, Apter, and Tiano (1991) have found that Ethiopian adolescents hospitalized following suicide attempts suffered from dissociative states and somatization disorders. Arieli, Gilat, and Aycheh (1994) interviewed the relatives of 44 Ethiopian Jews who committed suicide between 1983 and 1992 in order to chart the "profile" of high-risk individuals. It was found that the typical victim was a young married male who displayed the clinical picture of depression, behaved oddly prior to the suicide act, but did not express his wish to kill himself.

When immigrants from Ethiopia succumb to the pressures of *aliya,* they often articulate their inchoate experiences of distress through cultural idioms that render the administration of mental health care particularly challenging. In many cases, the psychological basis of the patients' complaints may be hard to trace, given the cultural prescription of emotional restraint and concealment of hurt and the tendency toward somatization. The cultural construction of distress is lucidly displayed in cases of *zar* possession recently reported among the newcomers (Arieli & Aycheh, 1994; Grisaru & Witztum, 1995). In this culture-specific syndrome, based on the belief in the *zar* spirits as agents of affliction, women are far more susceptible to the attack of the spirits, which is manifested in a wide variety of dissociative symptoms. The traditional therapy is not exorcistic but symbiotic: The healing rituals are not designed to expel the invading spirits but to transform them into allies through institutionalizing a lifelong relationship with them within the *zar* cult (see Bourguignon, 1979).

Zar-related behavioral problems were found in about 10% of the admissions to two outpatients clinics in Israel (Arieli & Aycheh, 1994; Grisaru & Witztum, 1995). Since other variants of possession illness, specific to other Jewish groups, had rapidly attenuated following immigration and modernization (see Bilu, 1980, 1985), the future vicissitudes of the *zar* spirits in Israel may serve as an index of the pace of enculturation of Ethiopian Jews in Israel. In any case, the readiness of Israeli mental health practitioners to view the *zar* illness behavior within its cultural context and to incorporate the rituals of the *zar* cult into their therapeutic arsenal (see Grisaru & Witztum, 1995) is an important step in the direction of building a culturally sensitive system for providing mental health care to the immigrants from Ethiopia. In this vein, culturally attuned screening devices are being developed to assist mental health workers in the early identification of signs of emotional distress among the newcomers (Youngmann & Minuchin-Itzighson, 1993).

The Shadow of the Holocaust

The extermination of 6 million Jews by Nazi Germany during World War II, probably the most systematic genocide ever committed in human history, has left an indelible impact on Jewish individuals and communities all over the world. This impact is particularly vivid in the State of Israel, the establishment and existence of which have been politically and morally tied to the complex Holocaust heritage. No less than 300,000 survivors lived in the country in 1993, and the loss of relatives and kin casts a shadow on almost every Israeli family of European origin. On the collective level, the Holocaust has become, after years of denial and repression, a major tenet of Israel's civil religion (Liebman & Don Yehiya, 1983), inscribed on its "sacred space" (in the form of national monuments for commemoration) and embedded in its "sacred time" (in the form of the Holocaust Day, a festive day for remembrance). As a major formative experience in the construction of the Israeli national identity, with continuous reverberations in all the arenas of Israeli public discourse, the Holocaust has far-reaching bearings on the mental health of Israelis. This review is limited to the impact on survivors and their descendants.

According to clinical studies in Israel and abroad, Holocaust survivors were subject to a "massive cumulative trauma" (Keison, 1992) that had long-lasting effects on their mental health, which manifested, among other things, in depression, nervousness and irritability, sleep problems, disturbed vitality, fatigue, and memory problems (e.g., Eitinger, 1964; Matussek, 1975). The configuration of symptoms displayed by survivors, designated "concentration camp syndrome," was assigned a special category in the International Classification of Diseases and Related Health Problems, 10th edition, referred to as "enduring personality changes after catastrophic experience" (World Health Organization, 1992). In terms of the current psychiatric classification, post-traumatic stress disorder and pathological grief reaction appear to cover together most of the symptoms of the survivors.

Given the methodological pitfalls of clinical studies, epidemiological community studies in which matched nonclinical populations survivors and controls are examined in a context that is not manifestly related to the Holocaust constitute the best means for assessing the effects of massive psychic trauma. Levav (1994) carefully reviewed seven such studies conducted 25 to 40 years after the Holocaust. In all of the studies it was found that survivors had significantly higher levels of psychological distress. To illustrate, the most recent of these studies (Fening & Levav, 1991) found that survivors had a 70% rate of demoralization compared with 16% among the comparison group. The data strongly support the dose–effect hypothesis (the greater the trauma, the more severe the psychopathology) and the priority of trauma-enhancing stressors over premorbid personality variables in accounting for the symptoms. The main variable responsible for not succumbing to psychopathological distress among survivors was social support (Antonovsky, 1979). Contrary to a suggested "hardening effect" (Shuval, 1957–58) with advanced age, late effects increase rather than abate (Dasberg, 1987). The potential vulnerability of the survivors became especially apparent when they were exposed to renewed trauma, such as threat of cancer (Baider, Peretz, & Kaplan De Nour, 1992, 1993) and SCUD missiles attack during the Gulf War (Solomon & Prager, 1992).

Whereas the generation of survivors is gradually shrinking, the adverse effects of Nazi persecutions might persist through the transgenerational transmission of psychopathological patterns. Many clinical studies conducted in Israel and abroad have supported this possibility, thus marking the offspring of the survivors, "the second generation," as an especially vulnerable group. Several mediating mechanisms that impaired parental abilities and family functioning were postulated, such as overinvolvement, withdrawal, emotional constriction, pathological grief, and excessive preoccupation with past traumas. In contrast to clinical studies, however, research based on matched groups has failed to reveal higher morbidity rates in the second generation in comparison with controls (e.g., Leon, Bucher, Kleinman, Goldberg, & Almagor, 1981; Schwartz, Dohrenwend, & Levav, 1994; Weiss, O'Connell, & Siiter, 1986; Zlotogorski, 1983). This does not mean that the impact of the Holocaust is being altogether abated with the demise of the survivors. Findings suggest that offspring of Holocaust survivors seem to have developed unique coping mechanisms that enabled them to deal with their parents' psychological burden (Keinan, Mikulincer, & Rybnicki, 1988). Thus, they appear less individuated from their parents (Brom, Kfir, & Dasberg, 1994; Halik, Rosenthal, & Pattison, 1990) and are less disposed to externalize aggression (Nadler, Kav-Venaki, & Gleitman, 1985). But the differences in coping style (Rose & Garske, 1987) and in character organization (Felsen & Erlich, 1990) should not be misinterpreted as indicating stronger susceptibility to psychopathology. There is some evidence, however, that offspring of Holocaust survivors suffered from higher rates of psychopathology in childhood, when the relations with their parents were intense and continuous, but the symptoms subsided later on (Levav, 1994).

Jewish survivors immigrated to other countries besides Israel, but very few studies sought to compare their mental health to that of Israeli survivors. Contrary to the view of Israel as a therapeutic venue (Schneider, 1988), Tabory and Weller (1987) found a greater degree of mental impairment among Israeli survivors in comparison with survivors in Montreal. It might well be that the perpetually tense military situation prevalent in the country together with the numerous memorials and ceremonies commemorating the Holocaust are triggers for retraumatization. The association between the Holocaust and the persistent military threat in Israel, abundant in both public and private discourse, brings us to the effects of war-induced stress on the mental health of Israelis.

The Shadow of War

The wearisome cycle of bloodshed and hostilities in which the State of Israel has been engulfed since its establishment has left its mark on various facets of Israeli collective experience. To what extent have these conditions of chronic tension affected the emotional well-being of Israeli citizens? We will focus on two recent lines of investigation, dealing with the psychological casualties of the Lebanon War in 1982 and the Gulf War in 1991.

Given the heroic ethos of the Israeli soldier and the critical importance (and concomitantly, the social prestige) accorded to the Israeli Defense Forces (IDF) in dealing with imminent military threats, it is no wonder that psychological breakdown in the battlefield was met with embarrassment, denial, and concealment. The psychological casualties of Israel's first wars were kept hidden from the public eye, as a recent historical research convincingly showed (Witztum, Levy, Granek, & Kotler, 1989). The traumatic 1973 Yom Kippur War, in which almost every third casualty suffered from some combat reaction, increased the awareness of war-related distress, but it was only in the 1982 Lebanon War that this awareness was translated into systematic research on the scope and long-term effects of combat stress reaction (CSR). The recently promulgated data on the psychological casualties of the Lebanon war (Solomon, 1993) are the most comprehensive depiction of the enduring toll of war among Israeli soldiers.

Nearly one quarter of the military casualties in the Lebanon War suffered from CSR, characterized by isolation and psychological numbness, anxiety, guilt feelings, loneliness and depression, vulnerability, loss of self-control, and disorientation. The overall rate of casualties almost doubled after the war, with the emergence of delayed stress reactions. Posttraumatic stress disorder (PTSD), the long-term sequela of CSR, was found in 59% of the casualties 1 year after the war and in 43% 3 years later. These stunning numbers are, in fact, a modest estimate of the phenomenon, since cases of PTSD were unexpectedly found in a control group of soldiers (i.e., veterans who did not succumb to CSR in Lebanon) at a rate of 9 to 19% during the 3-year follow-up. The disorder has adverse impact on the casualties' family relations, social life, and functioning in work. Furthermore, in a country where a considerable cultural pressure is exerted on men to be strong, the unfortunate result is a considerable decrease in perceived self-efficacy and self-esteem. The harsh reality of repeated wars is a fertile ground for reactivation of previous trauma, but the myth of the fearless, hardy soldier inhibits many veterans in need from seeking psychiatric help.

In addition to war veterans, certain groups in the civilian sector are dangerously exposed to war-related stress. Noted among them are the families of the 18,000 soldiers who fell in battle (Malkinson, Rubin, & Witztum, 1993). The painful task of living with the loss is particularly agonizing for bereaved parents, as reflected in high rates of psychopathology and mortality (Auslander, 1987). Survivors of terrorist attacks constitute another group at high risk (Dreman, 1989; Milgram, 1986).

The wide exposure of civilian groups to war-related stress was strongly noted and comprehensively studied during the Gulf War. This war gave rise to a unique set of stressors (Milgram, 1994): missile attacks on civilian targets, the persistent threat of chemical attack, the confinement of family members in sealed rooms during these attacks, and the blurring of wartime roles (soldier and civilian, adult and youth). A recent review (Milgram, 1994) summarized the effects of these stressors. The overall conclusion was that Israeli society as a whole coped well with the unfamiliar threat and losses, and the war has not produced any long-term changes in mood and coping abilities. However, relatively high levels of fear reactions, related to personality (e.g., trait anxiety) and background (e.g., Holocaust exposure) variables, were documented in the general population after the first attacks, and residual long-term stress reactions were detected in certain vulnerable groups, such as young children, disabled elderly, and people living in areas hit by SCUD missiles. Even though the quantified effects of the war, as documented by objective research, do not appear dramatic, the Gulf War undermined some cherished assumptions about civilian vulnerability, the deterrent power of the IDF, and Israel's offensive initiatives in war. This growing sense of vulnerability might deepen future traumas among the Israelis.

SUMMARY

The unfortunate dearth of comparative mental health research that examines matched groups of Israeli and Diaspora Jews has compelled us to deal separately with the two sectors of the Jewish people. Research outside Israel has been limited to North America and Western Europe. Compared with their non-Jewish neighbors, Jews in the Western world have been characterized by a consistent profile of psychopathology, marked by higher rates of affective disorders and (to a lesser degree) psychoneuroses, and lower rates of alcoholism, drug addiction, antisocial personality disorders, and (to a lesser degree) schizophrenia. In terms of health-seeking behaviors, Jews outside Israel have been noted by their relatively high willingness to use psychological help for emotional problems.

While it is extremely difficult, and perhaps altogether futile, to compare the mental health of Israelis as a whole to the mental health of other nations or Jewish groups, it is clear that Israeli Jews are exposed to the emotionally adverse effects of multiple stressors, some of which are unique to the Israeli setting. We concentrated on four sources of emotional distress present on the Israeli scene in the 1980s and 1990s: intra-Jewish ethnic diversity, recent immigrations from the ex-Soviet Union and Ethiopia, the Holocaust, and the recent wars in

Lebanon and the Persian Gulf. The psychic toll that these stressors exert on Israeli society reveals the naiveté of the Zionist dream of Israel as a therapeutic milieu for the Jews of the Diaspora, but it should not be taken as an indication that Diaspora Jews have lower levels of emotional distress than Israeli Jews. Given the different stressors, a comparison of the psychological gains and losses in the two milieus is hardly feasible.

REFERENCES

Antonovsky, A. (1979). *Health, stress, and coping.* San Francisco: Jossey-Bass.

Arieli, A. (1988). Persecutory experience and posttraumatic stress disorders among Ethiopian immigrants. In E. Chigier (Ed.), *Grief and bereavement in contemporary society* (pp. 70–76). London: Freund.

Arieli, A. (1992). Psychopathology among Jewish Ethiopian immigrants to Israel. *Journal of Nervous and Mental Diseases, 180,* 465–466.

Arieli, A., & Aycheh, S. (1993). Psychopathological aspects of the Ethiopian immigration to Israel. *Israel Journal of Medical Science, 29,* 411–418.

Arieli, A., & Aycheh, S. (1994). Mental disease related to the belief in being possessed by the "Zar" spirit (Hebrew). *Harefuah, 129,* 636–642.

Arieli, A., Gilat, I., & Aycheh, S. (1994). Suicide by Ethiopian immigrants in Israel (Hebrew). *Harefuah, 127,* 65–70.

Auslander, G. K. (1987). Bereavement research in Israel: A critical review of the literature. *Israel Journal of Psychiatry, 24,* 33–51.

Aviram, U., & Levav, I. (Eds.). (1981). *Community mental health in Israel* (Hebrew). Tel-Aviv: Gomeh, Cherikover.

Baider, L., Peretz, T., & Kaplan De Nour, A. (1992). Effect of the Holocaust on coping with cancer. *Social Science and Medicine, 34,* 11–15.

Baider, L., Peretz, T., & Kaplan De Nour, A. (1993). Holocaust cancer patients: A comparative study. *Psychiatry, 56,* 349–355.

Ben-Ezer, G. (1990). Anorexia nervosa or an Ethiopian coping style? *Mind and Human Interaction, 2,* 36–39.

Ben-Ezer, G. (1992). *Migration and absorption of Ethiopian Jews in Israel* (Hebrew). Jerusalem: Reuven Mass.

Bilu, Y. (1980). The Moroccan demon in Israel. *Ethos, 8,* 24–39.

Bilu, Y. (1985). The taming of the deviants and beyond: A psychocultural analysis of dybbuk possession and exorcism in Judaism. *The Psychoanalytic Study of Society, 11,* 1–32.

Bilu, Y. (1995). Culture and mental illness among Jews in Israel. In I. Al-Issa (Ed.), *Handbook of culture and mental health: An international perspective* (pp. 129–146). Madison, CT: International Universities Press.

Bourguignon, E. (1979). *Psychological anthropology.* New York: Holt, Rinehart and Winston.

Breen, B. (1968). Culture and schizophrenia: A study of Negro and Jewish schizophrenics. *International Journal of Social Psychiatry, 14,* 282–289.

Brom, D., Kfir, R., & Dasberg, H. (1994, November). *A controlled double-blind study on the offspring of the Holocaust survivors.* Paper presented at the Conference of the International Society for Traumatic Stress Studies, Chicago.

Budowski, D., David, Y., & Eran, Y. (1994). Characteristics of Jewish Ethiopian new immigrants. Unpublished report. JDC Israel: Betachin.

Calahan, D. (1970). *Problem drinkers: A national survey.* San Francisco: Jossey Bass.

Cooklin, R. S., Ravindram, A., & Carney, A. W. (1983). The pattern of mental disorder in Jewish and non-Jewish admissions to a general hospital psychiatric unit: Is manic depressive Illness a typically Jewish disorder? *Psychological Medicine, 13,* 209–212.

Dasberg, H. (1987). Psychological distress of Holocaust survivors and their offspring in Israel, 40 years later: A review. *Israel Journal of Psychiatry, 24,* 243–256.

Dreman, S. (1989). Children of victims of terrorism in Israel: Coping and adjustment in the face of trauma. *Israel Journal of Psychiatry, 26,* 206–220.

Durst, R, Minuchin-Itzighson, S., & Jabotinsky-Rubin, K. (1993). Brain-fag syndrome: Manifestation of transculturation in an Ethiopian Jewish immigrant. *Israel Journal of Psychiatry, 30,* 223–232.

Eaton, W. W., Lasry, J. C., & Sigal, J. (1979). Ethnic relations and community mental health among Israeli Jews. *Israel Annals of Psychiatry, 17,* 165–174.

Eaton, W. W., & Levav, I. (1982). Schizophrenia, social class, and ethnic disadvantage: A study of first hospitalization among Israeli-born Jews. *Israel Journal of Psychiatry, 19,* 289–302.

Eitinger, L. (1964). *Concentration camp survivors in Norway and Israel.* London: Allen & Anwin.

Epstein, A. (1992). *The impact of time and Jewish identity on the psychological adjustment on recent Soviet immigrants to Israel.* Unpublished doctoral dissertation, Yeshiva University, New York.

Felsen, I., & Erlich, H. S. (1990). Identification patterns of offspring of Holocaust survivors with their parents. *American Journal of Orthopsychiatry, 60,* 506–520.

Fenig, S., & Levav, I. (1991). Demoralization and social supports among Holocaust survivors. *Journal of Nervous and Mental Disorders, 179,* 167–172.

Fernando, S. J. M. (1975). A cross-cultural study of some familial and social factors in depressive illness. *British Journal of Psychiatry, 127,* 46–53.

Fishberg, M. (191911). *The Jew: A study of race and environment.* New York: W. Scott.

Gershon, E. S., & Leibowitz, J. L. (1975). Sociocultural and demographic correlates of affective disorders in Jerusalem. *Journal of Psychiatric Research, 12,* 37–50.

Gilman, S. L. (1993). *Freud, race, and gender.* Princeton, NJ: Princeton University Press.

Glassner, B., & Berg, B. (1984). Social locations and interpretations: How Jews define alcoholism? *Journal for the Study of Alcoholism, 45,* 16–25.

Glatt, M. (1975). Jewish alcoholics and addicts in the London area. *Mental Health and Society, 2,* 168–174.

Goldstein, E. (1984). *Homo Sovieticus* in transition: Psychoanalysis and problems of social adjustment. *Journal of the American Academy of Psychoanalysis, 12,* 115–126.

Grisaru, N., & Witztum, E. (1995). The Zar phenomena amongst Ethiopian new immigrants to Israel: Cultural and clinical aspects (Hebrew). *Sihot—Israel Journal of Psychotherapy, 9,* 209–220.

Halevi, H. S. (1963). Frequency of mental illness among Jews in Israel. *International Journal of Social Psychiatry, 9,* 268–282.

Halik, V., Rosenthal, D. A., & Pattison, P. E. (1990). Intergenerational effects of the Holocaust: Patterns of engagement in the mother–daughter relationship. *Family Process, 29,* 325–339.

Heinemann, I. (1939–40). The attitude of the ancient world toward Judaism. *Review of Religion, 4,* 385–400.

Hollingshead, A., & Redlich, F. (1958). *Social class and mental illness.* New York: John Wiley.

Keinan, G., Mikulincer, M., & Rybnicki, A. (1988). Perception of self and parents by second-generation Holocaust survivors. *Behavioral Medicine, 14,* 6–12.

Keison, H. (1992). *Sequential traumatization in children.* Jerusalem: Magness Press.

Keller, M. (1973). The great Jewish drink mystery. In A. Shilo & I. Selavan (Eds.), *Ethnic groups in America: Their morbidity, mortality, and behavior disorders.* Vol. 1. *The Jews.* Springfield, IL: Thomas.

Kohn, R., & Levav, I. (1994). Jews and their interethnic differential vulnerability to affective disorders, fact or artifact? I: An overview of the literature. *Israel Journal of Psychiatry, 31,* 261–270.

Landau, S. (1975). Pathologies among homicide offenders: Some cultural profiles. *British Journal of Criminology, 15,* 157–166.

Leon, G., Bucher, J. N., Kleinman, M., Goldberg, A., & Almagor, M. (1981). Survivors of the Holocaust and their children: Current status and adjustment. *Journal of Personality and Social Psychology, 41,* 503–516.

Lerner, Y., Mirsky, J., & Barasch, M. (1994). New beginnings in an old land: Refugee and immigrant mental health in Israel. In A. J. Marsella, T. Bornemann, S. Ekbland, & J. Orley (Eds.), *Amidst peril and pain: The mental health and well-being of world's refugees.* Washington, DC: American Psychological Association.

Levav, I., & Abramson, J. H. (1984). A community study of emotional distress in Jerusalem. *Israel Journal of Psychiatry, 21,* 19–35.

Levav, I., & Arnon, A. (1976). Emotional disorders in six Israeli villages. *Acta Psychiatrica Scandinavica, 53,* 387–400.

Levav, I., & Bilu, Y. (1980). A transcultural view of Israeli psychiatry. *Transcultural Psychiatric Research Review, 17,* 7–56.

Levav, I., & Kohn, R. (1995). The vulnerability of Jews to affective disorders. *Syllabus and proceedings summary. American Psychiatric 148 Annual Meeting.* Miami, Florida.

Levav, I., Kohn, R., Flaherty, J., Lerner, Y., & Eisenberg, E. (1990). Mental health attitudes and practices of Soviet immigrants. *Israel Journal of Psychiatry, 27,* 131–144.

Liebman, C. S., & Don Yehiya, E. (1983). *Civil religion in Israel.* Berkeley: University of California Press.

Malkinson, R., Rubin, S. S., & Witztum, E. (Eds.). (1993). *Loss and bereavement in Jewish society in Israel* (Hebrew). Jerusalem: Cana.

Malzberg, B. (1931). Mental disease among Jews. *Mental Hygiene, 15,* 766–774.

Malzberg, B. (1962). The distribution of mental disease according to religious affiliation in New York State, 1949–1951. *Mental Hygiene, 46,* 510–522.

Malzberg, B. (1963). *The mental diseases among Jews in Canada: A study of first admissions to mental hospitals, 1950–1952.* Albany, NY: Research Foundation for Mental Hygiene.

Maoz, B., Levy, S., Brand, N., & Halevi, H. S. (1966). An epidemiological survey of mental disorders in a community of newcomers in Israel. *Journal of the College of General Practitioners, 11,* 267–284.

Matussek, P. (1975). *Internment in concentration camps and its consequences.* New York: Springer-Verlag.

Milgram, N. (Ed.). (1986). *Stress and coping in time of war.* New York: Bruner/Mazel.

Milgram, N. (1994). Psychological research on Israel during the Gulf War (Hebrew). *Psychologia, 4,* 7–19.

Miller, L. (1976). Some data on suicide and attempted suicide in the Jewish population of Israel. *Mental Health and Society, 3,* 175–181.

Miller, L. (1979). Culture and psychopathology of Jews in Israel. *Psychiatric Journal of the University of Ottawa, 4,* 302–306.

Minuchin-Itzighson, S., & Hanegbi, R. (1988). Loss and mourning in the Ethiopian community: Anthropological and psychological approaches. In E. Chigier (Ed.), *Grief and bereavement in contemporary society* (Vol. 3, pp. 61–69). London: Freund.

Mirsky, J., Barasch, M., & Goldberg, C. (1992). Adjustment problems among Soviet immigrants at risk. *Israel Journal of Psychiatry, 29,* 1–16.

Mirsky, J., Ginat, Y., Perl, E., & Ritzner, M. (1992). The psychological profile of Jewish late adolescents in the USSR: A pre-immigration study. *Israel Journal of Psychiatry, 29,* 150–158.

Mirsky, J., & Kaushinsky, F. (1988). Psychological processes in immigration and absorption: The case of immigrant students in Israel. *Journal of American College Health, 36,* 329–335.

Mirsky, J., & Kaushinsky, F. (1989). Immigration and growth: Separation–individuation processes in immigrant students in Israel. *Adolescence, 24,* 725–740.

Monteiro, M. G., & Schuckit, M. A. (1989). Alcohol, drug, and mental health problems among Jewish and Christian men at a university. *American Journal of Drug and Alcohol Abuse, 15,* 403–412.

Murphy, H. B. M. (1982). *Comparative psychiatry.* Berlin: Springer-Verlag. Nadler, A., Kav-Venaki, S., & Gleitman, B. (1985). Transgenerational effects of the Holocaust: Aggression in second generation of Holocaust survivors. *Journal of Consulting and Clinical Psychology, 53,* 365–369.

Popper, M., & Horowitz, R. (1992). *Psychiatric hospitalization of immigrants, 1990–1991* (Hebrew). (Statistical Report No. 7). Jerusalem: Ministry of Health, Mental Health Services.

Rahav, M., Popper, M., & Nahon, D. (1981). The psychiatric case register in Israel: Initial results. *Israel Journal of Psychiatry, 18*, 251–267.

Ratzoni, G., Apter, A., Blumensohn, R., & Tiano, S. (1988). Psychopathology and management of hospitalized suicidal Ethiopian adolescents in Israel. *Journal of Adolescence, 11*, 231–236.

Ratzoni, G., Blumensohn, R., Apter, A., & Tiano, S. (1991). Psychopathology and management of hospitalized suicidal Ethiopian immigrants in Israel. *Israel Journal of Medical Science, 27*, 293–296.

Rose, S. L., & Garske, J. (1987). Family environment, adjustment, and coping among children of Holocaust survivors. *American Journal of Orthopsychiatry, 57*, 332–344.

Sanua, V. (1963). The sociocultural aspects of schizophrenia: A comparison of Protestant and Jewish schizophrenics. *International Journal of Social Psychiatry, 9*, 27–36.

Sanua, V. (1989). Studies in mental illness and other psychiatric deviances among contemporary Jewry: A review of the literature. *Israel Journal of Psychiatry, 26*, 187–211.

Schmidt, W., & Popham, R. (1976). Impressions of Jewish alcoholics. *Journal for the Study of Alcohol, 37*, 931–939.

Schneider, S. (1988). Attitudes toward death in adolescents offspring of Holocaust survivors: A comparison of Israeli and American adolescents. *Adolescence, 23*, 703–710.

Schreiber, S. (1995). Migration, traumatic bereavement and transcultural aspects of psychological healing: Loss and grief of a refugee woman from Begameder County in Ethiopia. *British Journal of Medical Psychology, 68*, 135–142.

Schwartz, S., Dohrenwend, B. P., & Levav, I. (1994). Non-genetic familial transmission of psychiatric disorders: Evidence from the children of the Holocaust. *Journal of Health and Social Behavior, 35*, 385–402.

Shuval, J. T. (1957–58). Some persistent effects of trauma: Five years after the Nazi concentration camps. *Social Problems, 5*, 230–243.

Shuval, J. (1982). Migration and stress. In L. Goldberg & S. Breznitz (Eds.), *Handbook of stress* (pp. 677–691). New York: Free Press.

Singer, J. (1958). Heritage of the ghetto on the second generation. In S. Georgene (Ed.), *Clinical studies in culture and conflict.* New York: Ronald Press.

Skolnick, J. H. (1958). Religious affiliation and drinking behavior. *Quarterly Journal of Alcoholism, 21*, 548–551.

Snyder, C. (1962). Inebriaty, alcoholism, and anomia. In M. Clinard (Ed.), *Anomia and deviant behavior.* New York: Free Press.

Snyder, C. R., & Palgi, P. (1982). Alcoholism among the Jews in Israel. *Studies on Alcoholism, 4*, 623–654.

Solomon, Z. (1993). *Combat stress reaction: The enduring stress of war.* New York: Plenum Press.

Solomon, Z., & Prager, E. (1992). Elderly Israeli Holocaust survivors during the Persian Gulf War: A study of psychological distress. *American Journal of Psychiatry, 149*, 1707–1710.

Strole, L., Langer, T., Michael, S., Opler, M., & Rennie, T. (Eds.). (1962). *Mental health in the metropolis: The Midtown Manhattan Study.* New York: McGraw Hill.

Tabory, E., & Weller, L. (1987). The impact of cultural context on the mental health of Jewish concentration camp survivors. *Holocaust and Genocide Studies, 2*, 299–305.

Yeung, P. P., & Greenwald, S. (1992). Jewish Americans and mental health: Results of the NIMH epidemiologic catchment area study. *Social Psychiatry and Psychiatric Epidemiology, 27*, 292–297.

Youngmann, R., & Minuchin-Itzighson, S. (1993). The development of a diagnostic instrument for early identification of emotional distress among Ethiopian immigrants in Israel (Hebrew). Unpublished report, JDC-Israel.

Weiss, E., O'Connell, A. N., & Siiter, R. (1986). Comparisons of second-generation Holocaust survivors, immigrants, and nonimmigrants on measures of mental health. *Journal of Personality and Social Psychology, 4*, 828–831.

Witztum, E., Levy, A., Granek, M., & Kotler, M. (1989). Combat reaction in Israel: 1948–1973. Part 1. *Sihot—Israel Journal of Psychotherapy, 4,* 60–64.

World Health Organization. (1992). *The ICD-10 classification of mental and behavioral disorders, clinical description and diagnostic guidelines.* Geneva: WHO.

Zlotogorski, Z. (1983). Offspring of concentration camp survivors: The relationship of perceptions of family cohesion and adaptability to levels of ego functioning. *Comprehensive Psychiatry, 24,* 345–354.

15

The Gypsies of Europe

From Persecution to Genocide

GABRIELLE TYRNAUER

INTRODUCTION

Gypsies, like Jews, were targeted for annihilation in Nazi Germany and its conquered territories. Men, women, and children were identified by bureaucrats and "racial scientists," rounded up by the police, incarcerated, and deported in cattle cars to concentration camps throughout the Third Reich, where they were exterminated in massive numbers by slave labor, hunger and disease, bullets and gas. Sometimes they were classified as "asocial," sometimes as "racially inferior," often as both. It made no difference whether they lived as "primitive" nomads or well-assimilated citizens.

Between 250,000 and 500,000 European Gypsies, approximately one fourth of those living in prewar Europe,[1] were murdered by the Nazis simply for the crime of existing. This genocide of an ancient European minority was carried out at the same time, by the same regime, and often the same government offices that were responsible for the Jewish Holocaust, though far less is known about it. In the Third Reich only Jews and Gypsies were targeted for total annihilation. They were very different peoples with different origins and

[1]This figure is derived from the estimates of Kenrick and Puxon (1972), recently revised downward. Some scholars and Gypsy political activists, on the basis of recent information, claim the figures should be much higher. The total given in the 1972 volume was 219,700 (p. 184).

GABRIELLE TYRNAUER • Refugee Research Project, McGill University, Montreal, Quebec, Canada H3A 2A5.

Ethnicity, Immigration, and Psychopathology, edited by Ihsan Al-Issa and Michel Tousignant. Plenum Press, New York, 1997.

histories, but in Hitler's Germany their destinies became one. The ideology on which Nazi policy toward both Jews and Gypsies was based derived in part from traditional prejudices, in part from the then-current "scientific" theories of eugenics and "racial hygiene." In this chapter, after providing a historical overview of the Gypsies' European diaspora, we will explore (1) traditional European prejudices as they combined with the "scientific racism" of Nazi ideology, providing the rationale for genocide; (2) the survivors' individual and collective responses to their persecution; and (3) the subsequent treatment accorded them by non-Gypsy societies in which they experienced the Nazi persecution.

HISTORICAL BACKGROUND

The "Gypsies"[2] first appeared in Europe in the late Middle Ages. From the beginning, they inspired wonder and fear. They told fortunes and had a special relation to the occult; many non-Gypsies believed it was to the devil, even when they seemed to profess Christian beliefs. They were talented musicians, entertaining the rulers and their subjects in the countries through which they passed. They came to fill an economic niche for the peasantry, sharpening knives and scissors, making cooking pots, and selling their wares to housewives door to door. They were rumored to steal children as well as chickens and nothing was more dreaded than a "gypsy curse" (for historical accounts, see Clébert, 1963; Kenrick & Puxon, 1972; and others listed in Tyrnauer, 1991).

The location of the original home of the Gypsies was a matter of considerable conjecture until the 18th century when a Hungarian theology student at Leyden noted the uncanny resemblance between the speech of some Indian fellow students and the Gypsies of his homeland. Subsequent linguistic studies convinced most scholars of the northwestern India origins of Gypsies, though the precise place and the Indian ethnic and social groups from which they derived remained a matter of dispute. As they produced no written history of their own and had preserved no clear "origin myths" even in their oral

[2]This term, like that of American "Indians," is based on a geographical misapprehension, as is another term sometimes applied to them in English and French, "bohemians." They came neither from Egypt nor Bohemia; nor did they belong to the Greek heretical sect, the Atsiganoi, which provided another name for them in many European languages (*Zigeuner* in German, *tsigane* in French, and many variations of the word in other European languages). While the term in all these languages has become charged with derogatory associations, no other word that covers the many subgroups—all of which have names for themselves—has replaced it. Among the educated and politicized, "Rom" has been used, but this is also the designation for a particular subgroup. In international circles, "Romani" is favored (as in "Romani Union," an organization with NGO status in the UN), but this is the term traditionally applied to English Gypsies. So, by default, the term "Gypsy" is still widely used, by the peoples themselves, and will be used here, but always in mental, if not physical (for the sake of convenience) quotation marks. Sometimes it will be used interchangeably with Romani.

traditions, the task of tracing their migration routes fell mainly to European linguists.

When the Gypsies left India, presumably in several waves, they traveled through the Middle East and on to southeastern Europe where the first record indicating their presence on the continent was found in Corfu and Greece, early in the 14th century. Nomadic Gypsies were recorded in Crete in 1322, "stopping only thirty days in one place" (Kenrick & Puxon, 1972, pp. 14–15). The Greeks called them by the name of a heretical sect, *atsiganoi,* from which derived the word used to designate them in most European languages i.e., the German *Zigeuner,* the Hungarian *Cigany,* the Italian *Zingari,* and so on.

After a relatively long sojourn in Greece—judging by the number of Greek loan words in Romanes, the Gypsy language—the nomads moved to Hungary and the Balkans, perhaps on the heels of the Turkish invasion. In some of these areas, in fact, they become associated with the invaders. During the 16th and 17th centuries, legislation was enacted in German and Czech areas expelling Gypsies as Turkish spies. At the Nuremberg trials, these beliefs were revived by some defendants to account for the roundups and deportations of Gypsies as "security risks." One of the early measures taken against them by the National Socialist regime was a prohibition against nomadism and the requirement of a fixed address. The "Gypsy as spy" image was at work here.

Gypsies appeared near the North Sea in 1417 carrying a safe-conduct letter from the Pope and calling themselves "Lords of little Egypt" (hence the name "Gypsy"). They explained their wandering through a number of pious stories, the best-known one being that they had refused sanctuary to the Holy family during its sojourn in Egypt, and were thus obliged to perform a nomadic penance for a number of years. This tale is said not only to have won over the Pope but also to have impressed King Sigismund of Hungary sufficiently for him to grant them a letter of safe conduct through his lands.

By the late 15th century, there are accounts of the Gypsies in the chronicles of almost every European country. The early curiosity and good will of the settled people were replaced by hostility. The dark strangers were accused of witchcraft, thievery, kidnapping, and murder. Both Church and State discriminated against them and devised a large repertory of punishments for real or imagined crimes. These ranged from banishment to whipping to execution; Gypsy slavery in the Rumanian lands was not abolished until 1856. In the 18th century, there was a well-known cannibalism trial of Gypsies in Hungary; after the torture of almost 200 of the defendants and the execution of 41, the alleged victims were found alive and well (Kenrick & Puxon, 1972, chap. 3). Gypsies were treated like wild game ("freiwild") and "open seasons" were declared. These popular traditions and pastimes prepared the way for the Nazi Gypsy hunters.

Harassment and stronger forms of persecution alternated with attempts at forced assimilation. The persistent nomadism and the cultivation of an ethnic and cultural distinctiveness made the Gypsies visible, if moving, targets of the integrators as well as the persecutors. Maria Therese of Austria and her successor, Joseph II, used both carrot and stick, giving Gypsies land and calling them "New Hungarians," while forbidding them the use of their language and taking away their children to be raised by peasant families.

In a parallel assimilation attempt, Carlos III of Spain issued a 44-article "pragmatica" for the Gitanos (Gypsies) of his country, whom, following the Austro-Hungarian lead, he renamed "*nuevos castellanos*" or "New Castillians." He too forbade them the use of their language, traditional dress, and occupations, and encouraged sedentary work and lifestyles (Vossen, 1983, p. 54). Various German princes also experimented with integration attempts in their territories during the 18th century.

But neither persecution nor forced assimilation had the desired effect, and 200 years later, Gypsies continued to observe their customs, speak their language, and draw sharp boundaries between themselves and outsiders. Nevertheless, in parts of the old Austro-Hungarian empire, Spain, and other areas Gypsy groups were at least partially sedentarized as the result of centuries of powerful pressures to assimilate.

At the same time that Gypsies were being imprisoned, expelled, and enslaved by the princes through whose territories they passed, they became an important part of the European cultural scene. Individual musicians and dancers, singers, and circus performers acquired legendary reputations. Gypsies became part of the entourage of princes and czars. With the advent of the Romantic movement, the unfettered lifestyle of the nomads became attractive to a restless young generation of poets, musicians, and painters. These helped to create a stereotype of Gypsies tinged by envy and nostalgia, at the same time that legislators throughout Europe were making laws to combat the "Gypsy menace."

In Nazi Germany, the European ambivalence toward the Gypsies expressed itself in the most bizarre ways. German scholars were encouraged to search for the Gypsies' "Aryan" origins and language by German officials whose bureaucratic colleagues defined Gypsies as vermin. This ambivalence, in its most malignant form, could permit SS soldiers to listen with pleasure to a Gypsy orchestra hours before sending its members to their death.

As Hohmann (1980, pp. 14–17) points out, the story of the Nazi persecution and mass murder of the Gypsies cannot be fully understood without grasping the continuity of stereotypes or of the ambivalence that underlay them. It is here that we find the link between the romantic operetta clichés of Gypsy Barons and the Gypsy violins of Auschwitz.

The "Gypsy Question" in Germany

The "Gypsy question" (*Die Zigeunerfrage*) in Germany, as in other European countries, was only formulated at the time of national unification in the 19th century. In feudal times, Gypsies had a clear niche in society as itinerant artisans, traders, entertainers, and practitioners of healing and occult arts, particularly fortune-telling. They may have been despised and persecuted as well as romanticized, but their existence was not called into question.

With the rise of the bourgeois nation–state and its central focus on national identity, the *Zigeunerfrage* was born, as was the "question" of other troublesome minorities, particularly the Jews. The older Gypsy image of heathen, swindler, songbird, and kidnapper, gave way to a more sinister picture of the "inner enemy," disloyal to the state (the Turkish spy image), a criminal element in society, and worst of all, in the Nazi catalogue of sins, a threat to racial purity.

Data collection on the Gypsies for "law enforcement" purposes began under the monarchy with the establishment in 1899 of a *Zigeunernachrichtsdienst* (Gypsy Information Service) in Munich. In 1905, the government of Bavaria issued a *Zigeunerbuch* (Gypsy book) in which acts and edicts related to Gypsies in the years 1816–1903 were compiled to serve as guidelines for the continuing battle against the *Zigeunerplage* (Gypsy plague). By 1904, the industrious workers of the Gypsy Information Service had collected 3340 protocols about Gypsy individuals and families. Methods were refined after World War I, when the practice of fingerprinting was introduced. Thus, through the united efforts of the police, scholars, and bureaucrats, the Gypsies of Germany became the most researched and easily identified in Europe.

The legal situation of Gypsies did not improve under the Weimar Republic. A variety of laws pertaining to "Gypsies, travelers, and malingerers" were passed. In 1926, a "Gypsy Conference" was held in Munich to bring uniformity to the legislation of the different provinces of the Republic. Draconian laws against nomadism, lack of identification papers, and so forth were introduced and centralization of technical innovations such as fingerprinting made them more effective. Streck (1979, p. 73) notes the irony that "the first democracy on German soil" left a legacy with respect to the Gypsies that permitted the Nazis to implement their policies for a number of years without changing a single law.

GYPSIES IN NAZI GERMANY

The Legal Basis

While the Weimar laws sufficed for the first few years of National Socialist rule, new legislation, consistent with Nazi racial ideology, was required. The earliest discriminatory laws were not specific to Gypsies but were applied to them; for instance, a 1933 law that permitted sterilization of mental defectives later applied to Gypsies of mixed blood; a 1934 law that permitted the deportation of undesirable aliens was applied to foreign Gypsies. In 1935, the Nuremberg race laws were passed. These were aimed primarily at Jews and banned intermarriage with Germans. Although the Gypsies were not mentioned in the original legislation, later commentaries referred to them explicitly. In the same year, a citizenship law was passed, which distinguished between first-class (German or related blood) and second-class (alien blood) citizens. The second-class category applied to Jews and Gypsies.

The Nazi Ministry of the Interior indicated its strong support of the activities of the newly established (1936) Vienna-based International Center for the Fight Against the Gypsy Menace. After the annexation of Austria in 1938, anti-Gypsy legislation began there, including a deportation decree that permitted the dispatch of 400 Sinti (the group to which most German Gypsies belong) and Roma to Dachau, and another law that forbade nomadism.

In 1936, Himmler, by then the supreme chief of the merged SS and security forces, took over the campaign against the "inner enemies." His first assault was the asocial action of 1937, which permitted arrest and preventive detention of all asocials, among whom the Gypsies were considered foremost.

In the same year a research center was established within the Ministry of Health, under Dr. Robert Ritter, a neurologist and pediatrician, The *Rassenhygienische und bevölkerungsbiologische Forschungsstelle* (Racial Hygiene and Population Biology Research Center) was to play a decisive role in the definition, apprehension, and annihilation of the Gypsy population of Germany and, later, of occupied Europe.

Thus, the two-pronged attack on the Gypsy question, one related to race, the other to criminality, was launched by the racial scientists under the personal patronage of Heinrich Himmler. They were to establish the relation between the two, primarily through the collection of genealogies, designed both to enrich knowledge and to facilitate the work of law enforcement officers.

Some of these officers had admitted to considerable confusion about Gypsies during the first few years of the "Thousand-Year Reich." Some had sent perplexed memos to their superiors requesting clarification as to whether the Gypsies in their custody should be treated as Aryans or *Untermenschen* (subhumans). An important assignment of the Racial Hygiene and Population Biology Research Institute was to resolve such doubts.

Genealogy and Genocide

Genealogical research was a favored activity in the Third Reich. Himmler himself was fascinated by it and was patron of the *Ahnenerbe*, the organization that researched the Aryan ancestry for SS members and lesser mortals in Nazi Germany. As we have noted, the Gypsy Information Service, established under the Imperial Second Reich, had started the work of collecting genealogies for purely practical purposes, the better to keep track of what had become, by definition, a "criminal element." The Gypsy Information Service's genealogies became the nucleus of the collection in Ritter's Berlin research center. They were expanded to include nearly every German Gypsy. The research was conducted by an interdisciplinary team of scholars, and the data they gathered, in addition to the genealogies, included fingerprints, ethnological descriptions, anatomical measurements, and psychological profiles. Under Dr. Ritter, the collection of these data became at once a scholarly and patriotic mission. A member of Ritter's research team, Adolph Würth, wrote in 1938:

> The Gypsy Question is today in the first place a racial question. Just as the National Socialist State has solved the Jewish Question, so it will have to fundamentally regulate the Gypsy Question. A start has already been made. In the regulations for the implementation of the Nuremberg Laws for the protection of German blood, Gypsies have been placed on an equal level with Jews in regard to marriage prohibitions. In other words, they count neither as of German blood nor related to it. (Hohmann, 1980, p. 201)

The well-known commentator on the Nuremberg laws, Hans Globke (a member of Konrad Adenauer's cabinet in the postwar years), translated the "scientific" data into legal philosophy in 1937: Of all European peoples, only Jews and Gypsies had alien (*artfremdes*) blood, and thus represented a mortal threat to German racial purity (Hohmann, 1981, p. 102).

It remained for the members of Dr. Ritter's institute to determine who was the carrier of that blood and in what proportions. By 1941, his team had assembled nearly 20,000 protocols on individual Gypsies who had been examined by them. Through genealogies, fingerprints, and anthropomorphic measurements, they attempted to establish the relationship between the two bases for discrimination and eventual extermination laid down by their rulers: racial inferiority and hereditary criminality.

As the racial scientists provided their data to the police and the SS, they also produced recommendations for sedentarization, sterilization, and deportation. While they did not openly recommend extermination, their research paved the way for it so directly that it is hard not to agree with Miriam Novitch's (1981) assessment that

> the central role played by the German "scientists" and "racial experts" must be understood, because they were as responsible for the genocide of the Gypsies as were the members of the Einsatzgruppen who murdered them with bullets or the SS men in the death camps who murdered them with gas.

Eva Justin, Ritter's student and assistant, wrote a doctoral dissertation (published in 1944) in which she studied Gypsy children who had been brought up in a Catholic orphanage at Mulfingen. She concluded that Gypsies could not be changed or integrated; therefore, all attempts at education should cease. Furthermore, since

> the German people do not need the multiplying weed of these immature primitives, [all] educated Gypsies and part-Gypsies of predominantly Gypsy blood, whether socially assimilated or asocial and criminal, should, as a general rule, be sterilized. Socially integrated part-Gypsies with less than half Gypsy blood can be considered as Germans. (Kenrick & Puxon, 1972, p. 68)

The Nazi's ideological dilemma, stemming from the presumed Aryan origin's of the Gypsies, was nowhere more clearly seen than in the conflicting recommendations made by racial scientists and those in authority. While Justin recommended sparing the more assimilated—those with "less than half Gypsy blood"—others, including her "doctor father," Ritter, and his boss, Himmler, showed a marked preference for the nomadic "pure" Gypsies and proposed special reserves where they could roam freely, speak their own language, preserve ancient Aryan customs, and multiply for the study of future German scientists. Those who were at first exempted from deportation to Auschwitz included both the traditional, nomadic, and racially "pure" Gypsies and the "socially adapted" sedentary ones. These exemptions derived from the two conflicting models of *Zigeunerpolitik* (Zimmermann, 1987, pp. 40–43), one based on "racial purity," the other on degree of assimilation.

The confusion of those in authority was matched by the bewilderment of their victims. One Sinti woman recalled being summoned to a local clinic with her whole family for examination by the racial scientists. Knowing a little about the racial classification of Jews, many of them, accustomed to improvisation and disguise in their relation with the *gajo* (non-Gypsy), hurriedly invented German ancestors when questioned in the hopes of achieving more Aryan identity, not suspecting that the guidelines for determining "purity" were the opposite of those applied to Jews.[3]

The distinctions and classifications worked out in the Berlin Racial Hygiene Research Center came to be identified as one more of Himmler's harebrained schemes by his Nazi colleagues. Himmler apparently deferred to them, and in January 1943, signed the infamous Auschwitz Decree, ordering the dispatch of all nearly 30,000 Gypsies, regardless of group or status or degree of assimilation, to the death camp. German Roma and Sinti were even demobilized from the army and sent to Auschwitz. Survivors recall seeing them arriving in uniform, greeting the SS guards with "Heil Hitler," and sometimes continuing to wear their military decorations in the camp.

Up to that time, "Aryan" or "pure" Gypsies, identified by the racial scholars as approximately 3% of the German Gypsy population, were allowed to serve in the army, although subject to sterilization laws and the requirement of a fixed residence. Military service did not protect the soldier's family, however, so there were many instances of Wehrmacht soldiers whose families were prisoners in Auschwitz and other concentration camps. Some identified themselves in order to be released to join their families, others were denounced by

[3]Unless otherwise noted, all Gypsy testimony is taken from audio- and videotaped interviews made in Germany by Gabrielle Tyrnauer between 1980 and 1992. The videotapes may be seen in the following archives: (1) Yale University: The Fortunoff Videoarchives for Holocaust Testimonies; (2) McGill University: Living Testimonies; (3) Concordia University: Montreal Institute for Genocide Studies; and (4) University of Vermont: Bailey-Howe Library.

fellow soldiers or officers. These soldiers came, for the most part, from families that had lived in Germany for many centuries and were partly or almost wholly assimilated.

One such was Alfred Lessing (1993), who describes the experience in his recently published memoir. He volunteered for the army in a desperate attempt to find an escape route. Subsequently, his ethnic affiliation was researched by an unfriendly officer and he was immediately arrested. But he escaped from his makeshift prison and managed to avoid deportation.

The Road to Extinction

The roads to extinction (Friedman, 1980) were approximately the same for Gypsies as for Jews. Beginning with a definition of the target group by ideologues and racial scientists, there followed the identification of individuals who fit the definition, and then came their social and finally physical isolation from the surrounding population. Through this process, Jews and Gypsies were placed outside the law and deprived of the protection of the state (Friedman, 1980, p. 215). This made all other measures possible.

At the time the war broke out in 1939, there were approximately 22,000 Gypsies and 375,000 Jews still living in Germany (Hohmann, 1981, p. 143). Their legal status, or lack of it, was, for all practical purposes, almost identical by this time. Both had been stigmatized, classified, and stripped of their former identities and possessions. After the fall of Poland, the first deportations to the conquered Polish territory began for both Jews and Gypsies. The Lodz Ghetto was erected in April 1940. Some 5000 Gypsies were incarcerated there and subsequently exterminated at Treblinka. In October of the same year, the order for the creation of the Warsaw Ghetto was issued, and many more were imprisoned there. As the eastern countries were overrun, one after the other, the dreaded *Einsatzkommandos* swept through them in the wake of the German army to "cleanse" the conquered lands of Jews, Gypsies, and political functionaries, often with the enthusiastic support of native Fascist organizations. The orders given both to army commanders and to SS troops in the east for the elimination of Gypsies always contained elements of both racial ideology and security considerations.

Final Solution at Auschwitz

Auschwitz was the last stop on the Gypsies' tragic journey in Nazi Europe. A special subcamp for Gypsies was established, the *Zigeunerlager.* There, they were incarcerated with their families. At first, they were permitted to wear their own clothes and keep a few musical instruments so as to feed the German *Zigeunerromantik,* even while they were being prepared for annihilation. "They were my favorite prisoners," Auschwitz Commandant Höss (1958) wrote in a Polish prison. He was particularly fond of the children, introduced a nursery school, and built them a playground with a merry-go-round a few months before he ordered their liquidation. Dr. Mengele never failed to produce candy from his pocket when he visited the Gypsy camp to select experimental subjects. The German contradictions and ambivalence toward the Gypsies did not cease at the gates of the death camps. In early August 1944, the entire *Zigeunerlager* was liquidated in order to make room for incoming Hungarian Jews. Some 4000 Gypsies were gassed on its final night.

THE GYPSY RESPONSE

The Gypsies' responses to this genocidal policy varied with their personalities and culture. Yet, there were certain responses and coping mechanisms that cut across linguistic, occupational, and lifestyle differences. These stemmed directly from the centuries of being a mobile, mythologized, and despised "visible minority" in Europe.

The most common responses were the traditional Gypsy ones: flight and subterfuge. Due to centuries of practice, being on the run and hiding or presenting a counterfeit identity was easier for them and caused less psychological damage than for most sedentary peoples. It should be noted that even sedentary Gypsies travel extensively during the summer months and on the occasions of weddings, funerals, and other important ceremonial occasions. Mobility is not an incidental activity; it represents a basic value.

Gypsy survivor accounts of wartime experiences always contain stories of repeated successful or failed escape attempts. Flight was the first response to danger. This is in contrast with the narratives of most Jewish survivors, particularly assimilated ones, whose first responses were to obey the orders of those in authority. They had lived in an orderly society and were slow to grasp the mortal threat of simple orders (e.g., to report to a railroad station or an assembly point).

Disguises, concealment, and subterfuge, like flight, were traditional defense mechanisms in Gypsy cultures. Alfred Lessing's (1993) memoir is entitled *My Life in Hiding*, and he recounts one disguise and hiding place after another: as a South American jazz guitarist, a circus worker, a soldier, an Italian "artiste," and so forth. While there is fear of discovery, there is little of the guilt or identity crisis revealed in Jewish testimonies of concealment, when the survivor, sometimes even a child survivor, must disown his or her name, family, nationality, and religion in the interest of survival. Concealment and disguises are culturally approved strategies when dealing with outsiders and Gypsies learn them at an early age. Thus, they cause no personal anguish or sense of separation from the community because they do not contradict the learned values or behavior.

Incarceration, on the other hand, particularly when it involved separation from families, was harder and made Gypsies more intractable as prisoners. Even the Nazis recognized this and it was presumed to be one of the principal reasons for setting up a "family camp" for them within Auschwitz–Birkenau. Survivors tell of the horror of captivity, even under better circumstances. One of the most painful aspects of it was the inability to observe the ritual cleanliness and taboos that are such a basic part of the Gypsy culture. The memories that seemed to evoke the most horror in the survivors are those that forced men and women, parents and children to undress and often eliminate in front of each other. The mass incarceration represented a destruction of the Gypsies' collective existence even before it destroyed them individually.

The survivors of the genocide remained rudderless after liberation until they could make contact with relatives. Gypsies cannot be "loners" and remain within the culture. The worst punishment that can be inflicted by the community is for an individual to be outcast or declared *marimé* (ritually impure). The extended family is essential to the individual's survival regardless of the subgroup to which he or she belongs. Family values in this culture are not at odds with the value of mobility, as in sedentary cultures. The extended family generally travels as a unit, in one or more trailers, today as they did in horse-drawn caravans in the past. They do not leave their community and culture behind when they migrate from society to society. They go to considerable lengths to maintain the distinction between *Rom* (human being, Gypsy male) or *Romni* (female) and *Gajo* (outsider) and to resist the forces of assimilation in all the societies through which they pass. They expect to be marginal in the new society as they were in the old. But they are marginal as a group, not as individuals; a considerable psychological difference.

Thus, as members of a tight-knit group, they often thrive when the larger society is in chaos. Many of my interviewees reported the immediate postwar period in occupied Germany to be the happiest of their lives; most non-Gypsy Germans report the opposite. It was a time of acute shortages, of lives, careers, and cities in ruins. But for the Gypsies the period of Allied occupation was very different; they felt protected, as victims of Hitler's criminal and defeated regime. There was no centralized bureaucracy that targeted them for persecution; they were once more permitted to travel and they often entertained the occupying troops: "For a few years until the Germans got on their feet again, we were happy. We would sing and perform for the Amis [Americans] and we felt free again," said a Sinti puppeteer–musician.

But when they were separated from their families and groups, the longing to rejoin them often overcame any material advantages they had in occupied Germany. Another Sinto recalls being befriended by a Russian soldier who wanted to adopt him. He was the sole survivor of his immediate family and traveled about with the Russian until he heard news of some surviving cousins, aunts, and uncles. He left immediately to search for them.

Still another, unaware that any member of his family had survived, married a German woman and "passed," not even revealing his Gypsy identity to his new family. One day, several years after the war, his widow recalled, a caravan of Gypsies came to the village where they lived. He visited them, found connections, and told his wife that night about his identity and wartime experiences (from an audiotaped interview, Montreal, 1990).

There were many such stories of concealed and revealed postwar identities. One of the most dramatic was that of a man, also a sole survivor and married to a German woman who, however, knew of his ethnic origins and experiences when she married him. They owned an inn in the Black Forest. A group of local German men used to come regularly. One night, after many beers, they were discussing their wartime experiences, exchanging stories about their military service, and one of them turned to him and asked: "And you Herr X, where did you serve?" The Sinto, unprepared, fumbled for words, "I was with the SS." Some of the others had been too. They talked and laughed and sang the old Nazi songs late into the night, then left.

The Gypsy could not sleep that night. The next evening the group returned to their reserved table. Herr X confronted them and alluded to the previous night's conversation. "Gentlemen, I must tell you, it is true that I spent the war with the SS. But as a prisoner." His words were greeted with silence. Soon the men left, never to return.

His business declined so much that, within less than a year, he had to sell his hotel. But, as he said, his conscience was free. Eventually, this man became a leader within the German Gypsy political movement, participating in a hunger strike at the former concentration camp of Dachau and a sit-in demonstration in the Tübingen University library, where were stored the archives of the former Racial Hygiene Institute, which had measured and classified his relatives, providing the police and SS with the information that had led to their deaths.

His description of opening a filing cabinet 35 years after his liberation to find a complete genealogy of his murdered family was a wrenching experience to the listener. In the 1980s, he emigrated to Canada with his German wife and children and their families. At my request, he came to a gathering of Holocaust survivors, testified before a United States congressional committee investigating the whereabouts of the notorious Dr. Mengele, whose activities he had observed as a child in Auschwitz, and participated in events at the newly established US Holocaust Memorial Commission (precursor of the museum) in Washington, DC. He attributed his political activism in part to the experience at his inn in the Black Forest. It was his "coming out."

Most of the leaders of the political movement had some coming-out experience such as this. The puppeteer related a story of working at a carnival, where he passed as an Italian. Two of his German hired helpers were drunk and fighting. One called the other *ein dreckiger Zigeuner* (dirty Gypsy). He could not contain himself and began to shout at them: "You besotted dirty shits, you are not Gypsies, but I am!" They were stunned by the revelation, as was he himself. Thereafter, he also became a political activist. His wife recalled encountering a self-professed Nazi customer at the shooting gallery they owned: She drove him away, threatening to shoot him in the name of her murdered family.

These coming-out scenes were generally related by individuals who had some connection with the political movement or were assimilated in larger degree to the dominant society, often through intermarriage, in which confession of one's true identity to others is an essential part of integrity and self-respect. Traditionally, a life in hiding, at least with respect to the *gajo*, did not compromise an individual's self-esteem.

The younger brother of the puppeteer, on the other hand, who spent his working life among *gaje*, was concerned with concealment, not revelation. He was a well-known operetta singer who had studied at the conservatory. He had adopted an Italian name and was in constant fear of being uncovered. Disguise for him was a career as well as a life decision. Yet, he never severed his close connections with his family, and when on tour in the summer, he camped in his trailer with all his relatives instead of staying in a hotel with his colleagues. His wife and daughter went *hausieren* (peddling from door to door) in the villages outside of Vienna while he sang in the baroque Baden opera house.

Many of the men and women wore gold Stars of David, passing as Jewish traders. Why should they have chosen this identity, as despised as their own in Germany's past, I asked some of them, puzzled. One replied that it made them feel safer; the police would no longer dare persecute a Jew in Germany, "because there is an Israel."

But for the Gypsies of Germany, there was hardly a break in their persecution. There was a far greater sense of negative continuity. They did not emigrate en masse after the war. In fact, many returned to Germany from hiding or displaced persons camps elsewhere in search of relatives and because they had no other place to go. They would even return to the same towns and cities familiar to them from before the war. They told stories about being harassed by the same policeman who had arrested them during the Nazi period. One woman told the horrifying tale of being examined, after she had applied for reparations, by the doctor who had sterilized her during the Nazi period (Interview, 1992). The first book that grew out of the new political movement emphasized this continuity: A collection of essays by German scholars and journalists as well as Romani political activists was entitled "Gassed in Auschwitz, Persecuted until This Day" (Zülch, 1979).

While a large literature exists on the psychological problems of Jewish Holocaust survivors, their children, and even their grandchildren, there is no comparable body of research on Gypsy survivors. It is urgent that such research be done before these survivors of "the forgotten Holocaust" disappear without a historical trace. I have found in my interviews with the Sinti survivors many of the same psychological reactions to their experiences that have been described by Jewish Holocaust survivors. While the search for meaning has been less intense and there is a greater acceptance of the role of chance or luck in survival (which has also been reported by most Jewish survivors), there are nonetheless traces of survivor guilt in many of the testimonies. Symptoms of postraumatic stress disorder are reported, and can be observed, in many of the Gypsy survivor interviewees. There are examples of the same sense of inner isolation from community and family and of problems with their children related to the wartime experiences. "They don't want to hear about it any more; they can never understand what we went through," one woman said.

However, there is an important difference here. While many Jewish survivors never spoke about their experiences to their children in the hopes of sparing them a burden that might make adjustment to the new societies to which their parents had fled more difficult, Gypsy survivors did not hesitate to tell even the youngest about their experiences in great detail. The children were not expected to assimilate. The suffering of their people became a part of the oral tradition they passed on to them; they sang songs about them over campfires, but they were not expected to reveal them to outsiders. This was done only after some of them became involved in the Romani political movement. One activist Auschwitz survivor only began speaking publicly after the dramatic 1980 hunger strike in the former concentration camp at Dachau.

The Historical Urgency

The closed character of Gypsy society and the great fear that its members have of government officials, police, bureaucrats, and scholars, at whose hands they have experienced so much suffering in the past, make the gathering of these data the more urgent and the more difficult. It will fill the blank spaces in Holocaust history, supplementing and confirming Jewish testimony, and providing information to combat the already multiplying Holocaust deniers. The details of the regime in Auschwitz and the activities of Dr. Mengele and other SS functionaries are provided by the Gypsy survivors independently and in considerable detail. Ideally, this research should be conducted by an interdisciplinary team, including social scientists, oral historians, and psychologists. Interviewers must be trained in the techniques of oral history and must be knowledgable about Gypsies and World War II. They must have experience in interviewing survivors of traumatic events. Analysis of the data can be postponed but gathering it cannot. It is already the 11th hour.

THE PRESENT SITUATION OF GYPSIES IN EUROPE

For the Gypsies of Europe, times are again getting worse. The survivors of the Nazi genocide and their families are terrified by the rapid growth of neo-

Nazism. It binds their present to their past. The puppeteer, who collects ultranationalist newspapers, once said, "If they come to power again, I will not wait to be deported. I will sooner kill myself and all my family" (Interview, 1992). Their fears are well founded. Along with foreign asylum applicants, they have become the special targets of skinheads and other varieties of neo-Nazis.

One of my informants told me: "When I go into a tavern, I am often taken for a Turk. But if I open my mouth, my German is too good and they recognize me as a Gypsy. Then things get even worse" (Interview, 1992). Shortly after the destruction of the Berlin Wall, some of his relatives traveled to an East German city to sell their wares. As they slept, local skinheads poured a ring of gasoline around their trailer and struck a match. The family was incinerated. No one was punished. There were many stories of police turning their backs on crimes against Gypsies, particularly in former East Germany. Those who had the courage to ask for a small pension or reparations were forced into long, drawn-out bureaucratic wrangles.

At the highest levels of the German government, Gypsy asylum seekers from Romania were used as trial balloons for Chancellor Kohl's tough new antirefugee policy, in violation of international law. In other formerly Communist countries where Gypsies form a sizable minority, conditions for them have steadily deteriorated. In Romania, anti-Gypsy violence is widespread and has led to the exodus of hundreds of thousands of Gypsy refugees to the countries of Western Europe where they are increasingly unwelcome. In 1992, Germany entered into a treaty to return more than 40,000 Romanian Gypsy asylum seekers to their country in which, according to a Helsinki Watch report (1991), they were beaten by mobs and by the police, their homes were vandalized and burned down, and they were driven out of one village after the other. Helsinki Watch (1992) protested to German Chancellor Helmut Kohl in a letter dated September 24, 1992, in the following terms: "The German government's decision to single out Romanian Gypsies for deportation is discriminatory treatment that violates Germany's obligations 'to engage in no practice of racial discrimination' as established by international law."

In Hungary, new Fascist organizations that identify themselves as the heirs of the Arrow Cross, the Hungarian Fascist organization that murdered untold numbers of Jews and Gypsies during the final stages of World War II, vie with "New Age" skinheads in attacking Gypsies and foreigners (lacking sufficient indigenous Jews on whom to vent their xenophobic rage), while police stand idly by when they are not perpetrating violence of their own (Helsinki Watch, 1993).

At a 1994 Council of Europe meeting, it was reported that, since the last conference on the situation of Gypsies in Europe in 1991, their situation has grown steadily worse: "There is no group in Europe which is so systematically attacked and humiliated as the Gypsies," one speaker said (*O Drom*, 1994, p. 28). Unemployment in Slovakia is nearly 80% among the Roma, while infant mortality is three times higher than among the non-Gypsy population (*O Drom*, 1994, p. 12). In the Czech republic, despite support from President Havel for Roma aspirations, 80–90% of Roma living on Czech territory have been denied Czech nationality since the country was divided and are registered as Slovak (*O Drom*, 1994, p. 14). After the fall of Communism, government programs to control and assimilate the Roma have been replaced by official neglect and the unleashing of populist prejudices in societies making painful transitions to capitalism, if not always to democracy. In Austria, where the Nazi extermination of most of the 7000 Roma who lived in the Burgenland is still a burning memory, terrorists killed several in February 1995.

Once again the twisted road from ethnic stereotype to persecution and even murder is being followed. Some Romani activists are predicting new genocides in their "liberated" homelands. Thus, the Gypsy survivors of the Holocaust and their families in many parts of Europe are living between the nightmare of the past and a dread of the future.

REFERENCES

Clébert, J.-P. (1963). *The Gypsies*. London: Vista Books.

Friedman, P. (1980). *Roads to extinction: Essays on the Holocaust*. New York: Jewish Publication Society of America.

Helsinki Watch. (1991). *Destroying ethnic identity: The persecution of Gypsies in Rumania*. New York: Human Rights Watch.

Helsinki Watch. (1992). *"Foreigners out": Xenophobia and right wing violence in Germany*. New York and Washington, DC: Helsinki Watch.

Helsinki Watch. (1993). *Struggling for ethnic identity: The Gypsies of Hungary*. New York, Washington, Los Angeles, London: Helsinki Watch.

Hohmann, J. S. (1980). *Zigeuner und Zigeunerwissenschaft: Ein Beitrag zur Grundforchung und Dokumentation des Voelkermord im Dritten Reich* [Gypsies and Gypsy lore: A contribution to basic research and documentation of genocide in the Third Reich]. Marburg/Lahn: Guttandin and Hoppe.

Hohmann, J. S. (1981). *Geschichte der Zigeunerverfolgung in Deutschland* [The history of Gypsy persecution in Germany]. Frankfurt: Campus.

Höss, R. (1958). *Kommandant in Auschwitz*. Stuttgart: Deutsche Verlags-Anstalt. [First published in Polish in 1951; many subsequent translations and editions.]

Kenrick, D., & Puxon, G. (1972). *The destiny of Europe's Gypsies*. New York: Basic Books.

Lessing, A. (1993). *Mein Leben im Versteck* [My life in hiding]. Düsseldorf: Zebulon Verlag.

Müller-Hill, B. (1984). *Tödliche Wissenschaft. Die Aussonderung von Juden, Zigeunern und Geisteskranken 1933–1945* [Murderous science: The selection of Jews, Gypsies and the mentally ill 1933–1945]. Reinbeck bei Hamburg: Rowohlt. [Translated in 1988; New York: Oxford University Press]

Musmanno, M. A. (1961). *The Eichmann Kommandos*. Philadelphia: McCrae Smith.

Novitch, M. (1981). *The extermination of the Gypsies*. Paper presented at the Romani Union's Third World Congress, Göttingen.

O Drom: Magazine for and about *Roma and Sinti in Europe*. (1994). (Special English language edition, September). Amsterdam.

Streck, B. (1979). Die "Bekämpfung des Zigeunerunwesens": Ein Stück moderner Rechtsgeschichte [The struggle against the Gypsy nuisance: A piece of the modern history of law]. In

T. Zülch (Ed.), *In Auschwitz vergast, bis heute verfolgt* (pp. 64–87). Reinbek bei Hamburg: Rohwohlt Verlag.

Tyrnauer, G. (1980–1992). Audio and video oral history interviews.

Tyrnauer, G. (1991). *Gypsies and the Holocaust: A bibliography and introductory essay* (2nd ed.). Montreal: Montreal Institute for Genocide Studies.

Vossen, R. (1983). *Zigeuner, Roma, Sinti, Gitanos, Gypsies zwischen Vervolgung und Romantiesierung* [Gypsies: Roma, Sinti, Gitanos, Gypsies between persecution and romanticization]. Hamburg: Ullstein Sachbuch.

Zimmermann, M. (1987, April 8). Die nationalsozialistische Vernichtungspolitik gegen Sinti und Roma [The National Socialist extermination policy against Sinti and Roma]. *Politik und Zeitgeschichte,* supplement to the weekly *Das Parliament,* pp. 31–45.

Zülch, T. (Ed.). (1979). *In Auschwitz vergasst, bis heute verfolgt* [Gassed in Auschwitz, persecuted until this day]. Reinbek bei Hamburg: Rohwohlt Verlag.

VI

Epilogue

16

General Issues and Research Problems

IHSAN AL-ISSA

Clinical psychology and psychiatry are Western enterprises. Theory, research, and treatment of mental illness reflect the worldview of Western civilization. Until recently, the presumed universality and superiority of the Western model of normal and abnormal behavior has been accepted all over the world. However, with the influx of migration to Western countries from Africa, Asia, and Latin America during the second half of this century, many assumptions of clinical psychology and psychiatry have been challenged. This volume raises many conceptual problems and practical issues in dealing with the mental health of immigrants, refugees, and ethnic groups that are culturally different from the mainstream of Western society. Early conclusions based on poorly designed studies and faulty statistics have been questioned. This chapter will comment on some selected common themes and general research problems in the study of minority groups.

THE SELECTION OF STUDY SAMPLES

In intercultural and cross-cultural studies, the definition of ethnicity and the methods used for selecting samples tend to vary from one study to another. It is important that the ethnicity be defined and specified by researchers. Often,

IHSAN AL-ISSA • Department of Psychology, University of Calgary, Calgary, Alberta, Canada T2N 1N4.

Ethnicity, Immigration, and Psychopathology, edited by Ihsan Al-Issa and Michel Tousignant. Plenum Press, New York, 1997.

subjects may be selected on the basis of self-identification where individuals assign themselves to an ethnic category. However, ethnicity may be defined either in terms of concrete criteria (such as skin color or birth place) or simply based on the consensus of the in-group or out-group. With the process of acculturation of immigrants, the question is to what extent individuals are representative of their own ethnic groups. Members of the same ethnic group may have quite different attitudes, experiences, and background. The immigrants who have arrived recently may not share the same sense of ethnicity as second- or third-generation persons. When using a broad category for an ethnic group such as Hispanics or Southeast Asians, studies tend to combine subjects from different countries. Even whites as a category may be as varied as other ethnic groups.

In recent years, there has been a shift from the use of external criteria in defining ethnicity to a more subtle and internal criteria. Ethnic membership may be inferred from involvement in various activities and rituals, language use, and other signs that indicate identification with the group (Draguns, 1996; Sodowsky, Lau, & Plake, 1991). This approach takes into consideration the degree of acculturation of ethnic groups. Draguns (1996) suggested that it would be desirable to go beyond categorical labels of ethnic membership by including standardized and quantitative indicators of the person's adaptive functioning in both his or her own ethnic group and the multicultural host culture setting.

Samples of convenience such as students or institutionalized psychiatric patients may not represent the whole group. Ethnic groups differ in their access to mental health services. Thus, when these patients are used in research, they may not be representative of the mentally ill in the ethnic populations. How samples from ethnic populations may be biased is expressed by Robins and Regier (1991) in one of the most extensive epidemiological studies of mental illness:

> None of the sites included many Asian-American or American Indian respondents. As a result there were too few to study either ethnic group separately, and in analyses, they are combined with whites. There is a substantial Hispanic sample, but because most of these reside in Los Angeles, they are largely of Mexican heritage; Cubans and Puerto Ricans are underrepresented. Blacks came predominantly from areas to which they had migrated from the rural and urban south, and consequently, blacks of West Indian origin are few. (p. 17)

MODERATOR VARIABLES IN THE STUDY OF ETHNICITY

Gender

Ethnic minority women may be exposed to stresses related to adaptation to Western culture where sex roles are more liberal (Salgado de Snyder, Cervantes, & Padilla, 1990). Olmedo and Parron (1981) noted that the self-concepts of minority women are influenced by racial and ethnic stereotyping, which makes them feel unacceptable according to white standards of beauty. They experience high levels of anxiety and depression as a result of acculturation (Salgado de Snyder, 1987) and are twice as likely to die from diabetes and three times more likely to die from hypertension than white women (Olmedo & Parron, 1981). A variety of mental health problems of ethnic women (ranging from lower self-esteem, depression, and anxiety to alcohol and substance abuse, psychosomatic symptoms, and psychosis) were discussed by La Fromboise, Heyle, and Ozer (1990).

Socioeconomic Status

There is a significant gap between the socioeconomic status of ethnic groups and whites in the United States (Aponte & Crouch, 1995). This is particularly true for African Americans, Hispanics, and Native Americans. Although Asian Americans tend to closely match whites in socioeconomic status, some of the newly arrived groups such as Vietnamese, Laotians, and Cambodians are disproportionately represented in the low stratum.

The criteria for socioeconomic status (income or education) may sometimes pose specific problems in the study of ethnic groups. Income may be incompatible with educational level: A highly qualified professional may have low-status occupation and low income. On the other hand, pooling financial resources of family members may result in high income with low educational level. Thus, using either income or education in assessing socioeconomic status of ethnic groups is quite deceptive.

The effects of socioeconomic status that involves the distribution of power, privileges, and opportunities should not be confused with those of ethnicity (Draguns, 1996). Socioeconomic status may explain differences between ethnic groups in psychopathology and the utilization of mental health services. Chapter 6 and 14 (this volume) indicate how differences in schizophrenia between African Americans and whites in the United States and between the Sephardim and Ashkenazim in Israel disappear when socioeconomic status is controlled. Lower socioeconomic status of ethnic groups and immigrants may in part reduce their utilization of the mental health services, influencing epidemiological data.

Social Support

Support from the family and other social networks may have moderating or mediating effects on the stress experienced by ethnic groups. Ethnic groups are more likely to rely heavily on the social support of the extended family for assistance with personal problems rather than on friends, neighbors, or co-workers (Al-Issa & Ismail, 1994; Keefe, Padilla, & Carlós, 1979). In the study of southeast Asian refugees (Chapter 3, this volume), it was found that having social support and confiding relationships tended to modify the effects of the premigration trauma experiences on mental health. Similarly it was found that Chinese immigrants who are received by large and established communities in Canada had significantly less risk for depression than the Vietnamese, Laotians, and Cambodians who did not have such support. Both African Americans (Miller, 1992) and Hispanics (Kitano, 1989) rely on the extended family where many generations live in the household. However, since 1970 there has been an increase in the number of families with single parents among African Americans (McAdoo, 1991) and Hispanics (US Bureau of the Census, 1990). Turkish and North African "guest workers" in Europe also leave the extended family, including the spouse, in the home country, which adds to the difficulties of adaptation in the new environment (see Chapters 9 and 10, this volume). The comment of Sachdev (Chapter 12, this volume) on the effects of urbanization on the social networks of the Maori may apply to most non-Western immigrants who come from rural to urban European and North American environments:

> The change due to urbanization is quite fundamental even when not associated with a cultural change. In the case of the Maori, the move to a city also involves a move into a *Pakeha*-dominated culture. The traditional fabric of society, with the extended family (*Whanau*) as the basic unit, is broken, taking away the support system and the controls on behavior that are so important for the young Maori. Maori from different tribes are thrown together by chance, and the role of the *tangata whenua* (people of the land) becomes quite different. Because of the separation from the kin, traditional child-rearing practices are disrupted. The city, being modeled on a European society, demands a much greater acceptance of the *Pakeha* culture than that necessary in the countryside. To this demanding environment, the Maori brings a relatively poor education and job skills, thereby compounding the disadvantage. (Sachdev, Chapter 12, p. 196, this volume)

Unemployment

Refugees and immigrants tend to have a high rate of unemployment on arrival, a condition that increases their mental health risk (Chapter 3, this volume). For these refugees and immigrants, unemployment is not simply a loss of social status or restriction of social contact, but it is related to material deprivation and failure to meet family obligations. Examples of the relationship between unemployment and psychopathology are given in Chapters 3 and 4, this volume.

MODES OF ADAPTATION OF ETHNIC GROUPS AND IMMIGRANTS

It has been suggested that adaptation of ethnic groups and immigrants to acculturation may take four forms: assimilation, integration, separation, and marginalization (Berry & Kim, 1988; Chapter 1, this volume). The experience of Native Indians and Gypsies clearly shows the failure of policies of assimilation of these groups in North America and Germany, respectively (Chapters 11 and 15, this volume). During the first half of this century, Gypsies were forbidden to use their own language and their children were taken away to be raised by peasant families. However, neither persecution nor forced assimilation were successful in eliminating the cultural identity of Gypsies; they continued to observe their customs, speak their language, and remain isolated from the majority group. Gypsies in Europe are marginalized as a group, not as individuals (see Chapter 15, this volume). Similar policies of forced assimilation were practiced in Canada where children of Native Indians were placed in residential schools in which they were taught in English and forced to adopt a Western lifestyle (see Chapter 12, this volume, concerning similar treatment of the Maori children in New Zealand).

Experiences of immigrants and ethnic groups described in the present volume do not support the view that a certain mode of adaptation (such as integration, which is associated with multiculturalism) is more favorable for the mental health of immigrants and refugees (Berry, 1992; Berry & Kim, 1988). Gypsies seem to adjust to marginalization and separation as a group from European society. The isolation of Gypsies or the hiding of their identity described in Chapter 15 (this volume) does not seem to compromise their self-esteem.

In contrast, attempts to assimilate into the majority group may not be protective against prejudice and discrimination. Regardless of their degree of assimilation, Gypsies were sent to the death camps. The integration of Jewish people into German society did not prevent Nazi persecution. Attempts by North African youth to integrate into French society do not seem to result in full acceptance by the French population. East Indian and Haitian women who chose assimilation into French Canadian society tended to suffer from more symptoms than other groups who remained traditional. All these data reported in the present volume support the view that each ethnic group tends to adopt its unique style of adjustment, making generalization to all groups quite difficult.

MISDIAGNOSIS OF ETHNIC GROUPS AND IMMIGRANTS

Misdiagnosis of mental illness is higher among patients from minority groups than the majority population (Good, 1993). African Americans and Hispanics are more likely to be diagnosed as schizophrenics compared with whites (Chapter 6, this volume; Jones & Gray, 1986; Mukherjee, Shukla, Woodle, Rosen, & Olarte, 1983). Mukherjee et al. (1983) found that the diagnosis of schizophrenia is more likely when African Americans are young and experience hallucinations associated with affective disorders. As a result of the oppression of minorities, the differentiation between "healthy paranoia" or delusion of persecution and pathological delusions is rather problematic (Di Angi, 1976; Jones, 1990).

Could diagnostic error be attributed to prejudice and discrimination? British psychiatry has been accused of being racist in the overdiagnosis of schizophrenia among African Caribbeans and that psychiatrists may be prejudiced personally or theoretically against this group (Littlewood, 1993). In the United States, however, it has been suggested that systematic errors in diagnosis are more the result of the way psychiatrists process information than due to prejudice and discrimination against minorities (Draguns, 1996; López, 1989). It is therefore suggested that the training of clinicians should be directed toward general processes that lead to judgmental errors. Cognitive theories of prejudice discussed in Chapter 2 (this volume) seem to suggest that the tendency to attribute severe psychopathology to ethnic groups may be related to the general cognitive tendency to stereotype people of other races and to evaluate them more extremely than members of the in-group. Diagnostic bias may indicate that professionals are not immune from such cognitive judgmental bias.

Cochrane (1995) argued against both the stress and selection hypothesis in explaining high rates of schizophrenia among Afro-Caribbeans. He also rejected socioeconomic status, which was found to explain the overdiagnosis of schizophrenia among the Sephardim and African Americans in Israel and the United States, respectively (Chapters 6 and 14, this volume). Although he cited several studies in Britain supporting the misdiagnosis hypothesis, results of a study by Harrison, Owens, Holton, Neilson, and Boot (1988) is against such a hypothesis. Harrison et al. (1988) applied an increasingly restrictive definition of schizophrenia based on the International Classification of Diseases and Related Health Problems, ninth edition coding for certainty of diagnosis in hospitalized schizophrenic patients. Levels of certainty of the diagnosis of schizophrenia of Afro-Caribbeans and the general population were found to be quite similar, giving evidence against the misdiagnosis hypothesis. It may be that the hallucinations and delusions of the Afro-Caribbeans may not be indicative of schizophrenia if viewed in their cultural context. The study by Harrison et al. (1988) did not consider the cultural meaning of the symptoms of the two groups studied. Adebimpe (Chapter 6, this volume) reported many symptoms that could lead to the diagnosis of schizophrenia among Afro-Americans if they were assessed out of their cultural context: paranoia, abnormal speech, atypical hallucinations, and belief in witchcraft. Psychosis may also be secondary to sleep deprivation and prolonged fasting among members of certain churches in the black community. In addition to the cultural context of symptomatology, it is useful to consider the interactive stance taken by Cochrane (1995) to explain the high rate of schizophrenia and other mental illnesses among ethnic groups and immigrants:

> Kohn suggested that it was necessary for three independent factors to coincide in an individual for schizophrenia to appear: genetic predisposition, high levels of stress, and values related to "conceptions of reality" which are produced by the day-to-day experiences of the family and the individual in their contact with others and the institutions of society. Repeated exposure to discrimination and consequent lack of instrumental efficacy can produce an external locus of control, lowered self-esteem, helplessness, "and a fatalistic belief that one is at the mercy of forces and people beyond one's control ..." (Kohn, 1972, p. 300). This orientation is antipathetic to an effective response to stress which is, in any case, likely to be greater in a disadvantaged minority. Where these factors impinge on a person with a genetic predisposition, then schizophrenia will be manifested. Thus two populations with identical genetic vulnerability may show different rates of schizophrenia depending on their exposure to the other variables in Kohn's equation. (pp. 356–357)

SOMATIZATION AND CULTURE-SPECIFIC IDIOMS OF DISTRESS

Somatization

It has been argued that in the expression of emotions such as depression or anxiety, non-Western people (Southeast Asians and Latin Americans discussed in this volume) tend to somatize instead of expressing these emotions in psychological terms (Leff, 1973, 1988). Most of the studies on cross-cultural somatization are based on clinical observations and assessments. However, Guarnaccia (Chapter 5, this volume) reported that among Mexicans, data from factor analysis indicate a combined affective and somatic factor, supporting the expression of distress by somatic idioms. On the other hand, Beiser and Hyman (Chapter 3, this volume), in a study of Southeast Asians, found two independent factors—somatic distress and depressive affect—a result against the stereotype of the inability of Asians to "psychologize" in their expression of emotions. Whether somatic expression is an independent factor from affect or whether it is used to replace it among non-Western people is still an unresolved issue.

The interpretation of somatic expression of distress in terms of linguistic and emotional deficit or lack of psychological sophistication among non-Western people tend to involve value judgment (Leff, 1973, 1988). Draguns (1996) argued that culture may encourage sensitivity to either psychological or physiological processes, and the report of somatic symptoms may reflect "a genuine skill in attending to and reporting somatic processes" (p. 25). Draguns pointed out that in dealing with ethnic groups in North America, the cultural context in which the cultural background of the therapist, predominantly white, is widely different from the patient, and this situation could encourage communication of physical rather than psychological symptoms. Draguns (1996) stated that

> the contextual aspects of symptom presentation should be considered, especially as they occur across cultural lines. Encounters between a mental health professional

> who represents the mainstream American culture and a patient of a different cultural background may be conducted across a gap or even a chasm that many culturally different help seekers find difficult to cross. Under these circumstances, bodily distress becomes an easily communicated and perhaps a readily relieved component of a vague tangle of adverse experiences that defy being put into words to a stranger and in an imperfectly mastered language. (p. 25)

Another argument against the deficit hypothesis of somatization is that many traditional theories of medicine (e.g., in India, Southeast Asia, natives in North America and in Australia and New Zealand) take a holistic approach in which somatopsychic rather than psychological aspects of disease are emphasized (Al-Issa, 1995; Chapters 11 and 12, this volume). Koss (1990) argued that physical complaints may have an adaptive social function and may form a link between the individual, the social, and the political spheres. Kawanishi (1992) also argued how physical complaints of Asians have been decontextualized by being studied within a Western frame of reference. He suggested that in many Eastern cultures, the display of emotions in social interactions is not desirable. The expression of somatic symptoms may also reduce the stigma of mental illness and legitimize entry into health care. Thus, the expression of somatic rather than affective symptoms among non-Western patients seems to be related to many cultural factors rather than to an intrinsic deficit. It is estimated that in the general population in North America, three fourths of patients' visits to primary health care physicians are associated with somatization (Al-Issa, 1995), except that symptoms of non-Western patients tend to take a dramatic form (Ebigo, 1982).

Culture-Specific Idioms of Distress

Ethnic groups and immigrants may manifest culture-specific idioms of distress that do not fit within the Western classification system. One example is *nervios*, a Hispanic idiom of expression of anxiety symptoms. Symptoms such as headache, insomnia, lack of appetite, depression, fear, anger, trembling, disorientation, and other symptoms of *nervios* are socially acceptable expressions of being out of control and are precipitated by social life events such as disrupted family relationships (Low, 1981). Guarnaccia and Farias (1988) have shown that the social meaning of *nervios* may include family and work issues, fear of relatives left in the home country, as well as social commentary on racism and problems of adjustment in the United States. Similar to *nervios, ataque de nervios* also usually occurs following a stressful life event relating to the family (death, separation or divorce, conflict with spouse or children). It is characterized by uncontrollable shouting, crying, trembling, heat in the chest arising in the head, and verbal or physical aggression. *Ataque de nervios* closely fits the *Diagnostic and Statistical Manual of Mental Disorders,* fourth edition (DSM-IV) [American Psychiatric Association (APA), 1994] description of panic attack, except that its association with a precipitating event distinguishes it from panic disorder (Barron, 1994).

Another idiom of distress found among lower-class African Americans who are members of the Pentecostal church is "spiritual heart trouble." Its symptoms are those seen in anxiety and depressive disorders (Camino, 1992). It is related to role confusion and may result in "spiritual death." The patient may experience a wide range of symptoms such as "heavy heart," "heart beating fast," "saying things I shouldn't," and "loss of spiritual joy and desire" (Camino, 1992). It seems to be related to Pentecostal beliefs and is mediated by social life events. For other culture-specific idioms of distress, the reader is referred to Al-Issa and Oudji (in press) and Good and Kleinman (1985). Specific idioms of distress should be dealt with within the sociocultural context of the ethnic group.

TREATMENT

Sociocultural factors may play a major role in access to and the utilization of mental health services by ethnic groups and immigrants. These groups can also find their way to the mental health system through different pathways. They also may not utilize the health system because they have access to family, social networks, and native healers (Rogler, 1993; Rogler & Cortes, 1993; Chapter 3, this volume).

Pathways of help-seeking behavior of ethnic groups were investigated by Lin, Tardiff, Donetz, and Goresky (1978) among Chinese, Anglo-Saxons, Middle Europeans, and Native Indians in Vancouver, Canada. They were able to assess the extent of family involvement, medical intervention, and social and legal agency involvements in the entry into the mental health system. It was found that among Chinese patients, medical intervention occurred only when the family could not resolve the problem. Intervention by the legal or social agencies was quite rare. For example, psychotic symptoms were often tolerated as long as the patient was not aggressive or socially disruptive. Family loyalties and obligations played a major part in looking after the mentally sick. Unless it was necessary, family and community help was sought to avoid the shame associated with seeking mental health agencies' assistance. In contrast, Anglo-Saxons and Middle European families tended to refer their patients early to social agencies or outpatient and inpatient treatment. As compared with the Chinese, social services, medical facilities, and mental health agencies were contacted at much earlier stages, reflecting less tolerance of patients. Failure to refer a disturbed family member was conceived as disloyal, uncaring, and neglectful behavior. Finally, Native Indians' pathway to the mental health system tended to be an early legal and social agency intervention prompted by individuals other than family members. The social context and the type of problems presented, such as drug and alcohol problems associated with suicidal behavior, tended to play a larger part than in the case of the other ethnic groups. The picture of native utilization of health service reported by Waldram and Sachdev (Chapters 11 and 12, this volume, respectively) provides more support to the data by Lin et al. (1978). Indians and Metis in Canada experience less outpatient therapy and higher admission rates, suggesting that professionals consider them as more pathological and less compliant to the treatment regimen (Chapter 11, this volume). Similar to Native Indians (Somervell, Manson, & Shore, 1995), the Maori of New Zealand are also more often admitted involuntarily under the criminal law (Chapter 12, this volume).

There are many problems that may interfere with the treatment of ethnic minorities. Misdiagnosis may result in higher rate of unnecessary hospitalization and inappropriate medication (Friedman, Paradis, & Hatch, 1994; Williams & Chambless, 1994). *In vivo* exposure during behavior therapy is hindered by the frequent encounter of prejudice and discrimination during treatment sessions when clients carry out exposure sessions on their own (in grocery stores, restaurants, and department stores).

Another factor that contributes to the difficulties of the therapy of ethnic minorities is the racial mismatch between therapist and client, which may influence outcome. On the positive side, however, the involvement of the extended family in the treatment and the use of community support are expected to improve outcome (Friedman et al., 1994). Language barriers pose a serious problem in communicating meaning and affective experience in the newly acquired language (Sciarra & Ponterotto, 1991). The training of ethnic and native therapists and the use of indigenous treatment procedures with ethnic groups indicate promising progress.

CONCLUSIONS

In this volume, the authors have attempted to increase understanding of the factors involved in the etiology and treatment of mental illness among ethnic groups and immigrants. Although it is shown that there are general problems facing all these groups, each group has its own unique problems as well. The authors have taken into consideration historical and premigration experience, the migration experience, and the reaction of the host country, in addition to individual vulnerabilities. Data that expose diagnostic biases and faulty methodology in early research seem to challenge the stereotype of higher rates of mental illness among ethnic groups and immigrants. Gypsies and Jewish people in Nazi Germany, North Africans and Turks in Europe, native peoples in New Zealand and North America, refugees and immigrants in Canada, and East German migrants provide the reader with excellent examples of human adaptation and survival in the face of various adversities. These groups bring with them family and network systems and religions and other beliefs that provide a buffer against mental illness. Future research should delineate more clearly these potentials and their interaction with stressors in the dominant culture.

In North America, the 1990s have witnessed an awareness of cultural diversity and the need of teaching material related to ethnic groups during training in clinical psychology (APA, 1993). The DSM-IV has also paid attention to culture-specific syndromes, religious or spiritual problems, and problems related to acculturation (APA, 1994). Yet, we are still far from achieving a culturally fair mental health system, and it is hoped that the present contributions will move us a step farther in the direction of culturally sensitive theory, research, and treatment of mental illness.

REFERENCES

Al-Issa, I. (1995). Culture and mental illness in an international perspective. In I. Al-Issa (Ed.), *Culture and mental illness: An international perspective* (pp. 3–49). Madison, CT: International Universities Press.

Al-Issa, I., & Ismail, S. J. (1994). Social support and depression of male and female students in Kuwait: Preliminary findings. *Anxiety, Stress and Coping, 7,* 253–262.

Al-Issa, I., & Oudji, S. (in press). Culture and anxiety disorders. In S. S. Kazarian & D. Evans (Eds.), *Cultural clinical psychology: Theory, research and practice.* New York: Oxford University Press.

American Psychiatric Association. (1994). *Diagnostic and statistical manual of mental disorders* (4th ed.). Washington, DC: Author.

American Psychological Association. (1993). Guidelines for providers of psychological services to ethnic, linguistic and culturally diverse populations. *American Psychologist, 48,* 45–48.

Aponte, J. F., & Crouch, R. T. (1995). The changing ethnic profile of the United States. In J. F. Aponte, R. Y. Rivers, & J. Wohl (Eds.), *Psychological interventions and cultural diversity* (pp. 1–18). Boston: Allyn and Bacon.

Barron, D. L. (1994). DSM-IV: Making it culturally relevant. In S. Friedman (Ed.), *Anxiety disorders in African-Americans* (pp. 15–39). New York: Springer.

Berry, J. W. (1992). Acculturation and adaptation in a new society. *International Migrations, 30,* 69–85.

Berry, J. W., & Kim, V. (1988). Acculturation and mental health. In P. R. Dasen, J. W. Berry, & N. Sartorius (Eds.), *Health and cross-cultural psychology: Toward applications* (pp. 207–236). Newbury Park, CA: Sage.

Camino, L. A. (1992). The cultural epidemiology of spiritual heart trouble. In J. Kirkland, C. W. Sullivan, & K. Baldwin (Eds.), *Herbal and magical medicine: Traditional healing today* (pp. 118–136). Durham, NC: Duke University Press.

Cochrane, R. (1995). Mental health among minorities and immigrants in Britain. In I. Al-Issa (Ed.), *Culture and mental illness: An international perspective* (pp. 347–360). Madison, CT: International Universities Press.

Di Angi, P. (1976). Barriers to the black and white therapeutic relationship. *Perspectives in Psychiatric Care, 14,* 180–183.

Draguns, J. G. (1996). Multicultural and cross-cultural assessment: Dilemmas and decisions. In J. Impara & G. R. Sodowsky (Eds.), *Multicultural assessment in counseling and clinical psychology* (pp. 1–48). Hillsdale, NJ: Lawrence Erlbaum.

Ebigo, P. O. (1982). Development of a culture-specific (Nigeria) screening scale of somatic complaints indicating psychiatric disturbance. *Culture, Medicine and Psychiatry, 6,* 29–43.

Friedman, S., Paradis, C. M., & Hatch, M. L. (1994). Issues of misdiagnosis in panic disorder with agoraphobia. In S. Friedman (Ed.), *Anxiety disorders in African Americans* (pp. 128–146). New York: Springer.

Good, B. J. (1993). Culture, diagnosis, and comorbidity. *Culture, Medicine and Psychiatry, 16,* 427–446.

Good, B. J., & Kleinman, A. M. (1985). Culture and anxiety: Cross-cultural evidence for the patterning of anxiety disorders. In A. H. Tuma & I. D. Maser (Eds.), *Anxiety and anxiety disorders* (pp. 297–323). Hillsdale, NJ: Lawrence Erlbaum.

Guarnaccia, P. J., & Farias, P. (1988). The social meaning of *nervios*: A case study of the Central American woman. *Social Science and Medicine, 26,* 1223–1231.

Harrison, G., Owens, D., Holton, A., Neilson, D., & Boot, D. (1988). A prospective study of severe mental disorder in Afro-Caribbean patients. *Psychological Medicine, 18,* 643–657.

Jones, B. E., & Gray, B. A. (1986). Problems in diagnosing schizophrenia and affective disorders among blacks. *Hospital and Community Psychiatry, 37,* 61–65.

Jones, N. S. (1990). Black/white issues in psychotherapy: A framework for clinical practice. *Journal of Social Behavior and Personality, 5,* 305–322.

Kawanishi, Y. (1992). Somatization of Asians: An artifact of Western medicalization? *Transcultural Psychiatric Research Review, 29,* 5–36.

Keefe, S. E., Padilla, A. M., & Carlós, M. L. (1979). The Mexican-American extended family as an emotional support system. *Human Organization, 38,* 144–152.

Kitano, H. H. L. (1989). A model for counseling Asian Americans. In P. B. Pedersen, J. G. Draguns, W. J. Lonner, & J. E. Trimble (Eds.), *Counseling across cultures* (3rd ed., pp. 139–151). Honolulu: University of Hawaii Press.

Kohn, M. L. (1972). Class, family and schizophrenia: A reformulation. *Social Forces, 50,* 295–304.

Koss, J. D. (1990). Somatization and somatic complaint syndromes. *Transcultural Psychiatric Research Review, 27,* 5–29.

La Fromboise, T. D., Heyle, A. M., & Ozer, E. J. (1990). Changing and diverse roles of women in American Indian culture. *Sex Roles, 22,* 455–476.

Leff, J. (1973). Culture and the differentiation of emotional states. *British Journal of Psychiatry, 243,* 299–306.

Leff, J. (1988). *Psychiatry around the globe.* London: Gaskell.

Lin, T. Y., Tardiff, K., Donetz, G., & Goresky, W. (1978). Ethnicity and pattern of help-seeking. *Culture, Medicine and Psychiatry, 2,* 3–13.

Littlewood, R. (1993). Ideology, camouflage or contingency? Racism in British psychiatry. *Transcultural Psychiatric Research Review, 30,* 243–290.

López, S. R. (1989). Patient variable biases in clinical judgement: Conceptual overview and methodological considerations. *Psychological Bulletin, 106,* 184–203.

Low, S. M. (1981). The meaning of *nervios*: A sociocultural analysis of symptom presentation in San José, Costa Rica. *Culture, Medicine and Psychiatry, 5,* 25–48.

McAdoo, H. P. (1991). Family values and outcomes for children. *Journal of Negro Education, 60,* 351–365.

Miller, F. S. (1992). Network structural support: Its relationship to the psychosocial development of black females. In A. K. H. Burlow, W. C. Banks, H. P. McAdoo, & D. A. Azibo (Eds.), *African-American psychology: Theory, research and practice* (pp. 105–126). Newbury Park, CA: Sage.

Mukherjee, S., Shukla, S. S., Woodle, J., Rosen, A. M., & Olarte, S. (1983). Misdiagnosis of schizophrenia in bipolar patients. A multiethnic comparison. *American Journal of Psychiatry, 140,* 1571–1574.

Olmedo, E. L., & Parron, D. L. (1981). Mental health of minority women: Some special issues. *Professional Psychology, 12,* 103–111.

Robins, L. N., & Regier, D. A. (Eds.). (1991). *Psychiatric disorders in America: The Epidemiologic Catchment Area Study.* New York: Free Press.

Rogler, L. H. (1993). Culturally sensitizing psychiatric diagnosis: A framework for research. *Journal of Nervous and Mental Disease, 181,* 401–408.

Rogler, L. H., & Cortes, D. E. (1993). Help seeking pathways: A unifying concept in mental health care. *American Journal of Psychiatry, 150,* 554–561.

Salgado de Snyder, V. N. (1987). Factors associated with acculturative stress and depressive symptomatology among married Mexican immigrant women. *Psychology of Women Quarterly, 11,* 475–488.

Salgado de Snyder, V. N., Cervantes, R. C., & Padilla, A. M. (1990). Gender and ethnic differences in psychosocial stress and generalized distress among Hispanics. *Sex Roles, 22,* 441–453.

Sciarra, D. T., & Ponterotto, J. G. (1991). Counseling the Hispanic bilingual family: Challenges to the therapeutic process. *Psychotherapy, 28,* 473–479.

Sodowsky, G. R., Lau, E. W. M., & Plake, B. (1991). Moderating effects of sociocultural variables on acculturation attitudes of Hispanics and Asian Americans. *Journal of Counseling and Development, 70,* 194–204.

Somervell, P. D., Manson, S. M., & Shore, J. H. (1995). Mental illness among American Indians and Alaska Natives. In I. Al-Issa (Ed.), *Culture and mental illness: An international perspective* (pp. 315–329). Madison, CT: International Universities Press.

US Bureau of the Census. (1990). *Fertility of American women: June 1990. Current population reports.* Series P-20, No. 454. Washington, DC: US Government Printing Office.

Williams, K. E., & Chambless, D. L. (1994). The results of exposure-based treatment in agoraphobia. In S. Friedman (Ed.), *Anxiety disorders in African Americans* (pp. 149–165). New York: Springer.

Index

CPSIA information can be obtained at www.ICGtesting.com
Printed in the USA
LVOW010002090812

293584LV00002B/59/A

9 780306 484322